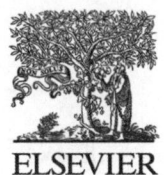

A THERANOSTIC AND PRECISION MEDICINE
APPROACH FOR FEMALE-SPECIFIC CANCERS

针对女性特异性肿瘤的精准治疗

主　编　[印] RAMA RAO MALLA
　　　　[美] GANJI PURNACHANDRA NAGARAJU
主　审　孟元光
主　译　李立安　叶明侠

中华医学电子音像出版社
CHINESE MEDICAL MULTIMEDIA PRESS
北　京

版权所有　　侵权必究

图书在版编目(CIP)数据

针对女性特异性肿瘤的精准治疗 /（印）拉玛·拉奥·马拉，（美）甘吉·普纳查恩德拉·纳加拉朱主编；李立安，叶明侠译. --北京：中华医学电子音像出版社，2025. 8. --ISBN 978-7-83005-424-3

Ⅰ. R737.305

中国国家版本馆 CIP 数据核字第 2025YC8732 号

北京市版权局著作权合同登记章图字：01-2025-1971 号

针对女性特异性肿瘤的精准治疗

ZHENDUI NVXING TEYIXING ZHONGLIU DE JINGZHUN ZHILIAO

主　　编：［印］RAMA RAO MALLA　　［美］GANJI PURNACHANDRA NAGARAJU
主　　译：李立安　叶明侠
策划编辑：薛瑞华　鲁　静
责任编辑：赵文羽
责任印刷：李振坤
出版发行：中华医学电子音像出版社
通信地址：北京市西城区东河沿街 69 号（中华医学会宣武门办公区）
邮　　编：100052
E - mail：cma-cmc@cma.org.cn
购书热线：010-51322635
经　　销：新华书店
印　　刷：廊坊市佳艺印务有限公司
开　　本：720mm×1020mm　1/16
印　　张：21.25
字　　数：433 千字
版　　次：2025 年 8 月第 1 版　2025 年 8 月第 1 次印刷
定　　价：180.00 元

购买本社图书，凡有缺、倒、脱页者，本社负责调换

A Theranostic and Precision Medicine Approach for Female-Specific Cancers，1E
Rama Rao Malla，Ganji Purnachandra Nagaraju
ISBN：9780128220092
Copyright © 2021 Elsevier Inc. All rights reserved，including those for text and data mining，AI training，and similar technologies.
Authorized Chinese translation published by Chinese Medical Multimedia Press.

《针对女性特异性肿瘤的精准治疗》（第1版）（李立安　叶明侠　译）
ISBN：9787830054243
Copyright © Elsevier Inc. and Chinese Medical Multimedia Press. All rights reserved. No part of this publication may be reproduced or transmitted in any form or by any means，electronic or mechanical，including photocopying，recording，or any information storage and retrieval system，without permission in writing from Elsevier Inc. Details on how to seek permission，further information about the Elsevier's permissions policies and arrangements with organizations such as the Copyright Clearance Center and the Copyright Licensing Agency，can be found at our website：www.elsevier.com/permissions.
This book and the individual contributions contained in it are protected under copyright by Elsevier Inc. and Chinese Medical Multimedia Press（other than as may be noted herein）.

This edition of A Theranostic and Precision Medicine Approach for Female-Specific Cancers is published by Chinese Medical Multimedia Press under arrangement with ELSEVIER INC.
This edition is authorized for sale in China only，excluding Hong Kong，Macau and Taiwan. Unauthorized export of this edition is a violation of the Copyright Act. Violation of this Law is subject to Civil and Criminal Penalties.

本版由ELSEVIER INC授权中华医学电子音像出版社在中国大陆地区（不包括香港、澳门以及台湾地区）出版发行。
本版仅限在中国大陆地区（不包括香港、澳门以及台湾地区）出版及标价销售。未经许可之出口，视为违反著作权法，将受民事及刑事法律之制裁。
本书封底贴有Elsevier防伪标签，无标签者不得销售。

注意

本书涉及领域的知识和实践标准在不断变化。新的研究和经验拓展我们的理解，因此须对研究方法、专业实践或医疗方法作出调整。从业者和研究人员必须始终依靠自身经验和知识来评估和使用本书中提到的所有信息、方法、化合物或本书中描述的实验。在使用这些信息或方法时，他们应注意自身和他人的安全，包括注意他们负有专业责任的当事人的安全。在法律允许的最大范围内，爱思唯尔、译文的原文作者、原文编辑及原文内容提供者均不对因产品责任、疏忽或其他人身或财产伤害及/或损失承担责任，亦不对由于使用或操作文中提到的方法、产品、说明或思想而导致的人身或财产伤害及/或损失承担责任。

编委会

主　审　孟元光
主　译　李立安　叶明侠
副主译　闫志风　杨　雯　李　震　翟青枝
　　　　李明霞　付　蒙　王　岳
译　者　（按姓氏笔画排序）
　　　　丁佳佳　解放军总医院第七医学中心
　　　　王　岳　解放军总医院第七医学中心
　　　　叶明侠　解放军总医院第七医学中心
　　　　付　蒙　北京市海淀区妇幼保健院
　　　　闫志风　解放军总医院第七医学中心
　　　　李　震　北京大学第一医院
　　　　李立安　解放军总医院第七医学中心
　　　　李明霞　解放军总医院第七医学中心
　　　　杨　华　解放军总医院第七医学中心
　　　　杨　雯　解放军总医院第七医学中心
　　　　张妮娜　解放军总医院第七医学中心
　　　　陈　珂　解放军总医院第七医学中心
　　　　陈梦雨　解放军总医院第七医学中心
　　　　武雅雯　解放军总医院第七医学中心
　　　　周嘉璐　解放军总医院第七医学中心
　　　　孟穆阳　解放军总医院第七医学中心
　　　　赵路阳　解放军总医院第七医学中心

胡甲琳	解放军总医院第七医学中心
高　原	解放军总医院第七医学中心
董明理	解放军总医院第七医学中心
解　冰	解放军总医院第七医学中心
翟青枝	解放军总医院第七医学中心
翟鑫宇	解放军总医院第七医学中心

原著作者

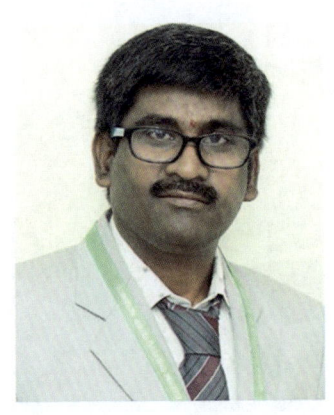

Rama Rao Malla 教授是印度安得拉邦维沙卡帕特南甘地技术与管理学院（认定具有大学资质）科学研究所生物化学与生物信息学系的教职人员。他在印度安得拉邦维沙卡帕特南的安得拉大学获得生物化学硕士和博士学位，并曾在美国伊利诺伊大学医学院进行博士后研究，其研究重点是探索四跨膜蛋白 CD151 作为治疗靶点及其候选 miRNA 或外泌体 CD151 作为三阴性乳腺癌早期诊断标志物的潜力；同时致力于研究 CD151 在肿瘤微环境中的作用及其介导的耐药机制。Malla 博士在国际同行评审期刊上发表了超过 85 篇研究论文，在国内外学术会议上发表了 100 余篇摘要，并参与编写了 20 余部由国际出版社出版的书籍。Malla 博士担任多家国际期刊的编委顾问及编委成员，并曾获得一项研究卓越奖和一项学术卓越奖。

原著作者

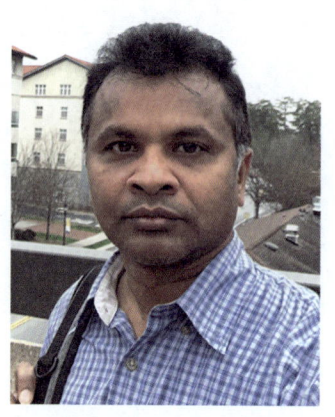

Ganji Purnachandra Nagaraju 博士是美国埃默里大学医学院血液学与肿瘤内科学系的教职人员。Nagaraju 博士在印度安得拉邦蒂鲁帕蒂的斯里文卡特斯瓦拉大学获得生物技术硕士和博士学位，并于印度奥里萨邦贝汉布尔的贝汉布尔大学获得科学博士学位。Nagaraju 博士的研究重点是与胃肠道恶性肿瘤相关的转化项目，已在国际知名期刊上发表 90 余篇研究论文，并在各种国内和国际会议上发表了 50 余篇摘要。Nagaraju 博士是多本出版物的作者和编辑，包括 *Role of Tyrosine Kinases in Gastrointestinal Malignancies*, *Role of Transcription Factors in Gastrointestinal Malignancies*, *Breaking Tolerance to Pancreatic Cancer Unresponsiveness to Chemotherapy*, *Theranostic Approach for Pancreatic Cancer* 和 *Exploring Pancreatic Metabolism and Malignancy*。他是很多国际公认学术期刊的编辑委员会成员，也是温希普（Winship）癌症研究所发现及发展治疗研究项目的准成员。Nagaraju 博士曾获得包括美国临床化学协会会士（FAACC）在内的多个国际奖项。他还是美国印度裔科学家协会、综合与比较生物学会、科学顾问委员会、RNA 协会、美国临床化学协会和美国癌症研究协会的会员。

贡献者

Phaniendra Alugoju
Department of Biochemistry and Molecular Biology, School of Life Sciences, Pondicherry University, Puducherry, India

Dinakara Rao Ampasala
Centre for Bioinformatics, School of Life Sciences, Pondicherry University, Puducherry, India

Neelakantan Arumugam
Department of Biotechnology, School of Life Sciences, Pondicherry University, Puducherry, India

Dariya Begum
Department of Biosciences and Biotechnology, Banasthali University, Banasthali, Rajasthan, India

L. V. K. S. Bhaskar
Department of Zoology, Guru Ghasidas Vishwavidyalaya, Bilaspur, Chhattisgarh, India

Ishita Bhattacharyya
Centre for Bioinformatics, School of Life Sciences, Pondicherry University, Puducherry, India

Narayan P. Burte
Department of Pharmacology, Viswabharathi Medical College, Kurnool, Andhra Pradesh, India

Nyshadham S. N. Chaitanya
Department of Animal Biology, School of Life Sciences, University of Hyderabad, Gachibowli, Hyderabad, India

V. Dixit
Department of Botany, Guru Ghasidas Vishwavidyalaya, Bilaspur, Chhattisgarh, India

Bhavya Kavitha Dwarapureddi
Department of Environmental Science, GITAM Institute of Science, GITAM (Deemed to be University), Visakhapatnam, Andhra Pradesh, India

Mohan Krishna Ghanta
Department of Pharmacology, SRMC & RI, Sri Ramachandra Institute of Higher Education and Research, Chennai, Tamil Nadu, India

Manoj Kumar Gupta
Department of Biotechnology and Bioinformatics, Yogi Vemana University, Kadapa, Andhra Pradesh, India

Santosh C. Gursale
Department of Pharmacology, BKL Walawalkar Rural Medical College, Sawarde, Ratnagiri, Maharashtra, India

Pavan Kumar Kancharla
Department of Biotechnology, School of Life Sciences, Pondicherry University, Puducherry, India

Manoj Kumar Karnena
Department of Environmental Science, GITAM Institute of Science, GITAM (Deemed to be University), Visakhapatnam, Andhra Pradesh, India

V. K. D. Krishna Swamy
Department of Biochemistry and Molecular Biology, School of Life Sciences, Pondicherry University, Puducherry, India

Rama Rao Malla
Cancer Biology Lab, Department of Biochemistry and Bioinformatics, Institute of Science, GITAM (Deemed to be University), Visakhapatnam, Andhra Pradesh, India

Neha Merchant
Department of Hematology and Medical Oncology, Winship Cancer Institute, Emory University, Atlanta, GA, United States

Mathavan Muthaiyan
Centre for Bioinformatics, School of Life Sciences, Pondicherry University, Puducherry, India

Ganji Purnachandra Nagaraju
Department of Hematology and Medical Oncology, Winship Cancer Institute, Emory University, Atlanta, GA, United States

Leimarembi Devi Naorem
Centre for Bioinformatics, School of Life Sciences, Pondicherry University, Puducherry, India

Jayshree Nellore
Department of Biotechnology, School of Bio and Chemical Engineering, Sathyabama Institute of Science and Technology, Chennai, Tamil Nadu, India

Kiranmayi Patnala
Department of Biotechnology, Institute of Science, GITAM (Deemed to be University), Visakhapatnam, Andhra Pradesh, India

Sujatha Peela
Department of Biotechnology, Dr. BR Ambedkar University, Srikakulam, Andhra Pradesh, India

P. S. Pradeep
Centre for Laboratory Animal Technology and Research, Sathyabama Institute of Science and Technology, Chennai, Tamil Nadu, India

Samrat Rakshit
Department of Zoology, Guru Ghasidas Vishwavidyalaya, Bilaspur, Chhattisgarh, India

A. Ram Sailesh
Department of Environmental Science, Institute of Science, GITAM (Deemed to be University), Visakhapatnam, India

Vadde Ramakrishna
Department of Biotechnology and Bioinformatics, Yogi Vemana University, Kadapa, Andhra Pradesh, India

K. Santhiya
Department of Biochemistry, Biotechnology and Bioinformatics, Avinashilingam Institute for Home Science and Higher Education for Women, Coimbatore, Tamil Nadu, India

S. Saxena
Department of Medical Laboratory Sciences, Lovely Professional University, Phagwara, India

S. Shinde
Department of Biotechnology, Guru Ghasidas Vishwavidyalaya, Bilaspur, Chhattisgarh, India

D. Shukla
Department of Biotechnology, Guru Ghasidas Vishwavidyalaya, Bilaspur, Chhattisgarh, India

Sreedevi Muttathuveliyil Sivadasan
Department of Biotechnology, School of Life Sciences, Pondicherry University, Puducherry, India

J. Sivaprabha
Department of Biochemistry, Biotechnology and Bioinformatics, Avinashilingam Institute for Home Science and Higher Education for Women, Coimbatore, Tamil Nadu, India

Nagarjuna Sivaraj
Department of Biochemistry and Bioinformatics, GITAM Deemed to be University, Visakhapatnam, Andhra Pradesh, India

D. Sivaraman
Centre for Laboratory Animal Technology and Research, Sathyabama Institute of Science and Technology, Chennai, Tamil Nadu, India

N. Srinivas
Department of Environmental Science, Institute of Science, GITAM (Deemed to be University), Visakhapatnam, India

S. Sumathi
Department of Biochemistry, Biotechnology and Bioinformatics, Avinashilingam Institute for Home Science and Higher Education for Women, Coimbatore, Tamil Nadu, India

K. Suresh Kumar
Department of Environmental Science, Institute of Science, GITAM (Deemed to be University), Visakhapatnam, India

A. K. Tiwari
Department of Zoology, Bhanwar Singh Porte Government Science College, Pendra, India

Saritha Vara
Department of Environmental Science, GITAM Institute of Science, GITAM (Deemed to be University), Visakhapatnam, Andhra Pradesh, India

Amouda Venkatesan
Centre for Bioinformatics, School of Life Sciences, Pondicherry University, Puducherry, India

K. Vijaya Rachel
Department of Biochemistry and Bioinformatics, GITAM Deemed to be University, Visakhapatnam, Andhra Pradesh, India

N. K. Vishvakarma
Department of Biotechnology, Guru Ghasidas Vishwavidyalaya, Bilaspur, Chhattisgarh, India

Soumya Vishwas
Department of Biotechnology, Institute of Science, GITAM (Deemed to be University), Visakhapatnam, Andhra Pradesh, India

原著前言

2002年，Funkhouser提出了"诊疗一体化"(theranostic)的概念，指通过分子检测、影像学检查和靶向治疗将诊断与治疗相结合，旨在根据每位肿瘤患者的具体情况制订个性化治疗方案，从而改善疾病诊断和预后。治疗诊断学可以早发现、早管理和靶向精准治疗，使女性特异性肿瘤(female-specific cancer，FSC)患者最终获得更好的疗效。我们全面、准确地汇总了FSC的前沿诊疗策略（即诊断、治疗和精准医学相结合），著成本书，以飨读者。

FSC涵盖乳腺癌、宫颈癌、卵巢癌和子宫内膜癌，这些肿瘤的致死性极高，并且会在短期内出现疾病进展，主要是由于缺乏有效的早期检测方法及对放化疗的抵抗。迄今为止，通过使用化疗药物等细胞毒性药物改善FSC预后的尝试均未取得理想效果，其主要挑战仍在于多数患者FSC细胞对化疗的原发性耐药。因此，改善FSC的预后依赖于引入能调节原发及获得性耐药机制的新型药物。

对FSC中遗传、表观遗传及分子通路失调认识的加深，揭示了肿瘤发展相关机制的复杂性，这些机制包括关键致癌性或肿瘤抑制性miRNA的表达改变、甲基化模式修饰及关键致癌激酶上调等。此类认知将推动新型生物标志物的开发，从而辅助这些致死性疾病的早期诊断与管理。同时，这也为设计靶向癌症进展期间上调的特异性信号通路的创新治疗性化合物奠定了一定基础。

本书精准聚焦于具有更广泛治疗选择的主题范畴。通过探索目前针对FSC开发的新型诊疗一体化（即诊断、治疗与精准医学相结合）策略，对此类信息进行全面且准确的整合。此外，本书对新确诊及转移性FSC患者面临的化疗耐药、现有治疗方案及前瞻性治疗方案进行了深度剖析。最后，本书探讨了如何将这些多维进展整合至精准化与个体化的诊疗中，最终提高管理患者的水平。

Rama Rao Malla
印度安得拉邦维沙卡帕特南甘地技术与管理学院（认定具有大学资质）科学研究所
生物化学与生物信息学系癌症生物学实验室

Ganji Purnachandra Nagaraju
美国佐治亚州亚特兰大市埃默里大学温希普癌症研究所
血液学和肿瘤内科学系

序 一

在当今医学领域,精准医疗正以前所未有的速度重塑肿瘤治疗的格局。女性特异性肿瘤(包括乳腺癌、卵巢癌、宫颈癌和子宫内膜癌)因其复杂的生物学特性、高复发率及治疗耐药性,始终是临床与科研攻关的焦点。这些肿瘤不仅威胁全球女性的健康,更因其异质性和个体化治疗需求的迫切性,呼唤着更具创新性和针对性的解决方案。在此背景下,《针对女性特异性肿瘤的精准治疗》一书的问世,恰逢其时。

本书由 Rama Rao Malla 教授和 Ganji Purnachandra Nagaraju 教授领衔,汇集多国专家的智慧,系统梳理了女性特异性肿瘤的前沿诊疗策略。全书以"精准治疗"为核心,从分子机制到临床实践,从基础研究到转化应用,构建了一座连接科学与临床的桥梁。书中不仅深入探讨了植物化学物、纳米技术、代谢重编程等新兴治疗手段,还聚焦于化疗耐药性这一长期困扰临床的难题,提出了药物再利用、靶向联合治疗等突破性思路。

本书的独特之处在于其"从实验室到病床"的全程视角。每一章均以扎实的实验数据支撑临床观点,辅以丰富的临床试验案例,使理论性与实用性并重。无论是从事癌症生物学研究的学者、临床肿瘤科医师,还是药物开发领域的从业者,均可从中获得启发。对于医学生与科研新手,书中详尽的机制图解与术语表亦能助其快速把握核心概念。

精准医疗之路道阻且长,但正如书中反复强调的——唯有深入理解肿瘤的分子本质,方能实现真正的个体化治疗。期待本书能激发更多创新思维,引领未来研究迈向更高的精准度与治愈率。

愿每一位翻开此书的读者,都能在字里行间感受到科学的力量,并以此为翼,在对抗女性特异性肿瘤的征途中,开辟新的可能。

解放军总医院第七医学中心妇产医学部主任

2025 年 7 月

序 二

在医学的长河中,肿瘤治疗始终是一个充满挑战的领域。随着科技的进步和研究的深入,我们逐渐认识到,肿瘤并非单一的疾病,而是由多种因素引起的复杂病理状态。特别是针对女性特异性肿瘤,精准治疗的理念应运而生,为无数患者带来了希望。

《针对女性特异性肿瘤的精准治疗》一书正是在这一背景下诞生的。本书不仅汇集了当前女性特异性肿瘤研究的最新成果,还深入探讨了精准医疗在这一领域的应用与前景。本书的编著者都是在各自领域有着深厚造诣的专家学者,他们的贡献使得本书内容丰富、权威,且具有极高的实用价值。

本书内容涵盖了乳腺癌、卵巢癌、宫颈癌等多种女性特异性肿瘤的病理机制、诊断方法和治疗策略,每一章都详细介绍了相关肿瘤的分子生物学特性、遗传学背景及临床表现,为读者提供了全面的疾病认知框架。更为重要的是,本书深入探讨了精准治疗的核心理念,包括个体化治疗方案的设计、靶向药物的应用、免疫治疗的最新进展,以及多学科综合治疗模式的实践等。

精准治疗不仅是技术的革新,更是医学理念的转变。本书不仅为临床医师提供了宝贵的参考资料,更为患者及其家属提供了科学、系统的疾病知识和治疗选择。通过阅读本书,读者将能够更好地理解精准治疗的科学依据,从而在面对疾病时做出更为明智的决策。

在未来的医学发展中,精准治疗无疑将成为主流。本书的出版恰逢其时,不仅为医学界同仁提供了宝贵的学术资源,更为推动精准医疗在女性特异性肿瘤治疗中的广泛应用奠定了坚实的基础。我们期待本书能够为相关领域的研究与实践带来新的启示,为更多患者带来康复的希望。

是为序。

中国医学科学院北京协和医学院
北京协和医院妇科肿瘤中心主任

2025 年 7 月

前 言

随着医学研究的不断深入，人们对抗癌症的办法越来越多，对癌症的发病机制也有了一定的了解，各种新兴技术、分子靶向药物的问世及应用为癌症的诊疗提供了新思路。但在临床工作中，癌症耐药、治疗药物毒性等难题仍然困扰着我们。女性特异性肿瘤包括乳腺癌、宫颈癌、卵巢癌和子宫体癌，是全球女性健康的严重威胁。流行病学数据显示，这类肿瘤约占女性所有肿瘤的40%。近年来，随着环境的持续恶化和人们生活方式的改变，女性特异性肿瘤的发病率和死亡率均呈现显著上升趋势。作为妇产科医师，我们肩负着为患者提供个体化、精准化诊疗方案的重要使命，这要求我们必须系统全面地掌握肿瘤的发病机制，并持续跟进最新的治疗策略。

A Theranostic and Precision Medicine Approach for Female-Specific Cancers 一书由印度甘地技术与管理学院的 Rama Rao Malla 教授和美国埃默里大学医学院的 Ganji Purnachandra Nagaraju 教授编撰。两位教授长期致力于肿瘤早期诊断、耐药机制及靶向治疗研究，并在国际期刊发表百余篇高水平学术论文。本书聚焦女性特异性肿瘤的前沿诊疗进展，系统梳理了精准医学与诊治一体化的最新策略，并深入探讨如何将以上研究个性化地整合到临床实践中。阅读此书后，我深受启发，对女性特异性肿瘤的发病机制、治疗挑战及未来方向有了更深刻的理解。

我们翻译此书旨在为临床医师和科研工作者提供一份全面、权威的参考资料，帮助读者深入理解肿瘤的分子机制、遗传学特征、流行病学、耐药机制及新兴诊疗技术，从而为临床实践提供科学依据和创新思路。

在翻译过程中，我们始终秉持"信、达、雅"的原则，力求在忠实原著的基础上，确保译文的准确性与可读性。针对存在学术争议的内容，我们广泛查阅了国内外相关领域的权威指南、最新文献和研究数据，并通过译者注的形式加以说明，以保障译著的科学严谨性和临床实用性。

衷心感谢原著作者 Rama Rao Malla 教授和 Ganji Purnachandra Nagaraju 教授的卓越贡献，他们的研究成果为女性特异性肿瘤的精准治疗提供了重要理论依据和实践指导。我们要特别感谢所有参与本书中译本翻译和审校的专家同仁，正是他们严谨的学术态度和宝贵的专业意见，才使得这部译著更加完善。同时，也衷心感谢中华医学电子音像出版社对本书出版工作的大力支持。

最后，我们诚挚希望本书能为临床医师、科研工作者及相关从业人员提供有价值的参考，共同推动女性肿瘤防治事业的进步。

主　译

2025 年 7 月

目录

第 1 章　特定植物化学物在妇科肿瘤中的作用 ································· 1
　　Dariya Begum，Neha Merchant，Ganji Purnachandra Nagaraju
　一、概述 ··· 2
　二、子宫体癌 ·· 3
　三、宫颈癌 ·· 8
　四、卵巢癌 ·· 13
　五、结论 ·· 19
　参考文献 ·· 19

第 2 章　筛选三阴性乳腺癌的潜在治疗药物 ·· 31
　　Leimarembi Devi Naorem，Mathavan Muthaiyan，Ishita Bhattacharyya，
　　Dinakara Rao Ampasala，Amouda Venkatesan
　一、概述 ·· 32
　二、材料与方法 ·· 33
　三、结果 ·· 35
　四、讨论 ·· 44
　五、结论 ·· 45
　参考文献 ·· 45

第 3 章　女性特异性癌症的化疗耐药性及相关处理 ····························· 49
　　S. Sumathi，K. Santhiya，J. Sivaprabha
　一、乳腺癌 ·· 51
　二、卵巢癌 ·· 55
　三、宫颈癌 ·· 59
　四、结论 ·· 62
　参考文献 ·· 62

第4章 女性癌症的流行病学 ········· 72
Saritha Vara, Manoj Kumar Karnena, Bhavya Kavitha Dwarapureddi

一、概述 ········· 72
二、乳腺癌 ········· 73
三、宫颈癌 ········· 76
四、卵巢癌 ········· 78
五、子宫体癌 ········· 80
六、结论 ········· 81
参考文献 ········· 82

第5章 基于量子点纳米抗体的三阴性乳腺癌治疗技术 ········· 94
Rama Rao Malla

一、概述 ········· 95
二、具有生物医学应用价值的量子点 ········· 95
三、量子点的构造 ········· 95
四、量子点的独特特性 ········· 97
五、用于生物标志物检测的量子点 ········· 98
六、前哨淋巴结显像技术 ········· 98
七、量子点在三阴性乳腺癌靶向成像中的应用 ········· 99
八、用于三阴性乳腺癌生物发光成像的自发光量子点 ········· 100
九、量子点在三阴性乳腺癌微转移检测中的应用 ········· 100
十、用于三阴性乳腺癌免疫疗法的量子点 ········· 100
十一、用于基因治疗的量子点 ········· 101
十二、用于三阴性乳腺癌光动力和光热疗法的量子点 ········· 101
十三、用于三阴性乳腺癌靶向治疗的纳米抗体 ········· 103
十四、结论 ········· 104
参考文献 ········· 104

第6章 纳米技术在卵巢癌领域的进展 ········· 108
Kiranmayi Patnala, Rama Rao Malla, Soumya Vishwas

一、概述 ········· 110
二、诊断和临床治疗现况 ········· 111
三、纳米技术在诊断和成像中的应用 ········· 112
四、化疗中的纳米技术 ········· 115
五、临床前研究 ········· 117

六、纳米技术在新疗法中的应用 …………………………………………………… 119
七、结论 ……………………………………………………………………………… 123
参考文献 …………………………………………………………………………… 124

第 7 章　乳腺癌的植物药疗法 ………………………………………………… 135
Phaniendra Alugoju, Nyshadham S. N. Chaitanya, V. K. D. Krishna Swamy, Pavan Kumar Kancharla

一、概述 ……………………………………………………………………………… 136
二、乳腺癌在印度的患病率 ………………………………………………………… 136
三、乳腺癌发生的危险因素 ………………………………………………………… 136
四、乳腺癌相关的分子机制 ………………………………………………………… 137
五、乳腺肿瘤发生的诱因 …………………………………………………………… 140
六、用于乳腺癌研究的细胞系 ……………………………………………………… 140
七、乳腺癌的治疗策略 ……………………………………………………………… 141
八、植物药疗法 ……………………………………………………………………… 141
九、结论 ……………………………………………………………………………… 169
参考文献 …………………………………………………………………………… 169

第 8 章　卡铂和紫杉醇在子宫内膜癌治疗中的作用 ………………………… 184
Sreedevi Muttathuveliyil Sivadasan, Pavan Kumar Kancharla, Neelakantan Arumugam

一、概述 ……………………………………………………………………………… 185
二、子宫内膜癌的主要危险因素 …………………………………………………… 185
三、子宫内膜癌的治疗方案 ………………………………………………………… 186
四、卡铂的作用机制和化学特性 …………………………………………………… 189
五、紫杉醇的作用机制及化学特性 ………………………………………………… 191
六、结论 ……………………………………………………………………………… 193
参考文献 …………………………………………………………………………… 193

第 9 章　女性特异性肿瘤 ………………………………………………………… 197
P. S. Pradeep, D. Sivaraman, Jayshree Nellore, Sujatha Peela

一、概述 ……………………………………………………………………………… 198
二、结论 ……………………………………………………………………………… 205
参考文献 …………………………………………………………………………… 205

第10章　宫颈癌的治疗方案 ·· 209
　　　　S. Shinde, N. K. Vishvakarma, A. K. Tiwari, V. Dixit, S. Saxena,
　　　　D. Shukla
　一、概述 ·· 210
　二、病理生理学 ·· 211
　三、风险因素 ·· 212
　四、治疗策略 ·· 216
　五、先进疗法 ·· 220
　六、治疗性 HPV 疫苗 ·· 221
　七、宫颈癌预防措施 ·· 222
　参考文献 ·· 222

第11章　通过计算方法识别宫颈癌靶向分子 ····················· 228
　　　　Manoj Kumar Gupta, Vadde Ramakrishna
　一、概述 ·· 229
　二、靶分子的鉴定 ··· 230
　三、药物鉴定 ·· 233
　四、结论 ·· 233
　参考文献 ·· 234

第12章　宫颈癌代谢：代谢途径和细胞能量产生的主要重编程 ········ 240
　　　　Vijaya Rachel, Nagarjuna Sivaraj
　一、概述 ·· 241
　二、糖酵解 ··· 242
　三、磷酸戊糖途径 ··· 243
　四、脂肪酸氧化 ·· 244
　五、肿瘤代谢和诊断成像 ··· 245
　参考文献 ·· 247

第13章　乳腺癌和宫颈癌相关治疗的药物经济学和成本效益 ········ 253
　　　　Mohan Krishna Ghanta, Santosh C. Gursale, Narayan P. Burte,
　　　　L. V. K. S. Bhaskar
　一、概述 ·· 254
　二、药物经济学 ·· 254
　三、乳腺癌 ··· 255

四、宫颈癌 ·· 258
五、结论 ·· 260
参考文献 ·· 260

第14章 针对女性特异性肿瘤的精准医疗：策略、挑战和解决方案 ·············· 265
Rama Rao Malla, Ganji Purnachandra Nagaraju

参考文献 ·· 267

第15章 环境致癌物及其对女性特异性肿瘤的影响 ······························ 269
N. Srinivas, Rama Rao Malla, K. Suresh Kumar, A. Ram Sailesh

一、概述 ·· 270
二、致癌因素 ·· 270
三、致癌物质 ·· 270
四、其他致癌因素 ·· 274
五、女性特异性肿瘤 ······································ 274
六、接触持久性有机污染物对女性健康的影响 ················ 276
七、持久性有机污染物的作用机制 ·························· 276
八、持久性有机污染物对癌症的影响 ························ 276
九、结论 ·· 277
参考文献 ·· 277

第16章 CYP1B1基因rs1056836位点多态性与子宫内膜癌风险的荟萃分析 ········· 285
Samrat Rakshit, L. V. K. S. Bhaskar

一、概述 ·· 286
二、材料和方法 ·· 287
三、结果 ·· 287
四、讨论 ·· 290
参考文献 ·· 291

第17章 纳米技术的发展在乳腺癌中的应用 ···································· 295
Kiranmayi Patnala, Soumya Vishwas, Rama Rao Malla

一、概述 ·· 296
二、纳米技术在癌症管理中的应用 ·························· 297
三、乳腺癌 ·· 299
四、纳米技术在化疗中的应用 ······························ 300

五、纳米技术在新型疗法中的应用 ………………………………………… 303
六、结论 ……………………………………………………………………… 306
参考文献 ……………………………………………………………………… 306

第 1 章
特定植物化学物在妇科肿瘤中的作用

Dariya Begum[a], Neha Merchant[b], Ganji Purnachandra Nagaraju[b]

[a] Department of Biosciences and Biotechnology, Banasthali University, Banasthali, Rajasthan, India
[b] Department of Hematology and Medical Oncology, Winship Cancer Institute, Emory University, Atlanta, GA, United States

摘要

妇科恶性肿瘤包括宫颈癌、子宫体癌和卵巢癌,其中宫颈癌是全球女性的第二大恶性肿瘤(译者注:仅次于乳腺癌)。妇科恶性肿瘤的治疗效果主要取决于疾病确诊时肿瘤的分级及分期。传统治疗方案包括手术切除、化学治疗和放射治疗,但存在肿瘤复发及不良反应等问题。以上治疗方法可导致原癌基因和抑癌基因失调,抑制细胞凋亡,促进转移,导致不良预后。因此,传统的治疗方法需要结合新型药物来预防不良反应的发生,同时增强肿瘤细胞对放化疗的敏感性。植物化学物质包括从植物中自然提取的生物活性化合物。这些生物活性化合物可以拮抗失调基因,联合使用可提高传统治疗的效果。在本章中,笔者研究了数种特定的植物化学物质,包括白藜芦醇、染料木素和姜黄素,这些植物化学物质目前已被广泛用于肿瘤单独治疗和与传统治疗结合的联合治疗中。此外,还探讨了这些生物活性化合物和新型纳米制剂的剂型,以提高所用药物的生物利用度、稳定性和药代动力学。

关键词

妇科癌症,预后,子宫体癌,卵巢癌,宫颈癌,植物化学物质,白藜芦醇,染料木素,姜黄素

缩略词

AgNP	银纳米颗粒
AHR	芳基烃受体
ATR	丝氨酸/苏氨酸蛋白激酶
COX-2	环氧合酶 2
CXCR4	趋化因子受体 4
DHA	二氢青蒿素
DHS	二羟基对称二苯代乙烯

EGCG	表儿茶素酸盐
EGFR	表皮生长因子受体
EMT	上皮-间充质转化
ER α,β	雌激素受体 α,β
ER	内质网
ERK	胞外信号调节激酶
FOXO3	叉头盒转录因子
GAL-3	半乳糖凝集素 3
HER	人表皮生长因子受体
HIF-1α	缺氧诱导因子-1α
HNPG	5-羟基 4′-硝基-7-丙酸-染料木素
HPV	人乳头状瘤病毒
IL	白介素
MK	肝素结合细胞因子
MMP	基质金属蛋白酶
mTOR	哺乳动物雷帕霉素靶蛋白
NF-κB	核因子 κB
NQO1	还原型辅酶
OCSLC	卵巢癌干细胞样细胞
P-gp	P 糖蛋白
PIK3	磷脂酰肌醇-4,5-二磷酸 3-激酶
PTEN	磷酸酶-张力蛋白基因（译者注：人第 10 号染色体缺失的磷酸酶及张力蛋白同源的基因）
STAT3	信号转导及转录活化因子 3
TGFA	转化生长因子
TPGS	d-α-生育酚聚乙二醇
VEGF	血管内皮生长因子

一、概述

妇科癌症是女性生殖系统恶性肿瘤，是女性第四大最常见癌症[1]。延误诊断的主要原因是人们对这些癌症的认知缺乏、病理鉴别不足和筛查机会短缺，导致这些癌症通常直到晚期才被发现。在妇科癌症中，子宫体癌、宫颈癌和卵巢癌最为常见，且对患者预后和临床结局有不良影响[1]。这些癌症的发病率和死亡率不同[2]。

据以往研究估计,2019年有10 900名女性被诊断患有妇科癌症,同年有33 100例死亡患者[3]。与妇科癌症相关的常见危险因素包括肥胖、高龄、使用促排卵药物、使用激素替代疗法、免疫抑制和吸烟。人乳头状瘤病毒(human papillomavirus,HPV)和衣原体等感染也是宫颈癌的危险因素[4]。此外,结直肠癌、乳腺癌和卵巢癌遗传史和家族史也与宫颈癌发生相关[1]。子宫切除术和输卵管结扎术可降低子宫体癌和卵巢癌风险[5]。因此,女性有察觉症状和体征的意识、进行规律的筛查及遵循预防策略非常重要[1]。此外,晚期及复发性肿瘤的治疗仍存在挑战。研究人员已多次尝试通过靶信号转导通路途径以控制癌细胞进展,并延长患者总生存期和改善预后。

基于恶性肿瘤的分期和分型,传统治疗方法包括化疗、放疗、免疫治疗和激素治疗等。常用于联合治疗的化疗药物包括紫杉醇、多柔比星和顺铂,但这些药物常伴随不良反应,并可能因为多药耐药性而导致疾病复发。耐药性通常是由信号通路失调引起的。因此,为实现更高的治疗目标,需要制订敏感和个性化的治疗策略。植物化学物质是从植物中获得的天然可用分子,具有多种生物活性。研究发现,这些化合物在拮抗导致恶性肿瘤的失调信号通路中发挥着关键作用。健康的饮食中很容易获得这些化合物,联合使用它们可以强化常规治疗的效果。此外,这些植物化学物质通常不会产生不良反应,还可靶向调节导致肿瘤增殖和进展的多种信号通路[6]。因此,这些植物化学物质具有抗癌特性,可用于癌症的治疗。

在本章中,笔者将重点介绍妇科癌症,以及特定植物化学物在控制肿瘤进展和诱导细胞凋亡信号通路中的作用。

二、子宫体癌

子宫是位于盆腔的一个中空器官,其功能是孕育胎儿。在解剖学上,子宫分为内层、外层和底层,分别称为子宫内膜、子宫肌层和子宫颈。子宫体癌是指子宫肌层细胞的异常生长。它发生在子宫的2个不同部位,据此可分为2类:①常见的发生于子宫内膜的子宫内膜癌;②少见的发生于子宫其他组织的子宫肉瘤。子宫体癌是预后较差的妇科肿瘤之一,其治疗方法为切除子宫。但肿瘤复发需要有效的治疗药物。培唑帕尼(译者注:一种血管生成抑制剂)和曲贝替定(译者注:一种烷化剂)最常用于子宫体癌的治疗,但对于肿瘤细胞因信号通路失调而产生耐药性的效果较差。例如,哺乳动物雷帕霉素靶蛋白(mammalian target of rapamycin,mTOR)信号通路常在妇科肿瘤患者中异常高表达[7]。类似的,子宫内膜样癌由DNA错配修复基因失调,以及磷酸酶-张力蛋白基因(phosphatase and tensin homolog,*PTEN*)和*KRAS*突变引起[8-10]。肿瘤蛋白53(tumor protein 53,*TP53*)基因突变、人表皮生长因子受体2(human epidermal growth factor receptor 2,*HER2*)基因异常扩增、钙黏蛋白 E 失活也会导致子宫内膜癌[11]。此外,子宫浆液性癌是由于 p53（译者注:原文有误,应为 TP53。该错误后文多次出现,为尊重原著,本版译文保留原著书写方式,请读者注意）、PIK3CA、HER2 和 PPP2R1A 基因突变、细胞周期调节蛋白 D1/E 过表达、钙黏蛋白和 p16 表达下调引起的[12,13]。因此,下调的抑癌基因和凋亡基因、上调的生存基因及信号通路共同导致了化疗耐药。发现这些失调基因并用活性植物化学物靶向作用它们可以增加化疗敏感性,获得更好的生存结局。

(一) 白藜芦醇

白藜芦醇是天然多酚类生物活性化合物,又称 3,5,4′三羟基二苯乙烯,存在于葡萄、花生、浆果和高浓度红酒中[14],因其抗氧化和抗癌特性而广受欢迎。作为一种抗炎物质,它可以调节某些促炎蛋白和酶的激活,如核因子 κB(nuclear factor kappa B,NF-κB)[15]和环氧合酶 2(cyclooxygenase-2,COX-2)[16]。白藜芦醇通过激活 AMPK 依赖的信号通路诱导自噬,但研究发现,自噬也会诱导癌症进展[17]。因此,Fukuda 等提出白藜芦醇和自噬抑制剂——氯喹可有效诱导子宫内膜癌细胞 Ishikawa 的凋亡[18],并可作为一种诱导细胞凋亡的治疗策略。但白藜芦醇诱导细胞自噬和凋亡的分子机制尚不明确。肾上腺髓质素存在于上皮细胞和间质中[19],在子宫内膜修复时表达上调,并通过诱导内皮细胞增殖和管腔形成以促进血管生成。此外,研究发现在缺氧条件下,通过激活缺氧诱导因子-1α(hypoxia inducible factor-1 alpha,HIF-1α),多种癌症中肾上腺髓质素 mRNA 和肽水平较高[20-23]。Evans 等进一步确定 HIF-1α 可诱导子宫内膜癌原代细胞分泌血管内皮生长因子(vascular endothelial growth factor,VEGF)[24]。他们还首次发现白藜芦醇和表儿茶素酸盐(epigallocatechin gallate,EGCG)抑制肾上腺髓质素分泌,从而降低癌症发病率。激活 Wnt 信号通路可诱导 β-联蛋白(β-catenin)积累,并将其转运至细胞核,随后激活 c-myc 和细胞周期蛋白 D(cyclin D)转录,从而促进各种肿瘤的发生[19]。白藜芦醇在胃癌和结直肠癌中可抑制 Wnt 信号通路。Sexton 等[25]发现,在子宫肿瘤细胞中,高剂量白藜芦醇可通过抑制 COX-2 诱导细胞凋亡,并在一组细胞系中验证其可影响肿瘤细胞增殖;在子宫肉瘤细胞中,白藜芦醇可抑制 β-catenin 和 c-myc 表达（译者注:全书多次出现 c-myc 和 c-Myc 混用,为尊重原著,本版译文保留原著书写方式,请读者注意）。因此,它通过使 Wnt 信号通路失活而抑制细胞增殖,诱导细胞凋亡[26]。随后,Chen 等[27]发现,白藜芦醇可抑制 β-catenin 进而抑制子宫肌瘤。子宫肌瘤是最常见的子宫肿瘤[28,29],可产生大量细胞外基质(extracellular matrix,ECM),包括胶原蛋白、纤维连接蛋白和蛋白聚糖[30,31]。此外,α-SMA、COL1A1 和 β-catenin 在 ECM 中表达上调,导致子宫肌瘤的发生、发展。体内外试验均表明,白藜芦醇降低了上述因子 mRNA 和蛋白的表达水平,但其所涉及的分子机制尚未明确[27]。综上所述，白藜芦醇可以作为癌症治疗的补充药物，但要确定这种化合物的具体功效，还需要进行进一步研究。

(二)姜黄素

姜黄素是一种活性植物化学物，源自一种治疗用途的印度香料——姜黄。它用于治疗多种癌症，如子宫平滑肌肉瘤。此前有研究表明，姜黄素通过下调 *MTOR*[32,33]等癌基因的表达来抑制肿瘤细胞生长。Wong 等[34]发现该生物活性化合物下调了子宫平滑肌肉瘤细胞中 mTOR(Ser2448)及其效应因子 p70S6 和 S6 的磷酸化；随后他们证实，经腹腔注射姜黄素可抑制体内子宫平滑肌肉瘤细胞的生长。它们通过抑制 mTOR 及诱导细胞凋亡来控制生长。低剂量姜黄素可抑制 mTOR，但对 Akt 无抑制作用。腹腔使用姜黄素可提高姜黄素抑制 Akt 和 mTOR 的生物利用度和效果。雄激素受体可诱导 Wnt 信号通路激活并导致耐药。在另一项研究中，Feng 等[35]发现，姜黄素在人子宫内膜癌细胞中通过下调 Wnt 信号通路中的 AR 和 β-catenin 表达而诱导细胞凋亡。姜黄素还以剂量依赖方式下调基质金属蛋白酶-2(matrix metalloproteinase-2，MMP-2)的 mRNA 和蛋白表达。此外，钙黏蛋白 E 与 MMP-2 成反比，而 MMP-2 在高浓度姜黄素暴露中表达上调[36]。既往研究发现，姜黄素在子宫内膜癌细胞中通过下调 MMP-2 和 MMP-9 介导的胞外信号调节激酶(extracellular signal-regulated kinase，ERK)通路来控制肿瘤细胞的迁移[37]。多种癌细胞中可检测到 Slit-2，它是一种分泌蛋白，是轴突引导分子，在抑制肿瘤细胞生长和新陈代谢、诱导细胞凋亡和细胞周期阻滞等方面起着至关重要的作用。Sirohi 等[38]检测到姜黄素诱导 Slit-2 表达，通过下调趋化因子受体 4[(C-X-C)chemokine receptor type 4，CXCR4]、MMP-2、MMP-9 和 SDF-1 来抑制肿瘤细胞的迁移。因此，姜黄素可以选择性地影响子宫内膜肿瘤细胞聚集和转移，但姜黄素的生物利用度和稳定性一直限制其应用。研究人员已经修改了姜黄素的结构以生产其类似物。例如，姜黄素类似物 HO-3867，在早期研究中可介导抑制信号转导及转录活化因子 3(signal transducer and activator of transcription 3，STAT3)磷酸化，并诱导各种癌细胞的凋亡[39,40]。Tierney 等[41]的研究发现，pSTAT3 Ser727 表达与子宫内膜肿瘤的生长和存活有关；并且 HO-3867 可以靶向 pSTAT3 Ser727，通过下调活性的 CDK5 和 ERK1/2 来抑制 Ishikawa 细胞的生长和增殖。此外他们还发现，HO-3867 可以上调抑癌蛋白 p53 表达、诱导 caspase-3 和 caspase-7 分裂，以及下调 Bcl-2 和 Bcl-xL 的表达；HO-3867 还可以诱导细胞周期阻滞在 G2/M 期。以上结果表明，HO-3867 有可能成为一种很有前景的癌症治疗药物。此外，纳米技术的发展提高了植物化学药物的疗效。例如，使用聚乙二醇(15)-羟基硬脂酸酯和 d-α-生育酚基聚乙二醇(tocopheryl polyethylene glycol, TPGS) 首次将姜黄素成功封装在混合胶束中。纳米设计的姜黄素胶束通过增强细胞内摄取及诱导细胞凋亡,从而具有更有效的抗癌特性,这是由于子宫内膜癌细胞系中表达下调。此外,其能调节 P 糖蛋白(permeability glycolprotein,P-gp)流出,防止肿瘤细胞产生耐药性,并下调肿瘤坏死因子-α(tumor necrosis factor-α,TNF-α)、白介素(interleukin,IL)-6 和 IL-10[42]的表达。同样,Xu 等[43]的研究证实,姜黄素包裹的脂质体在体内和体外均可有效抑制 NF-κB 对子宫内膜癌细胞的激活。研究还发现,其可以下调 MMP-9 的表达,说明姜黄素在纳米颗粒中具有治疗潜力和效果。姜黄素的临床试验记录见表 1-1。然而,有必要进一步探索该植物化学物的分子机制,评价其安全性和有效性。

表 1-1 植物化学物用于妇科肿瘤的临床试验记录

妇科肿瘤类型	植物化学物	干预药物	文章标题	阶段	临床试验标识号
宫颈癌、子宫体癌、子宫内膜癌	姜黄素(饮食补充)	帕博利珠单抗、放射治疗、阿司匹林、兰索拉唑、环磷酰胺、维生素 D	患者管理与"免疫鸡尾酒"疗法	Ⅱ期	NCT03192059
子宫内膜癌	姜黄素(饮食补充)	curcuphyt(译者注:药名,一种姜黄提取物补品)	姜黄素对子宫内膜癌患者有抑制肿瘤和诱导炎症的作用	Ⅱ期	NCT02017353
子宫内膜癌	染料木素	染料木素	染料木素预防健康绝经后女性罹患子宫内膜癌的有效性研究	Ⅰ期	NCT00099008
宫颈上皮内瘤变	姜黄素	姜黄素	姜黄素治疗宫颈鳞状上皮内瘤变的疗效观察	Ⅰ期早期	NCT02554344
肿瘤/子宫病变	姜黄素	姜黄素	局部应用姜黄素治疗宫颈癌前病变	Ⅱ期	NCT02944578

(三)染料木素

染料木素是一种从大豆产品中提取的天然异黄酮,因其雌激素作用而广为人知,是激素治疗的替代选择之一[44,45]。既往研究表明,染料木素具有抗氧化和抗转移的特性，可以在体内外调节负责细胞生长、血管生成和凋亡的多种基因的表达。染料木素因具有抗增殖作用而常用于治疗各种癌症的临床试验，包括结直肠癌、前列腺癌和膀胱癌。染料木素还可调节子宫肉瘤细胞的增殖。Hu 等[46]的研究发现，使用染料木素、香豆素、大豆黄酮等中草药产品和他莫昔芬可降低中国台湾省女性子宫内膜癌的发生风险。他莫昔芬常用于治疗雌激素受体阳性的乳腺癌，以减少复发。但持续使用会增加子宫内膜癌的发生风险，因此，联合使用植物雌激素中草药产品可以降低应用他莫昔芬者罹患子宫内膜癌的风险。有研究比较切除卵巢的大鼠立即应用和后期补充雌激素或染料木素发生子宫内膜癌的风险。结果显示，后期给予雌激素的大鼠出现增强的雌激素信号级联，由于 Ki67 和 VEGF-A 的激活导致细胞增殖，增加子宫内膜癌的风险。但在给予染料木素的大鼠中，无论何时补充，均未检测到这种细胞增殖。因此，与应用雌激素相比，应用染料木素的大鼠发生子宫内膜癌的风险较低[47]。此外，Naciff 等[48]通过比较其制备的同时暴露于染料木素和雌二醇的 Ishikawa 细胞的表达谱发现，染料木素的雌激素源性与雌二醇相似。他们还发现，染料木素以时间和剂量依赖的方式上调和下调多个与生物功能相关基因的表达，包括 FOS、EGFR1、FGFR2、SOX4、PTEN 和 TGFA，这些基因在人类子宫内膜中发挥着至关重要的作用。染料木素还可以通过上调 BAX 和 BAD 等促凋亡蛋白的表达和激活 caspase-3 来诱导 DNA 断裂和促进细胞凋亡[49]。同时，染料木素增强了 p27、p53 和 p21 的激活，降低了 β-catenin 的表达，以控制子宫内膜癌细胞的生长[49]。此外，染料木素还能诱导子宫内膜癌细胞凋亡，并对多柔比星产生耐药性。前期报道服用大剂量染料木素可以通过释放 TGF-β 来抑制酪氨酸激酶和 DNA 拓扑异构酶，诱导凋亡[50]。随后，Di 等[51]研究了染料木素通过 TGF-β 信号通路及其下游基因肌动蛋白 A（ACTINA）和 SMAD3 抑制子宫平滑肌瘤的生物学机制。研究结果表明，暴露于高剂量染料木素可下调 actin A 和 Smad3，有效控制子宫平滑肌瘤的生长。尽管染料木素因其抗增殖活性以拮抗肿瘤而闻名，但在胃肠道吸收不良，导致其使用受限。结构的改变会增强植物化学物的作用。Bai 等[52]测定了染料木素的一种类似物——5-羟基 4′-硝基-7-丙酸-染料木素（5-hydroxy-4′-nitro-7-propionyloxy-genistein，HNPG）。体外研究发现，HNPG 可诱导子宫内膜细胞的细胞周期阻滞在 G1 期。此外，HNPG 还下调了 cyclin D1、MMP-2、MMP-7、MMP-9、c-myc 和 β-catenin 的表达，使 Wnt/β-catenin 信号通路失活，同时提高了药物的稳定性和延长了药物的半衰期。确定染料木素疗效的临床试验见表 1-1。未来的研究重点在于提高染料木素的疗效和稳定性，以改进治疗策略。

三、宫颈癌

宫颈癌发生于与阴道相连的靠近子宫底部的子宫颈细胞。根据世界卫生组织（World Health Organization，WHO）的评估，宫颈癌是女性第四大易复发性癌症[53]。

宫颈癌在其侵袭前阶段没有任何症状，但细胞表现异常并侵入邻近组织，主要症状为月经间期的异常阴道出血或月经量异常增多。危险因素包括致癌的 HPV 的持续感染、吸烟和口服避孕药的使用[54]。鳞状细胞癌和腺癌是宫颈癌的 2 种主要病理类型，也是患者治疗方案选择和预后的决定性因素[55]。宫颈癌首选治疗方法仍为手术，但出现肿瘤复发和转移者通常预后不良[56]。化学治疗（简称"化疗"）是避免术后复发的选择，常用化疗药物主要以顺铂为基础，联合药物包括贝伐珠单抗、帕博利珠单抗和吉西他滨。然而，产生耐药性和药物不良反应往往影响治疗效果。因此，迫切需要探索对正常细胞毒性更小、疗效更持续的治疗策略。

（一）白藜芦醇

白藜芦醇是一种从浆果、花生和葡萄中获得的天然生物活性植物抗毒素[57]。研究表明，植物抗毒素具有多种生物学特性，如抗细胞增殖、抗转移、抗氧化和保护心脏[58,59]。早期相关研究显示，植物抗毒素对多种肿瘤具有抑癌和抗凋亡的作用。在宫颈癌方面，白藜芦醇通过诱导辐射增敏和凋亡效应而抑制多种肿瘤发生相关信号通路[60]。例如，白藜芦醇参与调控 STAT3、Notch 和 Wnt 这些宫颈癌相关肿瘤信号通路；白藜芦醇诱导 HeLa 和 SiHa 细胞株凋亡并抑制其进展，进一步抑制 JAK3-STAT3、Notch 和 Wnt 信号通路[61]。分析宫颈癌中 STAT3 的活性发现，SOCS3、SHP2 和 PIAS3 这 3 种蛋白抑制 STAT3 信号通路表达，而这 3 种蛋白在宫颈癌患者中表达下调。白藜芦醇通过影响上述 3 种蛋白从而抑制 STAT3 信号通路，进而控制宫颈癌的进展[62]。此外，研究发现，宫颈癌细胞中 PIAS3 和 SOCS3 表达降低[62]。应用白藜芦醇治疗后，PIAS3 表达增强为 SOCS3 的 3 倍，最终导致其在体内抑制 JAK1/2 酶活性，并显著抑制 STAT3 信号通路[62]。因此，PIAS3 激活可以预测白藜芦醇的治疗效果。Li 等[63]的研究发现，白藜芦醇可以激活线粒体凋亡信号通路，上调疏基蛋白酶-3 和疏基蛋白酶-9 表达、下调包括 Bcl-2 在内的抗凋亡蛋白表达。白藜芦醇通过下调细胞周期蛋白 D1（cyclin D1），使细胞周期阻滞在 G2 期。同组研究人员还发现，白藜芦醇可以增强 HeLa 细胞中肿瘤抑制因子 p53 的上调。E6 和 E7 基因激活使 p53 等多种肿瘤抑制蛋白失活，导致 HPV 感染，与约 55% 的宫颈癌有关。这些基因通过泛素化失活并被 E3 泛素连接酶(E6 相关蛋白)降解[64]。此外,当卤代烃等环境污染物与芳基烃受体(aryl hydrocarbon receptor,AHR)结合时,Mdm2 等 E3 泛素连接酶蛋白被激活[65]。研究人员推测这种 AHR 激活可能导致 p53 泛素化并促进宫颈癌的发生,但其与宫颈癌细胞增殖的关系尚不清楚。Flores 等[66]研究显示,白藜芦醇与 α-萘黄酮共同诱导细胞凋亡,抑制细胞增殖。它们通过共同激活 E2F4/5 诱导肿瘤抑制,并诱导细胞周期阻滞在 G1/S 期,延长了 p53 的半衰期。随后他们提出,AHR 的作用取决于细胞类型和细胞转化状态。他们发现,敲除 AHR 基因并不会抑制细胞增殖或促进细胞凋亡。可见 α-萘黄酮和白藜芦醇均能抑制 HeLa 细胞增殖并诱导细胞凋亡,对 AHR 无影响。同样,Mukherjee 等[67]使用一种联合植物化学药物 Tri-Curin,其中包括姜黄素、EGCG 和白藜芦醇,来抑制 HPV E6 和 E7 的表达。他们发现,在小鼠中皮下注射 TriCurin 无药物不良反应;同时,TriCurin 可以下调 HPV-18 E6 和 NF-κB 的表达,上调 p53 表达,激活巯基蛋白酶-3。此外,其使用的联合药物具有高稳定性且能抑制宫颈癌细胞的生长(80%~90%)。这种新型复合植物化学药物在未来治疗 HPV 相关肿瘤的前景十分可观。TRAIL 是非 p53 相关方式促进细胞凋亡的一种蛋白[68-70],也可以尝试作为控制宫颈癌细胞凋亡的治疗策略。Nakamura 等[71]发现,白藜芦醇通过磷酸化其转录因子 STAT3 来抑制凋亡抑制蛋白的表达;而抑制 STAT3 可以增强 TRAIL 表达,诱导细胞凋亡。他们用干扰小 RNA(small interfering RNA,siRNA)敲除宫颈癌细胞系凋亡抑制蛋白后,可以使细胞周期阻滞在 G2/M 期,同时钙黏蛋白 E 表达上调。因此,这是提高药物敏感性和诱导细胞凋亡的理想策略。与之相似,紫檀芪又称 3′,5′-二甲氧基白藜芦醇,具有如白藜芦醇的抗癌作用。研究发现,它通过破坏线粒体膜和抑制 mTOR/PI3K/Akt 通路诱导细胞凋亡[72]。植物抗毒素是一种有效的抗肿瘤药物,但其生物利用的局限性不利于进行进一步临床试验。近期,研究人员合成了一些增强生物利用度、提高药物稳定性和抗肿瘤疗效的类似物,包括 N-(4-甲氧基苯)-3,5-二甲氧基苯甲酰胺[73]和(E)-8-乙酰氧基-2-(3,4-二乙酰氧基苯)乙烯-喹唑啉[74],通过上调 Chk1/2-cdc25 和 p53/p21 肿瘤抑制蛋白诱导细胞周期阻滞在 G2/M 期。为提高药物疗效,研究人员还合成了胶囊化的白藜芦醇纳米颗粒。近期研究显示,绿色合成金纳米颗粒的白藜芦醇与多柔比星联合使用可以增强抑制宫颈癌的效果[75]。这种新型药物纳米载体提高药效的同时不会对健康细胞产生细胞毒性。因此,开发纳米复合物作为癌症诊断和治疗的先进应用至关重要。

(二)姜黄素

姜黄素是从长姜黄根中获得的天然酚类化合物。既往研究表明,姜黄素可以促进 p53 等肿瘤抑制蛋白表达,使各种促癌信号通路如 PI3K/Akt、Ras 和 β-catenin

失活。Nrf2 是一种靶向 NAD(P)H——醌氧化还原酶 1[NAD(P)H:(quinone oxidoreductase 1,NQO1)]的转录因子,NQO1 在诱导 p53 的稳定性中发挥关键作用,并可增强 Nrf2 的表达[76-79]。姜黄素可以促进 NQO1-p53 复合物的形成,也可以阻止 E6AP 等负调控因子在其启动子区域的结合[80]。姜黄素通过下调 β-catenin、叉头盒转录因子(forkhead box transcription factor,FOXO3)和 COX-2 等多种途径诱导其抗增殖作用,并降低 cyclin D1、Akt 和 HIF-1α 的表达。Ghasemi 等[81]发现,姜黄素可有效抑制 NF-κB 激活和 Wnt/β-catenin 信号通路,从而抑制宫颈癌细胞的进展和侵袭。失活的 NF-κB 可抑制 cyclin D1、MMP-9、前 MMP-2 和 COX-2 的表达[82]。姜黄素和氟尿嘧啶联合使用阻滞细胞周期停滞在 G2/M 期,使 G1 期前细胞凋亡。如前所述,HPV E6 和 E7 癌蛋白的过表达是导致宫颈癌的高危因素。这些病毒癌蛋白控制 PIRIN 的表达。PIRIN 对细胞上皮-间充质转化(epithelial-mesenchymal transition,EMT)和迁移过程中产生氧化应激传感器起着至关重要的作用。姜黄素可以下调 PIRIN 基因的表达,从而抑制 EMT。此外,该组研究者发现,使用 siRNA 敲减 PIRIN 可以显著增加钙黏蛋白 E 的表达,同时降低钙黏蛋白 N 的表达。当在细胞系和 PIRIN siRNA 中使用姜黄素时,也可获得类似结果[83]。在包括手术和放化疗在内的传统疗法中,光动力疗法在宫颈癌治疗中也具有一定优势,它并非完全切除肿瘤,但可缩小肿瘤体积,改善器官功能。He 等[84]将姜黄素与光动力疗法结合,通过靶向 Notch 信号通路来控制细胞侵袭。Notch 信号通路及其下游基因 VEGF 和 NF-κB 与宫颈癌的癌变相关。DAPT 是一种控制 Notch 信号通路的 γ-分泌酶复合物抑制剂,间接阻断了 Notch 信号通路。DAPT 与姜黄素和光动力疗法联合使用可以通过阻断 Notch 信号通路、抑制 NF-κB 和 VEGF 的表达,增强这种抑制作用。

显然,姜黄中含有的主要黄色生物活性化合物是姜黄素;还有其他相关化合物,如双脱甲氧基姜黄素和脱甲氧基姜黄素[85]。研究提示,这些化合物在多种癌症中均可通过线粒体功能障碍诱导细胞凋亡。研究发现,在宫颈癌中,这些化合物通过抑制 MMP-2 和 MMP-9 信号通路来抑制转移;还可调节参与促进转移蛋白的表达,包括钙黏蛋白 N、Ras、SNAIL、波形蛋白、β-联蛋白,ERK1/2 和 NF-κB 等均显著下调,PERK1/2 和钙黏蛋白 E 表达上调[86,87]。因此,这些化合物可以作为宫颈癌抗转移药物使用。目前,研究人员也在探索改变姜黄素的结构以增强化合物的动力学稳定性,提高其功效。Chaudhary 等[88]对在芳基环上被吡唑啉取代的 11 种新型姜黄素衍生物进行硅质分析。通过分子对接和模拟研究,确定所设计的类似物可与 IKκβ 蛋白有效的相互作用。4-溴-4′-氯类似物与 3 个氢键(对接分数为 -11.534 kcal/mol)相互作用,比原始化合物更有效(对接分数为 -7.12 kcal/mol)。该先导分子的共结晶结构直接连接到三磷酸腺苷(adenosine triphosphate,ATP)

结合袋上显示出较高的抑制作用。与原始化合物和紫杉醇相比,这种类似物增加了细胞毒性。但在体外试验中,由于巯基蛋白酶-3裂解增加,这种类似物导致细胞的凋亡率为70.5%,高于姜黄素本身的抑制作用(19.9%)。仍需要进一步的临床前和临床研究来确定姜黄素抗肿瘤药物的实际应用效果。此外,姜黄素在联合治疗中也显示出良好的效果。例如,当姜黄素和紫杉醇联合使用时可以上调p53表达,增强细胞药物敏感性并促进细胞凋亡。凋亡蛋白巯基蛋白酶(-3、-7、-8和-9)及PARP的裂解随着细胞色素c的释放而增强[89,90]。姜黄素可以逆转由紫杉醇引起的多药耐药性(multidrug resistance,MDR)。紫杉醇处理后,细胞内NF-κB、Akt[89]及其下游蛋白COX-2、cyclin D1[91]被激活,而使用姜黄素可抑制NF-κB和Akt。联合使用姜黄素和紫杉醇可通过抑制NF-κB、Akt而抑制XIAP、survivin和cIAP1等抗凋亡蛋白[90,92]。为提高其生物利用度和有效性,降低细胞毒性,目前研究者正在研发姜黄素胶囊化纳米技术。近期,研究者利用姜黄素衍生物ST06-Ag-NP设计了一种绿色合成的银纳米颗粒合成物(silver nanoparticle,AgNP),并在宫颈癌体外试验中应用[93],但现阶段主要数据与该研究尚无关联。Li等[94]比较了姜黄素和顺铂2种纳米载体的应用情况,根据其粒径、药物封装效率、药物释放量和Zeta电位(译者注:颗粒之间相互排斥或吸引力的强度的度量)对其进行了表征分析。这2种纳米载体分别为脂质聚合物杂化纳米颗粒和脂质聚合物纳米颗粒。体内外试验结果显示,含姜黄素和顺铂的脂质聚合物杂化纳米载体的细胞毒性比其他纳米载体更高,因此,脂质聚合物纳米颗粒可作为靶向肿瘤部位的有效药物载体。微泡介导的姜黄素也可以增强对宫颈癌的治疗效果。使用微泡可以提高药物稳定性及生物利用度,增加部分水溶性植物化学物的吸收。微泡与超声联合应用可以增强药物摄取,抑制肿瘤进展。Upadhyay等[95]研发了一种含有姜黄素的蛋白微泡,以牛血清白蛋白作为壳材料,全氟丁烷作为体外输送的核心气体。通过这种微泡,姜黄素的释放增加了4倍,肿瘤细胞的摄取增加了250倍,经3-(4,5-二甲基噻唑-2)-2,5-二苯基四氮唑溴盐(译者注:MTT法)检测,细胞活力下降71%。姜黄素对宫颈癌疗效的临床试验总结见表1-1,未来仍需开发更有效的药物系统提高给药效果和疗效。

(三)染料木素

既往流行病学研究认为,染料木素是一种从富含大豆的食物中获得的植物雌激素异黄酮,对预防宫颈癌等各种癌症都有积极作用。它具有抗增殖的特性,可以控制细胞周期和诱导细胞凋亡,更像是一种抗肿瘤药物。Hussain等提出,用染料木素促进染色质分裂和核聚集,使细胞凋亡[96],导致凋亡小体的积累以时间依赖的方式增加。通过流式细胞分析发现,使用染料木素可以诱导细胞周期阻滞在

G2/M 期。当应用染料木素时,降解 ECM 并促进肿瘤细胞迁移的 MMP,原本在宫颈癌细胞中下调的 TIMP、MMP 抑制剂表达上调。内质网应激在一定病理生理条件下可以诱导细胞凋亡,这种诱导反应源于内质网应激传感器释放 GRP78。染料木素显著增加了 GRP78 和 CHOP 蛋白的表达,可通过内质网应激诱导细胞凋亡[97]。DNA 甲基转移酶和组蛋白去乙酰化酶的激活导致异常的表观遗传修饰是宫颈癌的危险因素。染料木素还可使 DNA 甲基转移酶和组蛋白去乙酰化酶失活[98],增强 p21、钙黏蛋白 E、DAPK1 和 RARβ 等肿瘤抑制基因表达,而这些基因在宫颈癌中因甲基化酶在它们的启动子位点结合而被甲基化。此外,异黄酮化合物与多酚也具有抗癌特性。Dhandayuthapani 等[99]发现,染料木素单独或与白藜芦醇联合可使线粒体去极化和功能失调,激活巯基蛋白酶(-3 和-9)。巯基蛋白酶-3 依次裂解细胞和核成分,使 DNA 片段化并诱导细胞凋亡。此外,研究者还发现,这 2 种植物化学物均能抑制 HDM2 的表达,并促进 p53 的表达。既往发现,HDM2 基因在多种癌症中过表达,并与不良预后相关。它通过靶向 p53 降解该肿瘤抑制蛋白的蛋白酶,从而抑制细胞凋亡,诱导细胞增殖。早期研究发现,PI3K/Akt 信号通路促进肿瘤的发生[100,101],其下游 mTOR 促进肿瘤细胞的生长和存活[102]。mTOR 以 TORC1 和 TORC2 复合物的形式存在。它们被结合蛋白 4EBP1、翻译起始因子 eIF4E 和核糖体激酶 p70S6 激活,在多种癌症中表达上调。Sahin 等[103]发现,染料木素可增强 HeLa 细胞对顺铂的敏感性,表现为 mTOR 磷酸化减少、4E-BP1 和 p70S6 表达降低,而这些分子的水平通常会在初次使用顺铂后上调。顺铂已被证明可以上调 NF-κB[104]表达,应用染料木素共同处理 HeLa 细胞时,NF-κB 的表达下调。同样,Liu 等[105]发现,染料木素与顺铂联合使用可抑制 Erk1/2 磷酸化,降低 Bcl2 水平,增加 p53 和巯基蛋白酶-3 的表达,促进宫颈癌细胞系凋亡。研究人员正在努力通过开发类似物来提高染料木素的生物利用度并优化其药代动力学。Xiong 等[106]设计、合成并评估了 8 种染料木素类似物。他们发现,这些类似物具有高度抗增殖作用,并显示出更高的细胞毒性,在 C-5 和 C-7 中存在的 OH 组是导致其细胞毒性的原因。1-苄基-1H-吡唑-4-硼酸和吡啶 3-酰基是合适的生物异构体 4′-染料木素中存在的羟基苯基部分。类似的,染料木素类似物——7-二氟亚甲基-5,4′-二甲氧基染料木素也用于研究。它可以下调 c-myc 的 mRNA 和蛋白水平,进一步上调 Bax、巯基蛋白酶-9 和细胞色素 c 等凋亡蛋白,下调 Bcl-2[107]。近年来,纳米技术的应用提高了染料木素的抗癌特性,增强了药物在肿瘤部位的稳定性和负载性。例如,Cai 等[108]制备了一种新型的将叶酸与染料木素偶联的新型壳聚糖纳米颗粒。他们报道,FRs-α 在血液循环中的肿瘤细胞而非正常细胞中高度暴露。这些物质对叶酸很有吸引力,更容易靶向于与叶酸结合的纳米颗粒。他们将装载壳聚糖的纳米颗粒与叶酸纳米颗粒进行比较发现,后者同样显示出有效的促进细胞凋亡能力。与之类似,他们制备了一种可生物降解的 d-α-生育酚聚乙二醇 1000 琥珀酸 TPGS-b-PCL[聚(ε-己内酯)]纳米颗粒来封装染料木素治疗宫颈癌细胞系,在体外和体内可以更有效地抑制肿瘤进展,并增强细胞毒性[109]。上述研究结果显示了染料木素对抑制宫颈癌的优势作用。然而,进一步的临床研究及临床前研究对于确定该药物的疗效至关重要。

四、卵巢癌

卵巢是子宫两侧成对存在的生殖腺体,是雌激素和孕激素分泌的主要来源。据美国癌症协会统计,卵巢癌在女性癌症相关死亡中排名第五。每年约有新诊断患者 21 750 例,约有 13 940 例女性死亡与卵巢癌相关[5]。这是由于 4/5 的卵巢癌患者被发现时已是晚期。卵巢癌主要有 3 种类型,即卵巢上皮性癌(90%)、卵巢恶性生殖细胞肿瘤(3%)和卵巢性索间质肿瘤(2%)[110](译者注:《卵巢癌诊疗指南(2022 年版)》数据显示,卵巢上皮性癌约占卵巢恶性肿瘤的 80%,其次是卵巢恶性生殖细胞肿瘤和卵巢性索间质肿瘤,各约占 10% 和 5%)。卵巢癌相关的主要危险因素包括乳腺癌和卵巢癌家族史、绝经期激素治疗和肥胖[111-113]。此外,*BRCA1* 和 *BRCA2* 基因突变具有高度易感性,可导致约 40% 的卵巢癌发生[114]。卵巢癌的主要治疗方案为手术切除后进行辅助化疗。化疗与严重药物毒性和多药耐药相关。如前所述,使用植物化学物可以减少不良反应,并增强肿瘤细胞对化疗药物的敏感性。

(一)白藜芦醇

如前所述,白藜芦醇增强了各种癌细胞的抗癌特性,包括卵巢癌细胞。在卵巢癌 A2780 和 SKOV-3 细胞系中,白藜芦醇以时间和剂量依赖方式通过产生活性氧(reactive oxygen species,ROS)来抑制肿瘤细胞进展并诱导细胞凋亡。在人卵巢癌细胞系中,它以 ROS 依赖方式抑制 Notch1 信号通路表达,下调 Akt 的磷酸化促进 PTEN 表达[115]。有氧糖酵解在促进恶性肿瘤(包括卵巢癌)的生长中也有重要作用。白藜芦醇可抑制有氧糖酵解的过程。其通过减少对葡萄糖的摄取,诱导细胞凋亡,阻断 Akt 信号通路,调节卵巢癌细胞系中的 GLUT1 质膜转运。此外研究发现,白藜芦醇可以通过线粒体途径促进巯基蛋白酶-3 的分裂从而诱导细胞凋亡。除抑制糖酵解外,白藜芦醇还能激活 p-AMPK 信号通路,下调 mTOR。激活的 AMPK 进一步激活 TSC1/2 复合物,抑制 AMPK 下游 mTOR 蛋白,而该蛋白对肿瘤细胞增殖和存活起重要作用[116]。白藜芦醇与化疗药物表现相似。例如,白藜芦醇的作用类似于化疗药物奥沙利铂,促进癌细胞凋亡的同时还能促进免疫原性细胞死亡。Zhang 等[117]发现,白藜芦醇在体内和体外诱导免疫原性细胞死亡中发挥潜在作用。由化疗药物引起的免疫原性细胞死亡期间的信号提示也被证实与暴露于白藜芦醇时相似,包括 HMGB1 的分泌、细胞表面钙网蛋白的暴露和 ATP 的释放。他们发现,肿瘤微环境中存在成熟的树突状细胞和活性细胞毒性 T 细胞;进一步研究发现,TGF-β 的分泌减少,而 IFN-γ 和 IL-12p7 表达上调。这些均提示白藜芦醇可以联合程序性死亡受体配体 1(programmed death-ligand 1,PD-L1)和程序性死亡受体 1(programmed death-1,PD-1)抗体(免疫检查点抑制剂)为卵巢癌的治疗提供一种新方法。为确定白藜芦醇对卵巢癌细胞系的影响,Ferraresi 等[118]通过分析微 RNA(miRNA)组(microRNome)和转录组进行了与 IL-6 的比较研究。结果发现,当暴露于白藜芦醇和 IL-6 时,信使 RNA(mRNA)和 miRNA 表达发生相反的改变。此外,miRNA 的表观遗传修饰导致了基因表达改变。在 6 个 miRNA 中,hsa-miR486-3p(靶点 ULK2)和 hsa-miR21-5p(靶点 ATG10)通过 IL-6 的表达而上调,这些 miRNA 可以靶向作用于 STAT3,以促进肿瘤进展和转移。通过 IL-6 激活的 miRNA 也被发现可抑制卵巢癌细胞系中的肿瘤抑制因子 ARH-1,从而调节自噬,抑制细胞运动。在卵巢癌细胞中,miR-21 异常表达,与化疗耐药性和凋亡逃逸相关。白藜芦醇可以下调被 IL-6 激活的 STAT3,诱导 ARH-1 的合成,而 ARH-1 可以正向调节自噬。白藜芦醇通过与 BECLIN-1 结合,上调 ARH-1,诱导自噬。以上结果说明白藜芦醇在促进自噬和抑制肿瘤中也有一定作用。如前所述,并非所有 miRNA 都参与肿瘤的进展。例如,miR-424-3p 在 SKOV-3 和 OVCAR-3 卵巢癌细胞系中表达水平较低。研究发现,白藜芦醇可以诱导 miR-424-3p 的表达以控制肿瘤进展,由白藜芦醇激活的 miR-424-3p 可以诱导半乳糖凝集素-3(galectin-3,GAL-3)的降解,而 GAL-3 以 NF-κB 和 Akt 作为其上游诱导因子,可以促进肿瘤发生及促进药物耐药。白藜芦醇还通过降解 GAL-3、下调 Bcl-2 及上调巯基蛋白酶-3 以诱导细胞凋亡来增强对顺铂的敏感性[119]。尽管白藜芦醇具有很好的抗肿瘤特性,但由于其生物利用度低,与患者预后相关的临床疗效并不满意。然而,如前所述,已开发的白藜芦醇类似物在改善生物利用度方面表现出优势。例如,紫檀芪是一种去甲基化的类似物,已被研究人员广泛用于对抗卵巢癌细胞系。紫檀芪可以抑制卵巢癌细胞中的 STAT3 表达,使各种抗凋亡蛋白如 Bcl-2、Mcl-1 和 cyclin D1 下调,但其作用具有剂量和时间依赖性。其处于低浓度时,细胞周期阻滞在 S 期;处于高浓度时,细胞周期阻滞在 G0/G1 期。紫檀芪还可以提高顺铂等铂类药物对肿瘤细胞的敏感性[120]。4,4′-反式二羟基二苯乙烯(dihydroxystilbene,DHS)是白藜芦醇的另一种类似物,可以抑制核糖核苷酸还原酶(ribonucleotide reductase,RNR),比其原始化合物更有效。RNR 是一种催化 dNTPS 生物合成的酶,而 dNTPS 是 DNA 损伤修复和复制所必需的,由 RNR 的 M1 亚基

(M1 subunit of ribonucleotide reductase,RRM1)和 RRM2 2 个亚基组成。DHS 可以直接与 RRM2 结合,并通过细胞周期蛋白 F 引起泛素化。当其被蛋白酶体降解时可抑制 DNA 复制,诱导细胞周期阻滞在 S 期,并诱导细胞凋亡。此外,DHS 与 RRM2 结合增加 NF-κB 的活化,使胰腺癌细胞对吉西他滨、卵巢癌细胞对顺铂的敏感性增加[121]。此外,乙酰白藜芦醇可以抑制 NF-κB 激活,减少 VEGF 分泌,抑制血管生成[122]。近年来,研究人员开始研发对靶点开发新型的药物纳米载体。其中,草本纳米颗粒显示出类似于其他合成化学药物的治疗效果。Nam 等[123]使用朝鲜当归(Angelica gigas Nakai,AGN)及其提取的具有抗癌特性的苷苷和苦苷的提取物作为纳米颗粒。当与白藜芦醇结合使用时,AGN 显示强大的抗癌特性和在生理 pH 下有效释放白藜芦醇。Guo 等[124]开发了一种可使用铁蛋白(ferritin,FRT;pH 敏感的笼状纳米结构)和纳米级氧化石墨烯(nanoscale graphene oxide,NGO;具有巨大表面积的药物载体和高效的光热效应)。他们将白藜芦醇和 NGO 组合后与线粒体靶向分子 IR780 连接,封装为第二个载体 FRT。这样形成的 DDDs INR®FRT 在体内外卵巢癌细胞光热化疗中都是一种有效策略。它的设计是使药物在目标部位释放,不会对循环系统产生酸和热刺激。它针对线粒体释放白藜芦醇并与细胞器发生反应,进一步诱导细胞凋亡。这可能成为一种有效增强抗癌功能的药物传递系统。

(二)姜黄素

以前的多种研究中报道过这种黄色的膳食化合物,它对包括卵巢癌在内的几种癌症具有抗细胞凋亡的特性,研究发现其可诱导细胞凋亡[125]和自噬。然而,自噬激活不仅是死亡前期的信号,也是为了逃避细胞死亡以适应压力[126-128],进而对化疗产生耐药性。Liu 等[129]研究表明姜黄素通过增加 PARP 分裂和巯基蛋白酶-9 诱导卵巢癌细胞凋亡。同样,他们还发现姜黄素通过抑制 mTOR/Akt/p70S6K 信号通路诱导自噬,且具有时间和剂量依赖性。他们发现姜黄素抑制 mTOR 及其下游效应物的磷酸化,包括 4E-BP1 和 p70S6K,4E-BP1 和 p70S6K 的激活会促进血管生成和转移。此外,抑制这种级联反应进一步促进自噬,通过在肿瘤细胞中产生耐药性来削弱化疗的治疗效果。因此,他们将姜黄素与氯喹联合使用,以抑制自噬,同时抑制 Akt/mTOR/p70S6K 信号通路,以增强姜黄素的抗肿瘤活性。c-Myb 是另一种原癌基因,在多种癌症中诱导产生对顺铂的耐药性。Tian 等[130]发现 miR-520h 通过上调 TGF-β 和 c-Myb 促进 EMT 和转移。此外,在卵巢癌细胞中检测到它们的表达升高。另外,研究发现 c-Myb 上调 NF-κB 和 STAT3 的表达,而这两种蛋白会诱导 EMT。他们评估了使用 EGCG、姜黄素和萝卜硫素下调 c-Myb 表达和提高肿瘤细胞对顺铂的敏感性。其中 EGCG 对卵巢癌细胞的抑制作用更明显。因此,这些饮食因素作为中国传统饮食的一部分,将是一个有希望的抑制肿瘤的选择。同样,Zhao 等[131]也发现双氢青蒿素(dihydroartemisinin,DHA),它是青蒿素的活性代谢产物,从中草药青蒿中提取、具有药用价值、被用作抗疟剂[132]且具有抗肿瘤特性[133-137],它能诱导细胞凋亡和细胞周期阻滞,以抑制肿瘤进展。他们将 DHA 与姜黄素结合作为一种替代药物,通过抑制 midkine(MK)来加强卵巢癌的临床疗效。MK 具有肝素结合生长因子的特征,其在肿瘤中的过度表达与预后不良有关[138]。他们进一步发现,联合效应显示靶向 MK 的 miR-124 上调。miR-124 是诱导细胞凋亡的肿瘤抑制因子,在多种癌症中表达下调[139]。他们发现,单独 DHA 首先诱导细胞周期阻滞在 G2/M 期,姜黄素随后通过下调 Bcl-2 诱导细胞凋亡,而巯基蛋白酶-3 的表达未见明显变化。

此外,miR-124 的过表达和 MK 的表达沉默降低了编码 P-gp 表达的 MDR1 水平。另外,使用这种联合治疗显示无副作用且协同表现出有效的抗肿瘤活性,在体外和体内均可抑制肿瘤进展,诱导细胞周期阻滞。此外,研究发现 Wnt/β-catenin 信号通路在促进卵巢癌细胞增殖和 EMT 中起着至关重要的作用[140]。这种异常作用通路进一步上调其下游基因,包括 *cyclin D1*、*survivin*、c-*Myc* 和 *MMP*[141]。分泌型卷曲相关蛋白(secreted frizzled related protein,SFRP)是抑制 Wnt 信号通路的肿瘤抑制糖蛋白。然而,DNA 甲基转移酶存在下的 DNA 超甲基化导致 SFRP 失调,导致中国台湾省女性卵巢癌[142]。因此,Yen 等[143]将 DNA 甲基转移酶抑制剂 5-aza-2′-脱氧胞苷(5-aza-2′-deoxycytidine,DAC)与姜黄素联合使用,抑制 DNA 甲基化,诱导 SFRP5 表达,他们发现姜黄素抑制 DNMT 活性和 DNMT3a 蛋白表达。更进一步讲,这显著降低了 β-catenin 及其下游基因的表达。此外,这种佐剂组合还能抑制卵巢癌细胞的迁移,它们下调波形蛋白和纤连蛋白,上调钙黏蛋白 E。因此,姜黄素作为天然的 DNMT 抑制剂,增强了化疗药物疗效,可以应用于卵巢癌的表观遗传治疗。研究人员研发了姜黄素的衍生物,与原始化合物相比,它可以提高稳定性和生物有效性。例如 Koroth 等[144]合成了新的姜黄素化合物 ST03 和 ST08,具有诱导细胞凋亡和抑制迁移特性。本研究采用 PA1 卵巢癌细胞系和 MDA-MB-231 乳腺癌细胞系。姜黄素的两种衍生物对与癌症复发相关的干细胞样 PA1 癌型[145]和其他转移性 MDA-MB-231 细胞系均表现出有效的细胞毒性。此外,发现它们通过上调巯基蛋白酶-3 和巯基蛋白酶-9 来诱导内在凋亡途径。同样,有研究发现,另一种衍生物——二苯乙烯基哌啶酮(diarylidenylpiperidone)对卵巢癌细胞的抑制增殖和逆转 MDR 的效率优于原始化合物[39,146-149]。因此,这些化合物可作为新的抗肿瘤药物,以增强疗效和抑制癌症的转移和复发。纳米级的姜黄素颗粒也被开发用于克服 MDR。例如,用姜黄素包裹认为具有抗癌特性的 AgNP 可以使细胞敏感。对顺铂耐药细胞进行测试,将 cAgNP 进一步与顺铂联合应用并评估其抑制作用,结果显示,巯基蛋白酶-3/-9 和 p53 的上调增加、MMP9 基因下调,这表明诱导顺铂耐药细胞的凋亡效率升高[150]。同样,Zhao 等[151]融合聚乙烯亚胺[poly(ethylene imine),PEI]和硬脂酸作为纳米载体,通过磁共振成像证实,它们进一步装载姜黄素和紫杉醇,并靶向于卵巢癌细胞的 CD44 膜受体。植物化学物对妇科癌症化疗敏感患者的卵巢癌细胞 SKOV-3(译者注:为人卵巢腺癌细胞系)和 MDR SKOV3-TR30 最终产生抗癌作用。姜黄素通过逆转耐药和减少 P-gp 外排使细胞对紫杉醇敏感,证明了其分子机制。因此,这可能是一种很有前途的策略,没有不良反应,并且对耐药卵巢癌细胞具有有效的抗肿瘤特性。此外,设计一种新型的由液体驱动的共流聚焦,在聚乳酸-乙醇酸微颗粒中装载姜黄素,有利于腹腔内给药。这些化合物具有稳定性,姜黄素在离体培养基中的释放率达到 90%。药代动力学结果发现,通过腹腔注射,姜黄素能有效地释放到特定部位。因此,该研究将为卵巢癌等腹膜器官恶性肿瘤的治疗提供支持[152],纳米技术与药物联合使用是在克服多药耐药方面很有前景的一种卵巢癌治疗策略。

(三)染料木素

植物雌激素生物活性的染料木素是从大豆膳食中提取的,是一种异黄酮。早期流行病学研究发现,这些雌激素样化合物对治疗各种慢性疾病,如心血管疾病、糖尿病和癌症均有益。卵巢癌是激素相关性肿瘤。60%~100%的卵巢癌被认为与雌激素受体(estrogen receptor,ER)-α 和 ER-β 的失调相关,这 2 种受体因其配体结合特性和肿瘤进展程度而不同[153]。一般认为,ER-β 可以抑制肿瘤细胞增殖,而 ER-α 可以促进肿瘤进展[154]。Chan 等[155]研究了染料木素、大豆黄酮和 ERB-041(ER-β 合成激动剂)对卵巢癌细胞增殖、进展、凋亡、侵袭和增强 ER-β 活性的药理作用。研究者进一步确定染料木素诱导细胞周期阻滞在 S 期和 G2/M 期,而大豆黄酮诱导阻滞在 G1 期,这正是染料木素抑制 PI3K/Akt 磷酸化和上调 p21 表达的结果。FAK 的过表达与卵巢癌不良预后相关,同时发现这些生物活性化合物和激动剂起到抑制作用。化疗的局限性主要是卵巢癌细胞产生的耐药性。重要的是,卵巢癌干细胞样细胞(ovarian cancer stem-like cell,OCSLC)是一类由于其缓慢分裂特性而产生耐药性的细胞。它们无法被化疗药物靶向,而靶向这些细胞仍是临床应用的关键[156,157]。此外,激活 STAT3 的 IL-8 参与维持癌症干细胞(cancer stem cell,CSC)与肿瘤微环境之间的相互作用,这些与炎症和 ROS 产生、耐药性产生,以及肿瘤进展相关。为明确 IL-8/STAT3 的分子机制,Ning 等[158]将 SK-OV-3 细胞与 OCSLC 和巨噬细胞(THP-1)共培养。他们发现,干细胞是通过激活 IL-8/STAT3 活性而诱导[159],阻断 IL-8/STAT3 信号转导会延迟肿瘤相关巨噬细胞之间的通信。多项体外和体内研究表明,染料木素通过抑制各种肿瘤细胞中的

CSC 来抑制肿瘤发生[160]。Ning 等[158]发现,当染料木素暴露于 THP-1 处理的 OCSLC 中时,其通过阻断 STAT3/IL-8 信号级联中断它们之间的相互作用,并逆转极化。因此,染料木素抑制 SKOV-3 细胞的干性。综上所述,卵巢癌是雌激素应答性癌症之一,其进展和迁移是由 17β-雌二醇(E_2)激活的 EMT 所介导。此外,包括双酚 A(bisphenol A,BPA)和壬基酚(nonylphenol,NP)在内的内分泌干扰化学物质(endocrine disrupting chemical,EDC)在促进 EMT 引起癌症迁移中发挥主要作用[161]。Kim 等[162]研究显示,EDC-BPA 和 NP 上调波形蛋白、下调钙黏蛋白 E,促进 BG-1 卵巢肿瘤细胞的转移,这与 E_2 的作用相似,当使用阻断 ER 信号转导的 ICI 182780 拮抗剂时,进一步发现 E_2 的激活受到抑制。此外,他们还发现染料木素的作用类似于拮抗剂 ICI 182780,并在治疗时逆转卵巢癌肿瘤细胞的转移。它抑制由 BPA、E_2 和 NP 增强的 EMT。与拮抗剂一样,染料木素也激活 TGF-β 信号,其信号在卵巢癌细胞中被 ER 信号抑制。染料木素生物利用度低、稳定性差,限制了其应用。但结构修饰,如在染料木素中诱导 CF3 或 HCF2,会促进肿瘤细胞的抗肿瘤作用[163]。Ning 等[164]发现新合成的染料木素衍生物 7-二氟甲氧基-5,4'-二辛基染料木素(derivative 7-difluoromethoxyl-5,4'-di-n-octylygenistein,DFOG)能有效抑制体外 OVCSLC 的球形和集落形成,抑制 p-Akt、p-ERK1/2 和 NF-κBp65 的活性。此外,研究者还发现,该衍生物增强了 FOXO3a 和 FOXM1 表达的激活,这是抑制 NF-κB、PI3K 和 Akt 信号通路所必需的。同样,DFOG 也导致卵巢肿瘤细胞敏感,从而增强 let-7D(一种肿瘤抑制因子)的作用,进而导致与预后不良相关的 let-7D 与 c-Myc 表达下降;其下调可抑制 PI3K/Akt 信号通路,因此,let-7D 活性与 DFOG 对卵巢肿瘤细胞的致敏作用相关[165]。在另一项研究中,Bai 等[166]证实了一种新合成染料木素异黄酮 HNPG 的治疗效果。他们确定,HNPG 的体外抗肿瘤活性存在时间和剂量依赖性,其能抑制卵巢肿瘤细胞的增殖、转移和复制,并诱导细胞凋亡。他们发现,这种染料木素衍生物增加 ROS 积累并降低线粒体膜电位,并使 Bcl-2 下调和 Bax 蛋白上调的比例降低。此外,细胞色素 c 从线粒体膜释放,促进胱天蛋白酶裂解,诱导细胞凋亡。近期,Mittal 等[167]制备了染料木素,合成了负载染料木素的纳米结构脂质载体,以维持药物在卵巢癌肿瘤部位的有效释放。他们采用溶剂乳化和蒸发技术,以琥珀酸 TPGS 为表面活性剂,开发了纳米结构。生物分布和药代动力学研究均显示出有效的药物包埋率(94.27%)和更好的 Zeta 电位潜能(-20.21)。药物浓度在肿瘤部位保留时间较长,从而确定了染料木素的优良载体体系。未来的研究还需要根据癌症分期和类型来确定这些异黄酮的作用。

五、结论

妇科癌症是多种肿瘤抑制因子和致癌基因失调而引起的恶性肿瘤。传统治疗方法存在不良反应和肿瘤细胞对药物耐药的情况。因此，常规治疗方法外的优化治疗策略是必不可少的。生物标志物在妇科肿瘤的诊断和治疗中发挥着至关重要的作用，但缺乏精确的生物标志物一直是妇科肿瘤治疗的障碍。除此之外，对生物标志物分子机制的充分了解也是必不可少的，基因分型就是这样一种进步，其为根据疾病阶段制订个性化治疗方案奠定了基础。全面了解基因及分子途径涉及的基因失调和不良反应，才能消除肿瘤进展的威胁。植物化学物是自然提取的生物活性化合物，其有望消除这种威胁。此外，多项研究证明，膳食中植物化学物的摄入具有化学预防和肿瘤发生预防的作用。各种植物化学物的输注或与其他化疗药物的联合使用可增强治疗效果，以获得更好的临床结局。

此外，纳米颗粒作为药物载体的使用在各种体外和体内研究中被广泛探索。它们单独或与其他药物联合进行试验，以提高其疗效和药代动力学参数，同时增强化疗药物联合使用的治疗效果。本章主要关注各种失调基因及其在参与肿瘤进展不同信号通路中的作用，包括植物化学药物、化疗药物及纳米制剂在内的联合疗法的发展，有助于提高患者生存率，改善其生活质量，从而提高疗效并最大限度地减少不良反应。

参 考 文 献[*]

[1] Ledford LR, Lockwood S. Scope and epidemiology of gynecologic cancers: an overview. In: Seminars in oncology nursing. Elsevier; 2019.

[2] Centers for Disease Control and Prevention. Inside knowledge: get the facts about gynecologic cancer. CDC Publication; 2012.

[3] Siegel RL, Miller KD, Jemal A. Cancer statistics. CA Cancer J Clin 2019;69(1):7-34.

[4] Saslow D, et al. American Cancer Society, American Society for Colposcopy and Cervical Pathology, and American Society for Clinical Pathology screening guidelines for the prevention and early detection of cervical cancer. CA Cancer J Clin 2012;62(3):147-72.

[5] Torre LA, et al. Ovarian cancer statistics. CA Cancer J Clin 2018;68(4):284-96.

[6] Thangapazham RL, Sharma A, Maheshwari RK. Multiple molecular targets in cancer chemoprevention by curcumin. AAPS J 2006;8(3):E443.

[7] Dobbin ZC, Landen CN. The importance of the PI3K/AKT/MTOR pathway in the pro-

---

[*] 译者注：本书参考文献保留原著格式，以便读者查阅原始文献。

gression of ovarian cancer. Int J Mol Sci 2013;14(4):8213-27.

[8] Tashiro H, et al. Mutations in PTEN are frequent in endometrial carcinoma but rare in other common gynecological malignancies. Cancer Res 1997;57(18):3935-40.

[9] Enomoto T, et al. Alterations of the p53 tumor suppressor gene and its association with activation of the cK-ras-2 protooncogene in premalignant and malignant lesions of the human uterine endometrium. Cancer Res 1993;53(8):1883-8.

[10] Kim TH, et al. The synergistic effect of conditional Pten loss and oncogenic K-ras mutation on endometrial cancer development occurs via decreased progesterone receptor action. J Oncol 2010;2010:139087.

[11] Samarnthai N, Hall K, Yeh I. Molecular profiling of endometrial malignancies. Obstet Gynecol Int 2010;2010:162363.

[12] Catasus L, Gallardo A, Prat J. Molecular genetics of endometrial carcinoma. Diagn Histopathol 2009;15(12):554-63.

[13] Matias-Guiu X, Davidson B. Prognostic biomarkers in endometrial and ovarian carcinoma. Virchows Arch 2014;464(3):315-31.

[14] Biesalski HK. Polyphenols and inflammation: basic interactions. Curr Opin Clin Nutr Metab Care 2007;10(6):724-8.

[15] Rahman I, Biswas SK, Kirkham PA. Regulation of inflammation and redox signaling by dietary polyphenols. Biochem Pharmacol 2006;72(11):1439-52.

[16] Das S, Das DK. Anti-inflammatory responses of resveratrol. Inflamm Allergy Drug Targets 2007;6(3):168-73.

[17] Guo JY, Xia B, White E. Autophagy-mediated tumor promotion. Cell 2013;155(6):1216-9.

[18] Fukuda T, et al. Autophagy inhibition augments resveratrol-induced apoptosis in Ishikawa endometrial cancer cells. Oncol Lett 2016;12(4):2560-6.

[19] Maybin JA, et al. The expression and regulation of adrenomedullin in the human endometrium: a candidate for endometrial repair. Endocrinology 2011;152(7):2845-56.

[20] Cormier-Regard S, Nguyen SV, Claycomb WC. Adrenomedullin gene expression is developmentally regulated and induced by hypoxia in rat ventricular cardiac myocytes. J Biol Chem 1998;273(28):17787-92.

[21] Nakayama M, et al. Induction of adrenomedullin by hypoxia and cobalt chloride in human colorectal carcinoma cells. Biochem Biophys Res Commun 1998;243(2):514-7.

[22] Garayoa M, et al. Hypoxia-inducible factor-1 (HIF-1) up-regulates adrenomedullin expression in human tumor cell lines during oxygen deprivation: a possible promotion mechanism of carcinogenesis. Mol Endocrinol 2000;14(6):848-62.

[23] Nguyen SV, Claycomb WC. Hypoxia regulates the expression of the adrenomedullin and HIF-1 genes in cultured HL-1 cardiomyocytes. Biochem Biophys Res Commun 1999;265(2):382-6.

[24] Evans J, et al. Adrenomedullin interacts with VEGF in endometrial cancer and has varied modulation in tumours of different grades. Gynecol Oncol 2012;125(1):214-9.

[25] Sexton É, et al. Resveratrol interferes with AKT activity and triggers apoptosis in human uterine cancer cells. Mol Cancer 2006;5(1):45.

[26] Mineda A, et al. Resveratrol suppresses proliferation and induces apoptosis of uterine sarcoma cells by inhibiting the Wnt signaling pathway. Exp Ther Med 2019;17(3):2242-6.

[27] Chen H-Y, et al. Natural antioxidant resveratrol suppresses uterine fibroid cell growth and extracellular matrix formation in vitro and in vivo. Antioxidants 2019;8(4):99.

[28] Cramer SF, Patel A. The frequency of uterine leiomyomas. Am J Clin Pathol 1990;94(4):435-8.

[29] Baird DD, et al. High cumulative incidence of uterine leiomyoma in black and white women: ultrasound evidence. Am J Obstet Gynecol 2003;188(1):100-7.

[30] Arici A, Sozen I. Transforming growth factor-β3 is expressed at high levels in leiomyoma where it stimulates fibronectin expression and cell proliferation. Fertil Steril 2000;73(5):1006-11.

[31] Leppert PC, et al. Comparative ultrastructure of collagen fibrils in uterine leiomyomas and normal myometrium. Fertil Steril 2004;82:1182-7.

[32] Beevers CS, et al. Curcumin disrupts the Mammalian target of rapamycin-raptor complex. Cancer Res 2009;69(3):1000-8.

[33] Yu S, et al. Curcumin inhibits Akt/mammalian target of rapamycin signaling through protein phosphatase-dependent mechanism. Mol Cancer Ther 2008;7(9):2609-20.

[34] Wong TF, et al. Curcumin targets the AKT-mTOR pathway for uterine leiomyosarcoma tumor growth suppression. Int J Clin Oncol 2014;19(2):354-63.

[35] Feng W, et al. Curcumin promotes the apoptosis of human endometrial carcinoma cells by downregulating the expression of androgen receptor through Wnt signal pathway. Eur J Gynaecol Oncol 2014;35(6):718-23.

[36] Sun M, et al. Effects of curcumin on the role of MMP-2 in endometrial cancer cell proliferation and invasion. Eur Rev Med Pharmacol Sci 2018;22(15):5033-41.

[37] Chen Q, et al. Curcumin suppresses migration and invasion of human endometrial carcinoma cells. Oncol Lett 2015;10(3):1297-302.

[38] Sirohi VK, et al. Curcumin exhibits anti-tumor effect and attenuates cellular migration via Slit-2 mediated down-regulation of SDF-1 and CXCR4 in endometrial adenocarcinoma cells. J Nutr Biochem 2017;44:60-70.

[39] Selvendiran K, et al. Safe and targeted anticancer efficacy of a novel class of antioxidant-conjugated difluorodiarylidenyl piperidones: differential cytotoxicity in healthy and cancer cells. Free Radic Biol Med 2010;48(9):1228-35.

[40] Rath KS, et al. HO-3867, a safe STAT3 inhibitor, is selectively cytotoxic to ovarian cancer. Cancer Res 2014;74(8):2316-27.

[41] Tierney BJ, et al. Aberrantly activated pSTAT3-Ser727 in human endometrial cancer is suppressed by HO-3867, a novel STAT3 inhibitor. Gynecol Oncol 2014;135(1):133-41.

[42] Kumar A, et al. Enhanced apoptosis, survivin down-regulation and assisted immunochemotherapy by curcumin loaded amphiphilic mixed micelles for subjugating endometrial cancer. Nanomed Nanotechnol Biol Med 2017;13(6):1953-63.

[43] Xu H, et al. Liposomal curcumin targeting endometrial cancer through the NF-κB pathway. Cell Physiol Biochem 2018;48(2):569-82.

[44] Scambia G, et al. Clinical effects of a standardized soy extract in postmenopausal women: a pilot study. Menopause (New York, NY) 2000;7(2):105-11.

[45] Beck V, et al. Comparison of hormonal activity (estrogen, androgen and progestin) of standardized plant extracts for large scale use in hormone replacement therapy. J Steroid Biochem Mol Biol 2003;84(2-3):259-68.

[46] Hu Y-C, et al. Detection of a negative correlation between prescription of Chinese herbal products containing coumestrol, genistein or daidzein and risk of subsequent endometrial cancer among tamoxifen-treated female breast cancer survivors in Taiwan between 1998 and 2008: a populationbased study. J Ethnopharmacol 2015;169:356-62.

[47] Carbonel AF, et al. Soybean isoflavones attenuate the expression of genes related to endometrial cancer risk. Climacteric 2015;18(3):389-98.

[48] Naciff JM, et al. Dose-and time-dependent transcriptional response of Ishikawa cells exposed to genistein. Toxicol Sci 2016;151(1):71-87.

[49] Yeh C-C, et al. Genistein suppresses growth of human uterine sarcoma cell lines via multiple mechanisms. Anticancer Res 2015;35(6):3167-73.

[50] Polkowski K, Mazurek AP. Biological properties of genistein. A review of in vitro and in vivo data. Acta Pol Pharm 2000;57(2):135-55.

[51] Di X, et al. A high concentration of genistein down-regulates activin A, Smad3 and other TGF-β pathway genes in human uterine leiomyoma cells. Exp Mol Med 2012;44(4):281-92.

[52] Bai J, Luo X. 5-Hydroxy-4′-nitro-7-propionyloxy-genistein inhibited invasion and metastasis via inactivating Wnt/β-catenin signal pathway in human endometrial carcinoma Ji endometrial cells. Med Sci Monit 2018;24:3230.

[53] Ripon SH, Bhuiyan NQ. Cervical cancer risk factors: classification and mining associations. APTI-KOM J Comput Sci Inf Technol 2019;4(1):8-18.

[54] American Chemical Society. Cancer facts & figures 2019. vol. 2019. Atlanta: American Chemical Society; 2019.

[55] Bhatla N, Aoki D, Sharma DN, Sankaranarayanan R. Cancer of the cervix uteri. Int J Gynecol Obstet 2018;143:22-36.

[56] Touboul C, et al. Prognostic factors and morbidities after completion surgery in patients undergoing initial chemoradiation therapy for locally advanced cervical cancer. Oncologist

2010;15(4):405.

[57] Brisdelli F, D'Andrea G, Bozzi A. Resveratrol: a natural polyphenol with multiple chemopreventive properties. Curr Drug Metab 2009;10(6):530-46.

[58] Bollmann F, et al. Resveratrol post-transcriptionally regulates pro-inflammatory gene expression via regulation of KSRP RNA binding activity. Nucleic Acids Res 2014;42(20): 12555-69.

[59] Khurana S, et al. Polyphenols: benefits to the cardiovascular system in health and in aging. Nutrients 2013;5(10):3779-827.

[60] Chung T, et al. Expression of apoptotic regulators and their significance in cervical cancer. Cancer Lett 2002;180(1):63-8.

[61] Zhang P, et al. Biological significance and therapeutic implication of resveratrol-inhibited Wnt, Notch and STAT3 signaling in cervical cancer cells. Genes Cancer 2014;5(5-6):154.

[62] Zhang P, et al. PIAS3, SHP2 and SOCS3 expression patterns in cervical cancers: relevance with activation and resveratrol-caused inactivation of STAT3 signaling. Gynecol Oncol 2015;139(3):529-35.

[63] Li L, et al. Resveratrol suppresses human cervical carcinoma cell proliferation and elevates apoptosis via the mitochondrial and p53 signaling pathways. Oncol Lett 2018;15(6):9845-51.

[64] Stanley M. Pathology and epidemiology of HPV infection in females. Gynecol Oncol 2010; 117(2):S5-S10.

[65] Pääjärvi G, et al. TCDD activates Mdm2 and attenuates the p53 response to DNA damaging agents. Carcinogenesis 2005;26(1):201-8.

[66] Flores-Pérez A, Elizondo G. Apoptosis induction and inhibition of HeLa cell proliferation by alpha naphthoflavone and resveratrol are aryl hydrocarbon receptor-independent. Chem Biol Interact 2018;281:98-105.

[67] Mukherjee S, et al. Unique synergistic formulation of curcumin, epicatechin gallate and resveratrol, tricurin, suppresses HPV E6, eliminates HPV+ cancer cells, and inhibits tumor progression. Oncotarget 2017;8(37):60904.

[68] Pitti RM, et al. Induction of apoptosis by Apo-2 ligand, a new member of the tumor necrosis factor cytokine family. J Biol Chem 1996;271(22):12687-90.

[69] Zhang L, Fang B. Mechanisms of resistance to TRAIL-induced apoptosis in cancer. Cancer Gene Ther 2005;12(3):228-37.

[70] Wiley SR, et al. Identification and characterization of a new member of the TNF family that induces apoptosis. Immunity 1995;3(6):673-82.

[71] Nakamura H, et al. Therapeutic significance of targeting survivin in cervical cancer and possibility of combination therapy with TRAIL. Oncotarget 2018;9(17):13451.

[72] Bin WH, et al. Pterostilbene (3′,5′-dimethoxy-resveratrol) exerts potent antitumor effects in HeLa human cervical cancer cells via disruption of mitochondrial membrane po-

tential, apoptosis induction and targeting m-TOR/PI3K/Akt signalling pathway. J BUON 2018;23(5):1384-9.

[73] Lee K-W, et al. Resveratrol analog, N-(4-methoxyphenyl)-3, 5-dimethoxybenzamide induces G2/M phase cell cycle arrest and apoptosis in HeLa human cervical cancer cells. Food Chem Toxicol 2019;124:101-11.

[74] Kim J-Y, et al. Resveratrol analogue (E)-8-acetoxy-2-[2-(3, 4-diacetoxyphenyl) ethenyl]-quinazoline induces G2/M cell cycle arrest through the activation of ATM/ATR in human cervical carcinoma HeLa cells. Oncol Rep 2015;33(5):2639-47.

[75] Tomoaia G, et al. Effects of doxorubicin mediated by gold nanoparticles and resveratrol in two human cervical tumor cell lines. Colloids Surf B Biointerfaces 2015;135:726-34.

[76] Prasad S, et al. Curcumin, a component of golden spice: from bedside to bench and back. Biotechnol Adv 2014;32(6):1053-64.

[77] Theodore M, et al. Multiple nuclear localization signals function in the nuclear import of the transcription factor Nrf2. J Biol Chem 2008;283(14):8984-94.

[78] Stefanson AL, Bakovic M. Dietary regulation of Keap1/Nrf2/ARE pathway: focus on plant-derived compounds and trace minerals. Nutrients 2014;6(9):3777-801.

[79] Asher G, et al. Mdm-2 and ubiquitin-independent p53 proteasomal degradation regulated by NQO1. Proc Natl Acad Sci 2002;99(20):13125-30.

[80] Patiño-Morales CC, et al. Curcumin stabilizes p53 by interaction with NAD (P) H: quinone oxidoreductase 1 in tumor-derived cell lines. Redox Biol 2020;28:101320.

[81] Ghasemi F, et al. Curcumin inhibits NF-κB and Wnt/β-catenin pathways in cervical cancer cells. Pathol Res Pract 2019;215(10):152556.

[82] Shanmugam MK, et al. The multifaceted role of curcumin in cancer prevention and treatment. Molecules 2015;20(2):2728-69.

[83] Aedo-Aguilera V, et al. Curcumin decreases epithelial-mesenchymal transition by a Pirin-dependent mechanism in cervical cancer cells. Oncol Rep 2019;42(5):2139-48.

[84] He G, et al. Effects of notch signaling pathway in cervical cancer by curcumin mediated photodynamic therapy and its possible mechanisms in vitro and in vivo. J Cancer 2019;10 (17):4114.

[85] Paramasivam M, et al. High-performance thin layer chromatographic method for quantitative determination of curcuminoids in Curcuma longa germplasm. Food Chem 2009;113 (2):640-4.

[86] Liao C-L, et al. Bisdemethoxycurcumin suppresses migration and invasion of human cervical cancer hela cells via inhibition of NF-κB, MMP-2 and-9 pathways. Anticancer Res 2018;38(7): 3989-97.

[87] Lin C-C, et al. demethoxycurcumin suppresses migration and invasion of human cervical cancer HeLa cells via inhibition of NF-κB pathways. Anticancer Res 2018;38(5):2761-9.

[88] Chaudhary M, et al. 4-Bromo-4′-chloro pyrazoline analog of curcumin augmented antican-

cer activity against human cervical cancer, HeLa cells: in silico-guided analysis, synthesis, and in vitro cytotoxicity. J Biomol Struct Dyn 2019;38(5):1335-53.

[89] Bava SV, et al. Sensitization of taxol-induced apoptosis by curcumin involves down-regulation of nuclear factor-κB and the serine/threonine kinase Akt and is independent of tubulin polymerization. J Biol Chem 2018;293(31):12283.

[90] Dang Y-P, et al. Curcumin improves the paclitaxel-induced apoptosis of HPV-positive human cervical cancer cells via the NF-κB-p53-caspase-3 pathway. Exp Ther Med 2015;9(4): 1470-6.

[91] Bava SV, et al. Akt is upstream and MAPKs are downstream of NF-κB in paclitaxel-induced survival signaling events, which are down-regulated by curcumin contributing to their synergism. Int J Biochem Cell Biol 2011;43(3):331-41.

[92] Sreekanth C, et al. Molecular evidences for the chemosensitizing efficacy of liposomal curcumin in paclitaxel chemotherapy in mouse models of cervical cancer. Oncogene 2011;30 (28):3139-52.

[93] Murugesan K, et al. Effects of green synthesised silver nanoparticles (ST06-AgNPs) using curcumin derivative (ST06) on human cervical cancer cells (HeLa) in vitro and EAC tumor bearing mice models. Int J Nanomedicine 2019;14:5257.

[94] Li C, Ge X, Wang L. Construction and comparison of different nanocarriers for co-delivery of cisplatin and curcumin: a synergistic combination nanotherapy for cervical cancer. Biomed Pharmacother 2017;86:628-36.

[95] Upadhyay A, et al. Microbubble-mediated enhanced delivery of curcumin to cervical cancer cells. ACS Omega 2018;3(10):12824-31.

[96] Hussain A, et al. Inhibitory effect of genistein on the invasive potential of human cervical cancer cells via modulation of matrix metalloproteinase-9 and tissue inhibitiors of matrix metalloproteinase-1 expression. Cancer Epidemiol 2012;36(6):e387-93.

[97] Yang Y, et al. Genistein-induced apoptosis is mediated by endoplasmic reticulum stress in cervical cancer cells. Eur Rev Med Pharmacol Sci 2016;20(15):3292-6.

[98] Sundaram MK, et al. Genistein induces alterations of epigenetic modulatory signatures in human cervical cancer cells. Anti Cancer Agents Med Chem 2018;18(3):412-21.

[99] Dhandayuthapani S, et al. Induction of apoptosis in HeLa cells via caspase activation by resveratrol and genistein. J Med Food 2013;16(2):139-46.

[100] Vivanco I, Sawyers CL. The phosphatidylinositol 3-kinase-AKT pathway in human cancer. Nat Rev Cancer 2002;2(7):489-501.

[101] Wong AJ, et al. Increased expression of the epidermal growth factor receptor gene in malignant gliomas is invariably associated with gene amplification. Proc Natl Acad Sci 1987; 84(19):6899-903.

[102] Hay N, Sonenberg N. Upstream and downstream of mTOR. Genes Dev 2004;18(16): 1926-45.

[103] Sahin K, et al. Sensitization of cervical cancer cells to cisplatin by genistein: the role of NFkB and Akt/mTOR signaling pathways. J Oncol 2012;2012:461562.

[104] Solomon LA, et al. Sensitization of ovarian cancer cells to cisplatin by genistein: the role of NF-kappaB. J Ovarian Res 2008;1(1):9.

[105] Liu H, et al. Effects of genistein on anti-tumor activity of cisplatin in human cervical cancer cell lines. Obstet Gynecol Sci 2019;62(5):322-8.

[106] Xiong P, et al. Design, synthesis, and evaluation of genistein analogues as anti-cancer agents. Anti Cancer Agents Med Chem 2015;15(9):1197-203.

[107] Chen Y, et al. Effects of 7-difluoromethy-5,4′-dimethoxygenistein on proliferation and apoptosis of human cervical cancer cells and its mechanism. Zhong Nan Da Xue Xue Bao Yi Xue Ban 2016;41(5):463-70.

[108] Cai L, et al. Folate receptor-targeted bioflavonoid genistein-loaded chitosan nanoparticles for enhanced anticancer effect in cervical cancers. Nanoscale Res Lett 2017;12(1):509.

[109] Zhang H, et al. Fabrication of genistein-loaded biodegradable TPGS-b-PCL nanoparticles for improved therapeutic effects in cervical cancer cells. Int J Nanomedicine 2015;10:2461.

[110] Hussein MJ, Salai JS. Clinical and histopathological features of ovarian cancer in Rizgary Hospital/Erbil City from 2014 to 2017. Med J Babylon 2019;16(2):112-8.

[111] Beral V, Hermon C, Peto R, Reeves G, Brinton L, Marchbanks P, Negri E, Ness R, Peeters PHM, Vessey M, Gapstur SM, Patel AV, Dal Maso L, Talamini R, Chetrit A, Hirsh G, Lubin F, Sadetzki S, Allen N, Beral V, Bull D, Callaghan K, Crossley B, Gaitskell K, Goodill A, Green J, Hermon C, Key T, Moser K, Reeves G, Collins R, Doll R, Peto R, Gonzalez CA, Lee N, Marchbanks P, Ory HW, Peterson HB, Wingo PA, Martin N, Pardthaisong T, Silpisornkosol S, Theetranont C, Boosiri B, Jimakorn P, Virutamasen P, Wongsrichanalai C, Tjonneland A, Titus-Ernstoff L, Byers T, Rohan T, Mosgaard BJ, Vessey M, Yeates D, Freudenheim JL, Chang-Claude J, Kaaks R, Anderson KE, Folsom A, Robien K, Rossing MA, Thomas DB, Weiss NS, Riboli E, Clavel-Chapelon F, Cramer D, Hankinson SE, Tworoger SS, Franceschi S, Negri E, Magnusson C, Riman T, Weiderpass E, Wolk A, Schouten LJ, van den Brandt PA, Koetsawang S, Rachawat D, Palli D, Black A, Berrington de Gonzalez A, Brinton LA, Freedman DM, Hartge P, Hsing AW, Lacey Jr JV, Hoover RN, Schairer C, Graff-Iversen S, Selmer R, Bain CJ, Green AC, Purdie DM, Siskind V, Webb PM, McCann SE, Hannaford P, Kay C, Binns CW, Lee AH, Zhang M, Ness RB, Nasca P, Coogan PF, Palmer JR, Rosenberg L, Kelsey J, Paffenbarger R, Whittemore A, Katsouyanni K, Trichopoulou A, Trichopoulos D, Tzonou A, Dabancens A, Martinez L, Molina R, Salas O, Goodman MT, Lurie G, Carney ME, Wilkens LR, Hartman L, Manjer J, Olsson H, Grisso JA, Morgan M, Wheeler JE, Peeters PHM, Casagrande J, Pike MC, Ross RK, Wu AH, Miller AB, Kumle M, Lund E, McGowan L, Shu XO, Zheng W,

Farley TMM, Holck S, Meirik O, Risch HA. Ovarian cancer and body size: individual participant meta-analysis including 25,157 women with ovarian cancer from 47 epidemiological studies. PLoS Med 2012;9(4):e1001200.

[112] Collaborative Group on Epidemiological Studies of Ovarian Cancer. Menopausal hormone use and ovarian cancer risk: individual participant meta-analysis of 52 epidemiological studies. Lancet 2015;385(9980):1835-42.

[113] Lauby-Secretan B, et al. Body fatness and cancer—viewpoint of the IARC Working Group. N Engl J Med 2016;375(8):794-8.

[114] Alsop K, et al. BRCA mutation frequency and patterns of treatment response in BRCA mutation-positive women with ovarian cancer: a report from the Australian Ovarian Cancer Study Group. J Clin Oncol 2012;30(21):2654.

[115] Kim TH, Park JH, Woo JS. Resveratrol induces cell death through ROS-dependent downregulation of Notch1/PTEN/Akt signaling in ovarian cancer cells. Mol Med Rep 2019;19(4):3353-60.

[116] Liu Y, et al. Resveratrol inhibits the proliferation and induces the apoptosis in ovarian cancer cells via inhibiting glycolysis and targeting AMPK/mTOR signaling pathway. J Cell Biochem 2018;119(7):6162-72.

[117] Zhang Y, et al. Resveratrol induces immunogenic cell death of human and murine ovarian carcinoma cells. Infect Agents Cancer 2019;14(1):27.

[118] Ferraresi A, et al. Resveratrol inhibits IL-6-induced ovarian cancer cell migration through epigenetic up-regulation of autophagy. Mol Carcinog 2017;56(3):1164-81.

[119] El-kott AF, et al. The apoptotic effect of resveratrol in ovarian cancer cells is associated with down-regulation of galectin-3 and stimulating miR-424-3p transcription. J Food Biochem 2019;43(12): e13072.

[120] Wen W, et al. Pterostilbene suppresses ovarian cancer growth via induction of apoptosis and blockade of cell cycle progression involving inhibition of the STAT3 Pathway. Int J Mol Sci 2018; 19(7):1983.

[121] Chen C-W, et al. DHS (trans-4, 4′-dihydroxystilbene) suppresses DNA replication and tumor growth by inhibiting RRM2 (ribonucleotide reductase regulatory subunit M2). Oncogene 2019;38(13):2364-79.

[122] Tino AB, et al. Resveratrol and acetyl-resveratrol modulate activity of VEGF and IL-8 in ovarian cancer cell aggregates via attenuation of the NF-κB protein. J Ovarian Res 2016;9(1):84.

[123] Nam S, et al. Development of resveratrol-loaded herbal extract-based nanocomposites and their application to the therapy of ovarian cancer. Nanomaterials 2018;8(6):384.

[124] Guo X, Mei J, Zhang C. Development of drug dual-carriers delivery system with mitochondria-targeted and pH/Heat responsive capacity for synergistic photothermal-chemotherapy of ovarian cancer. Int J Nanomedicine 2020;15:301.

[125] Tork OM, Khaleel EF, Abdelmaqsoud OM. Altered cell to cell communication, autophagy and mitochondrial dysfunction in a model of hepatocellular carcinoma: potential protective effects of curcumin and stem cell therapy. Asian Pac J Cancer Prev 2015;16(18):8271-9.

[126] Aoki H, et al. Evidence that curcumin suppresses the growth of malignant gliomas in vitro and in vivo through induction of autophagy: role of Akt and extracellular signal-regulated kinase signaling pathways. Mol Pharmacol 2007;72(1):29-39.

[127] Kim JY, et al. Curcumin-induced autophagy contributes to the decreased survival of oral cancer cells. Arch Oral Biol 2012;57(8):1018-25.

[128] Li B, et al. Curcumin induces cross-regulation between autophagy and apoptosis in uterine leiomyosarcoma cells. Int J Gynecol Cancer 2013;23(5):803-8.

[129] Liu L-D, et al. Curcumin induces apoptotic cell death and protective autophagy by inhibiting AKT/mTOR/p70S6K pathway in human ovarian cancer cells. Arch Gynecol Obstet 2019;299(6):1627-39.

[130] Tian M, et al. Modulation of Myb-induced NF-κB-STAT3 signaling and resulting cisplatin resistance in ovarian cancer by dietary factors. J Cell Physiol 2019;234(11):21126-34.

[131] Zhao J, et al. Dihydroartemisinin and curcumin synergistically induce apoptosis in SKOV3 cells via upregulation of MiR-124 targeting midkine. Cell Physiol Biochem 2017;43(2):589-601.

[132] Zhang X-G, et al. A review of dihydroartemisinin as another gift from traditional Chinese medicine not only for malaria control but also for schistosomiasis control. Parasitol Res 2014;113(5):1769-73.

[133] Zhang CZ, et al. Dihydroartemisinin exhibits antitumor activity toward hepatocellular carcinoma in vitro and in vivo. Biochem Pharmacol 2012;83(9):1278-89.

[134] Lin R, et al. Dihydroartemisinin (DHA) induces ferroptosis and causes cell cycle arrest in head and neck carcinoma cells. Cancer Lett 2016;381(1):165-75.

[135] Lee J, Zhou H-J, Wu X-H. Dihydroartemisinin downregulates vascular endothelial growth factor expression and induces apoptosis in chronic myeloid leukemia K562 cells. Cancer Chemother Pharmacol 2006;57(2):213-20.

[136] Dong F, et al. Dihydroartemisinin targets VEGFR2 via the NF-κB pathway in endothelial cells to inhibit angiogenesis. Cancer Biol Ther 2014;15(11):1479-88.

[137] Wu B, et al. Dihydroartiminisin inhibits the growth and metastasis of epithelial ovarian cancer. Oncol Rep 2012;27(1):101-8.

[138] Ikematsu S, et al. Serum midkine levels are increased in patients with various types of carcinomas. Br J Cancer 2000;83(6):701-6.

[139] Zhang L, et al. Genomic and epigenetic alterations deregulate microRNA expression in human epithelial ovarian cancer. Proc Natl Acad Sci 2008;105(19):7004-9.

[140] Arend RC, et al. The Wnt/β-catenin pathway in ovarian cancer: a review. Gynecol Oncol

2013;131(3):772-9.

[141] Barbolina MV, Burkhalter RJ, Stack MS. Diverse mechanisms for activation of Wnt signalling in the ovarian tumour microenvironment. Biochem J 2011;437(1):1-12.

[142] Su HY, et al. An epigenetic marker panel for screening and prognostic prediction of ovarian cancer. Int J Cancer 2009;124(2):387-93.

[143] Yen H-Y, et al. Regulation of carcinogenesis and modulation through Wnt/β-catenin signaling by curcumin in an ovarian cancer cell line. Sci Rep 2019;9(1):1-14.

[144] Koroth J, et al. Investigation of anti-cancer and migrastatic properties of novel curcumin derivatives on breast and ovarian cancer cell lines. BMC Complement Altern Med 2019;19(1):1-16.

[145] Zeuthen J, et al. Characterization of a human ovarian teratocarcinoma-derived cell line. Int J Cancer 1980;25(1):19-32.

[146] Kálai T, et al. Synthesis of N-substituted 3,5-bis (arylidene)-4-piperidones with high antitumor and antioxidant activity. J Med Chem 2011;54(15):5414-21.

[147] Terlikowska KM, et al. Potential application of curcumin and its analogues in the treatment strategy of patients with primary epithelial ovarian cancer. Int J Mol Sci 2014;15(12):21703-22.

[148] Adams BK, et al. Synthesis and biological evaluation of novel curcumin analogs as anticancer and anti-angiogenesis agents. Bioorg Med Chem 2004;12(14):3871-83.

[149] Adams BK, et al. EF24, a novel synthetic curcumin analog, induces apoptosis in cancer cells via a redox-dependent mechanism. Anti-Cancer Drugs 2005;16(3):263-75.

[150] Ramezani T, et al. Sensitization of resistance ovarian cancer cells to cisplatin by biogenic synthesized silver nanoparticles through p53 activation. Iran J Pharm Res 2019;18(1):222.

[151] Zhao M-D, et al. Co-delivery of curcumin and paclitaxel by "Core-Shell" targeting amphiphilic copolymer to reverse resistance in the treatment of ovarian cancer. Int J Nanomedicine 2019;14:9453.

[152] Dwivedi P, et al. Core-shell microencapsulation of curcumin in PLGA microparticles: programmed for application in ovarian cancer therapy. Artif Cells Nanomed Biotechnol 2018;46(Suppl 3):S481-91.

[153] Anderl P, et al. Correlation between steroid hormone receptors, histological and clinical parameters in ovarian carcinoma. Gynecol Obstet Investig 1988;25(2):135-40.

[154] Leung Y-K, et al. Estrogen receptor (ER)-β isoforms: a key to understanding ER-β signaling. Proc Natl Acad Sci 2006;103(35):13162-7.

[155] Chan KK, et al. Estrogen receptor modulators genistein, daidzein and ERB-041 inhibit cell migration, invasion, proliferation and sphere formation via modulation of FAK and PI3K/AKT signaling in ovarian cancer. Cancer Cell Int 2018;18(1):65.

[156] Shibue T, Weinberg RA. EMT, CSCs, and drug resistance: the mechanistic link and

clinical implications. Nat Rev Clin Oncol 2017;14(10):611.

[157] Ma J, et al. Combination of a thioxodihydroquinazolinone with cisplatin eliminates ovarian cancer stem cell-like cells (CSC-LCs) and shows preclinical potential. Oncotarget 2018;9(5):6042.

[158] Ning Y, et al. Genistein inhibits stemness of SKOV3 cells induced by macrophages co-cultured with ovarian cancer stem-like cells through IL-8/STAT3 axis. J Exp Clin Cancer Res 2019;38(1):1-15.

[159] Ning Y, et al. Co-culture of ovarian cancer stem-like cells with macrophages induced SKOV3 cells stemness via IL-8/STAT3 signaling. Biomed Pharmacother 2018;103:262-71.

[160] Liu Y, et al. Genistein-induced differentiation of breast cancer stem/progenitor cells through a paracrine mechanism. Int J Oncol 2016;48(3):1063-72.

[161] Hwang K-A, et al. Anticancer effect of genistein on BG-1 ovarian cancer growth induced by 17β-estradiol or bisphenol A via the suppression of the crosstalk between estrogen receptor alpha and insulin-like growth factor-1 receptor signaling pathways. Toxicol Appl Pharmacol 2013;272(3):637-46.

[162] Kim Y-S, Choi K-C, Hwang K-A. Genistein suppressed epithelial-mesenchymal transition and migration efficacies of BG-1 ovarian cancer cells activated by estrogenic chemicals via estrogen receptor pathway and downregulation of TGF-β signaling pathway. Phytomedicine 2015;22(11):993-9.

[163] Ning Y, et al. Apoptosis induced by 7-difluoromethoxyl-5,4′-di-n-octyl genistein via the inactivation of FoxM1 in ovarian cancer cells. Oncol Rep 2012;27(6):1857-64.

[164] Ning Y, et al. Inactivation of AKT, ERK and NF-κB by genistein derivative, 7-difluoromethoxyl-5,4′-di-n-octylygenistein, reduces ovarian carcinoma oncogenicity. Oncol Rep 2017;38(2):949-58.

[165] Ning Y-X, et al. Let-7d increases ovarian cancer cell sensitivity to a genistein analog by targeting c-Myc. Oncotarget 2017;8(43):74836.

[166] Bai J, Yang BJ, Luo X. Effects of 5-hydroxy-4′-nitro-7-propionyloxy-genistein on inhibiting proliferation and invasion via activating reactive oxygen species in human ovarian cancer A2780/DDP cells. Oncol Lett 2018;15(4):5227-35.

[167] Mittal P, et al. Formulation and characterization of genistein-loaded nanostructured lipid carriers:pharmacokinetic, biodistribution and in vitro cytotoxicity studies. Curr Drug Deliv 2019;16(3):215-25.

第 2 章
筛选三阴性乳腺癌的潜在治疗药物

Leimarembi Devi Naorem, Mathavan Muthaiyan, Ishita Bhattacharyya,
Dinakara Rao Ampasala, Amouda Venkatesan
Centre for Bioinformatics, School of Life Sciences, Pondicherry University, Puducherry, India

摘要

三阴性乳腺癌（triple-negative breast cancer，TNBC）是一种缺乏雌激素受体（estrogen receptor，ER）、孕激素受体（progesterone receptor，PR）和人表皮生长因子受体（human epidermal growth factor receptor，HER）表达的乳腺癌亚型，约占确诊乳腺癌患者的 20%。TNBC 具有很强的侵袭性，其临床治疗具有挑战性，但开发新药耗时长且失败率高。为克服这些困难，人们提出药物再利用理论。药物再利用是为现有药物寻找新的治疗适应证，以提高药物生产力并充分利用其潜力的过程。本研究收集并使用了 1075 个 TNBC 的差异表达基因（differentially expressed genes，DEG）和重要 *Hub* 基因（译者注：*Hub* 基因与关键基因类似，但无明确包含关系）。使用药物基因组学数据库（Connectivity Map，CMap）、sscMap、SPIED3 和 LINCSL1000 CDS2 等药物再利用工具筛选 DEG 候选药物。随后，通过分子对接计算候选药物与 TNBC 相关 *Hub* 基因的结合亲和力。此外，对于入围药物，笔者收集了 STITCH 和 DrugBank 数据库中已知的靶基因，发现它们与 *Hub* 基因有少数的重叠。为研究 DEG 的重要功能和通路，进一步使用 Enrichr 工具进行了富集分析。根据所得分数，发现 31 种药物有希望重新用于癌症的治疗。从对接研究中可以明显看出，达拉非尼和丝裂原活化蛋白激酶 1（mitogen-activated protein kinase1，MAPK1）的最佳结合能为 -9.9 kcal/mol。在已报道文献中笔者注意到，上述多种治疗不同癌症的药物也可以用于其他癌症。通路和本体分析表明，DEG 在细胞分裂、增殖、DNA 复制和癌症相关通路等生物过程中高度富集。因此，本研究可能有助于发现现有癌症治疗药物的新适应证。

关键词
三阴性乳腺癌，药物再利用，对接研究

缩略词

ATC　　药物的解剖学、治疗学及化学分类法
BC　　乳腺癌
CMap　　药物基因组学数据库
CRC　　结直肠癌
DEG　　差异表达基因
DTI　　药物-靶标相互作用
GO　　基因本体论
STITCH　　化学物质相互作用的搜索工具
TNBC　　三阴性乳腺癌

一、概述

三阴性乳腺癌(TNBC)是一种与基底样乳腺癌(breast cancer,BC)非常相似的乳腺癌亚型[1]。它是一类缺乏 ER、PR 和 HER 表达的异质性肿瘤。由于 TNBC 对内分泌治疗和特异性靶向治疗均无反应,其治疗选择非常有限。TNBC 具有高侵袭性、高复发率和高转移率,且预后差[2],通常采用手术治疗、化学治疗(简称"化疗")和放射治疗(简称"放疗")相结合的方法进行治疗。最常见的治疗选择是新辅助化疗、多腺苷二磷酸核糖聚合酶抑制剂[poly(ADP-ribose)polymerase inhibitor,PARP inhibitor]、免疫治疗,以及使用细胞毒性药物化疗[3]。最近,美国食品药品管理局(Food and Drug Administration,FDA)加速批准阿替利珠单抗[atezolizumab(TECENTRIQ)]联合白蛋白紫杉醇用于程序性死亡受体配体 1(programmed death-ligand 1,PD-L1)阳性(PD-L1 阳性的肿瘤浸润性免疫细胞≥肿瘤面积的 1%)的成年 TNBC 患者[4]。然而,开发新药耗时长且失败率高。为克服这些困难,人们提出药物再利用理论[5]。

药物再利用或重新分析是一种策略,有助于确定已批准或正在研究的药物用于治疗原适应证之外的其他疾病的新用途。通常,药物再利用始于针对特定治疗靶点的已批准或已上市药物的计算机筛选;然后对筛选出的药物进行体外和体内试验验证;最后,这些化合物通过新适应证的临床试验,经 FDA 批准后上市。基因组学和计算方法的进步使药物开发和研究变得更加容易[6]。目前的计算机药物再利用技术主要集中于基因表达或药物-靶标相互作用(drug-target interaction,DTI)。各种已开发的计算方法使药物再利用的过程更加容易。例如,CMap 包含超过 7000 个表达谱,代表 1309 种化合物[7],用户可以输入基因与数据库进行比较。使用 Kolmogorov-

Smirnov 进行统计分析,关联度是其主要结果[8],负值越高,表示对应的扰动源抑制了基因通路的表达;正值越高,表示扰动源促进了基因通路的表达。CMap 包含具有药物的解剖学、治疗学及化学分类法(anatomical therapeutic chemical,ATC)代码的治疗性小分子,可用于寻找现有药物的新适应证。此外,还可使用 sscMap、SPIED3 和 LINCS-L1000 CDS2 等药物再利用工具[9-11]。同时,在 DrugBank、STITCH(化学物质相互作用的搜索工具)等公共数据库中也可找到不同水平的 DTI。

本研究的目的是利用计算机分析筛选治疗 TNBC 的候选药物。使用多种药物再利用工具查询 DEG,并根据其药理作用对筛选的 FDA 已批准药物和临床试验药物进行分析。这些药物与 TNBC 的 *Hub* 基因对接,以检查靶配体相互作用和复合物的稳定性。进一步对 DEG 进行通路和本体分析,研究其富集的功能和通路。确定的候选药物为 TNBC 患者的替代治疗方案提供了新的选择。

二、材料与方法

(一)数据收集

在 TNBC 的 1075 个 DEG 中,本研究纳入了 589 个上调的 DEG、486 个下调的 DEG,以及之前研究中产生的 12 个上调的 *Hub* 基因、4 个下调的 *Hub* 基

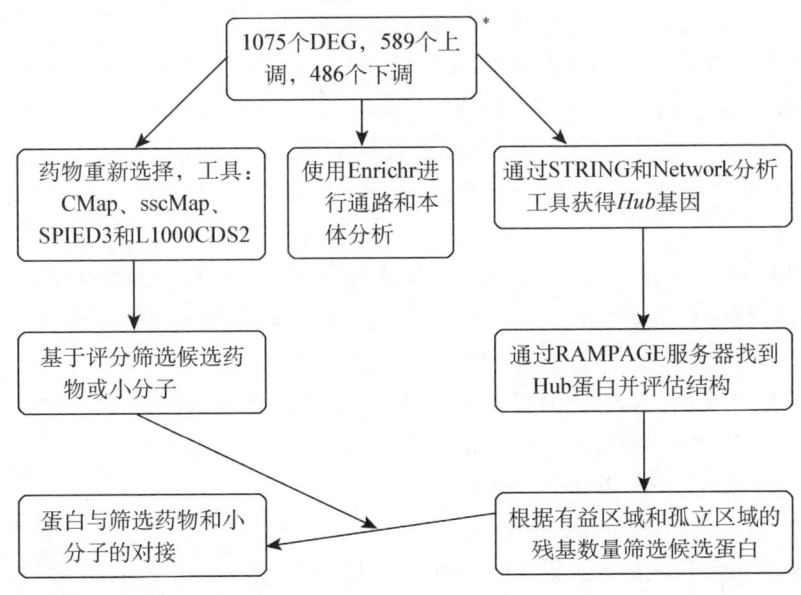

*译者注:此图在原著中为插图,无图序和图题。

因[14]*。上调的 Hub 基因是 AURKB、CCNB2、CDC20、DDX18、EGFR、ENO1、MYC、NUP88、PLK1、PML、POLR2F 和 SKP2，下调的 Hub 基因是 CCND1、GLI3、SKP1 和 TGFB3。

(二)利用 Network Analyst 进行 Hub 基因鉴定

将 DEG 上传到 NetworkAnalyst 中，研究蛋白质-药物相互作用网络。根据评分和相关度测量，筛选出 7 个基因(EGFR、AURKB、PLK1、AURKA、MAPK1、PNMT、GAMT)，其中上调基因 3 个，下调基因 2 个，EGFR、AURKB 和 PLK1 在既往研究中提取的 Hub 基因列表中较为常见[14]。

(三)对接研究的靶蛋白

笔者团队从既往研究[14]中收集了 20 个 Hub 蛋白，并使用 NetworkAnalyst 工具进行对接研究。随后，从 RCSB-PDB(www.rcsb.org)中检索人蛋白的结构，并使用 RAMPAGE(http://mordred.bioc.cam.ac.uk)进行分析。

(四)使用再利用工具筛选候选药物

使用多种生物信息学工具[CMap[15]、sscMap[9]、SPIED3(SPIEDw v2.0)[10] 和 LINCS-L1000CDS2[11]]筛选候选药物；用每个工具查询疾病特征，包括上调和下调的基因；为每个工具准备了所需格式的输入数据，用不同工具的结果筛选药物，考虑重新利用阴性标记的药物。具有 ATC 代码的扰动源是 FDA 已批准的药物，随机打乱结果和详细结果可从 CMap(https://portals.broadinstitute.org/cmap/)下载。此外，将前 100 名(按顺序排列)化学扰动源纳入 TNBC 潜在药物的候选名单。根据阴性平均关联度＜－0.199，富集评分＜－0.700，特异性＞0.50 的标准筛选候选药物。

sscMap 将结果保存为 .tab 文件，并根据 setsize＞5 和 setscore＜－0.085 标准选择潜在候选药物，仅考虑显著性值为 1 的药物(sscMap 中的 setsize 是指数据库中某一化合物重复参考图谱的数量)。共筛选出 10 种药物。

从 LINCS-L1000CDS2 中获得了 50 种反向模式扰动因子和 50 种模拟模式扰动因子，LINCS-L1000 的详细结果来自 Enrichment(https://amp.pharm.mssm.edu/Enrichr/)，并考虑 Z 评分＜－2.000 的药物。

SPIED3 是 SPIEDw(v2.0)的修改版本，具有独立的数据集，包括来自 CMap、LINCS 和 DrugMatrix 数据集的药物治疗。从 DRUGScmap 和 DRUGSlincs 中获

---

*译者注：原著参考文献出现顺序有误，为便于读者查阅，中文版保留原顺序，请读者注意。

取药物。在 CMap 结果中,51 种药物具有负相关评分。在 LINCS 结果中,有 50 种药物具有负相关评分。比较结果发现,CMap-SPIED3 中有 17 种药物,LINCS-L1000-SPIED3 中有 8 种药物,sscMap 中有 9 种药物,最终,31 种独特药物入围。

(五)入围药物已知靶基因及适应证的选取

从 DrugBank[12] 和 STITCH[13] 数据库中获取 31 种药物对应的靶基因。同时,从 DrugBank 和文献中获取了适应证和相关条件。

(六)分子对接研究

使用 PyRx[16] 虚拟筛选工具对筛选的药物与入围的 Hub 基因进行对接研究。使用 AutoDock Vina[17] 向导将这 15 种蛋白中的每一种与 31 种潜在的候选药物进行对接。首先使用 PyMOL 分子可视化系统观察蛋白质,去除配体和不必要的水分子,在链中添加缺失残基使结构完整,修饰后的蛋白质被上传到 WHAT IF web 界面,生成 PDB 文件。使用 MarvinSketch 将药物分子结构以 2D 和 3D 的形式绘制并清洗,生成 PDB 文件。对接为每种药物提供了不同的结构,并突出了它们与目标蛋白质的相互作用。结合能 < -5.0 kcal/mol 被认为是稳定的蛋白质-药物复合物。使用 PyMOL[18] 将复合物可视化。

(七)差异表达基因富集分析

1075 个 DEG 被上传到 Enrichr[19] 数据库进行分析,对人体的通路和本体进行解读。通路方面使用 KEGG(2019) 和 WikiPathways(2019) 数据库。本体方面下载并分析基因本体论(gene ontology,GO)过程(2018)、GO 分子功能(2018)和 GO 细胞成分(2018)的结果。

三、结果

(一)药物靶点

使用 NetworkAnalyst 工具研究药物-蛋白质相互作用网络(图 2-1)。基于程度和相关性测量,笔者前期研究中收集的 7 个基因(*EGFR*、*AURKB*、*PLK1*、*AURKA*、*MAPK1*、*PNMT* 和 *GAMT*)和 20 个 Hub 蛋白(AURKB、CCNB2、CDC20、DDX18、EGFR、ENO1、MYC、NUP88、PLK1、PML、POLR2F、SKP2、CCND1、GLI3、SKP1、AURKA、MAPK1、PNMT、GAMT 和 TGFB3)被列入候选名单[14],可以考虑进一步研究。

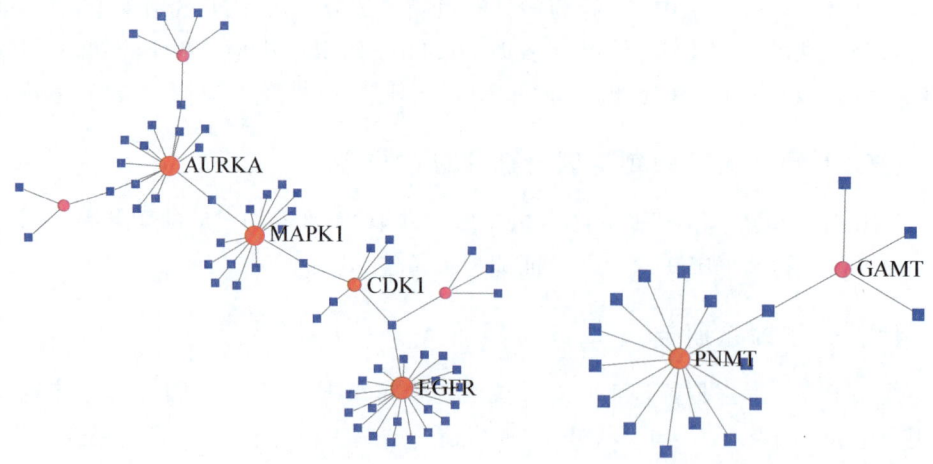

图 2-1 使用 NetworkAnalyst 的蛋白质-药物相互作用网络

随后，从 RCSB-PDB（www.rcsb.org）中检索这些人体蛋白的结构，并使用 RAMPAGE（http://mordred.bioc.cam.ac.uk）进行分析。根据允许区（＞95%）和离群区（＜1.5%）的百分比，甄选出 15 种蛋白质进行分子对接研究（表 2-1）。

表 2-1 分子对接研究入围 Hub 基因

Hub 基因	PDB ID	结合位点	RAMPAGE
AURKB	4AF3	83～88	93.8%（0.3%）
PLK1	3FC2	59～64	96.9%（0.0%）
CDC20	4GGA	183～188	97.1%（0.0%）
DDX18	3LY5	223～227	96.6%（0.0%）
EGFR	3GOP	718～723	97.2%（0.0%）
ENO1	3B97	7～11	96.8%（0.4%）
MYC	1NKP	903,906,907,910,913	97.2%（0.0%）
SKP2	1FS1	15,16,17,19,20	95.7%（1.3%）
AURKA	1MQ4	211～213	96.1%（0.4%）
MAPK1	1PME	31～35	96.3%（0.0%）
CCND1	2W96	15,16,17,18,20	91.3%（3.1%）
GLI3	4BLD	501～505	98.1%（0.0%）
TGFB3	1KTZ	34～38	95.1%（0.0%）
PNMT	1HNN	237,240,241,244,249	95.2%（0.8%）
GAMT	3ORH	18,19,20,23,24	96.7%（0.0%）

(二)使用再利用工具筛选和分析 TNBC 潜在候选药物

在每个工具中以不同格式搜索收集到的 DEG。对于本研究中使用的每种工具,负评分仅用于药物再利用。负评分表明该化合物具有抑制性,即它与基因标记负相关。此外,为找到现有药物的新适应证,纳入具有 ATC 密码子的扰动源。研究发现,只有治疗性小分子具有 ATC 密码子。

在 CMap 中发现了 396 个上调基因和 293 个下调基因,观察了 6100 个实例,其中 626 个正评分,1456 个负评分。SPIED3 发现了 579 个上调基因,472 个下调基因。根据每种工具设定的不同标准,共有 31 种药物进入下一步分析(表 2-2)。

表 2-2 入围药品 ATC 密码子及用途

序号	药品名称	ATC 密码子	用途(文献和 DrugBank)
1	达拉非尼[20]	L01XE23	黑色素瘤、甲状腺未分化癌
2	达沙替尼[21]	L01XE06	慢性髓细胞性白血病(chronic myelogenous leukemia,CML)
3	多韦替尼	—	正在进行多发性骨髓瘤、白血病、实体瘤的研究(Ⅲ期)
4	吐根碱	P01AX02	B 细胞淋巴瘤、急性髓系白血病
5	恩替司他(MS-275)[22]	—	晚期乳腺癌
6	芬地林	C08EA01	胰腺癌
7	氟维司群	L02BA03	激素受体阳性转移性乳腺癌
8	拉氧头孢[23]	J01DD06	癌症患者的厌氧菌感染
9	LY-294002[24]	—	增强奥沙利铂对胃癌的抗癌作用(实验)
10	甲氟喹	P01BC02	疟疾,在结直肠癌中被重新利用
11	甲麦角林	G02CB05	精神活性药物,作为血清素和多巴胺受体的配体
12	米托蒽醌	L01DB07	多发性硬化症、转移性乳腺癌
13	哌柏西利	L01XE33	晚期和转移性乳腺癌
14	哌克昔林	C08EX02	冠状血管扩张剂——心绞痛
15	丙氯拉嗪[25]	N05AB04	精神分裂症(抗精神病药)、恶心、眩晕,被用来治疗肺癌
16	普罗替林	N06AA11	抗抑郁药(神经系统)
17	嘌呤霉素	—	抗生素(正在研究中)

续表

序号	药品名称	ATC 密码子	用途（文献和 DrugBank）
18	乙胺嘧啶	P01BD01	文献用于肝细胞癌的抗疟疾药物
19	醌类他汀[26]	—	白血病
20	白藜芦醇	—	在临床前研究中，白藜芦醇已被发现具有潜在的抗癌特性
21	利福布汀	J04AB04	晚期艾滋病、结核病、晚期结核病
22	HDAC 抑制剂	—	肝细胞癌
23	司美替尼	—	正在研究（Ⅲ期）乳腺癌、肺癌
24	西罗莫司[28]	S01XA23，L04AA10	癌症治疗
25	坦内霉素	—	治疗多种类型癌症、实体瘤，或者慢性髓细胞性白血病
26	硫利达嗪	N05AC02	抗精神病药物
27	曲美替尼[29]	L01XE25	未分化甲状腺癌、转移性黑色素瘤
28	曲古抑素 A	—	抗癌治疗（正在研究中）
29	丙戊酸	N03AG01	癫痫，正在研究用于治疗艾滋病和各种癌症
30	伏立诺他	L01XX38	皮肤 T 细胞淋巴瘤
31	渥曼青霉素	—	黑色素瘤

注：HDAC. 组蛋白去乙酰化酶；—. 无内容。

这些药物的药理作用和用途已在文献、DrugBank、PubChem[30]、ChEMBL[31,32]中进行了研究。使用网络生物学方法发现曲美替尼可用于 TNBC[33]。甲氟喹是一种公认的抗疟疾药物，被重新定位于治疗结直肠癌（colorectal cancer，CRC）[34]。达拉非尼、达沙替尼、多韦替尼、米托蒽醌和司美替尼是批准或正在进行Ⅲ期临床试验的药物，用于治疗不同类型的癌症。有研究显示，HDAC 抑制剂[27]和喹诺他汀（quinostatin）具有抗癌活性，正在进行临床试验，但尚无任何已确定靶点。

同时，利用 STITCH 和 DrugBank 数据库，获得了这 31 个化合物已建立的靶基因（表2-3）。可以看出，这些基因与 TNBC 的 *Hub* 基因仅有少数重叠，初步表明 TNBC 中药物相关靶基因的表达并无显著差异。

表 2-3 筛选药物的可用靶点

序号	药品名称	靶基因
1	达拉非尼	$BRAF,RAF1,SIK1,NEK11,LIMK1,EIF2AK3,MDK$
2	达沙替尼	$ABL1,SRC,EPHA2,LCK,YES1,KIT,PDGFRB,STAT5B,ABL2,FYN,BTK,NR4A3,BCR,CSK,EPHA5,EPHB4,FGR,FRK,HSPA8,LYN,ZAK,MAPK14,PPAT,HCK$
3	多韦替尼	$NR1I2,FGFR2,FGFR1,FGFR3,FLT3,PDGFRB,YES1,KIT,LCK,FGR$
4	吐根碱	$MAPK14,FOS,SNRPA,TIMP3,PARP1$
5	恩替司他（MS-275）	$ROCK1,ERBB2,CDH1,HDAC2,HDAC1,STAT3,HSP90AA1,HSP90AB1,CFLAR,INPP5J$
6	芬地林	$HRAS$
7	氟维司群	$ESR1,AR,ESR2,PRL,IGFR1,CYP19A1,TFF1,PGR,CCND1,RB1$
8	拉氧头孢	$ELANE$
9	LY-294002	$PIM1,PIK3CG,MAPK3,CASP3,MTOR,RPS6KB1,PIK3CA,PIK3CD,AKT1,GSK3B$
10	甲氟喹	$HBA1,ADORA2A,JUN,CALR,ABCC1,ABCC4,DHFR$
11	甲麦角林	$SCN2A,HTR2C,HTR2A,HTR2B,HTR7,HTR6,HTR1A,HTR1B,HTR1D,HTR1F,HTR1E$
12	米托蒽醌	$TOP2A,TOP2B,ABCB1,ABCC1,ABCG2,PIM1,ATM,PTPN2,FAS,CASP3$
13	哌柏西利	$CDK2,CDK4,CDK6,CDKN2B,TP53,RB1,CCND1,CDKN2A,DRD2,CCNE1$
14	哌克昔林	$CPT1A,CPT2,KCNH2,ERBB3,CYP2D6,TMPRSS1D$
15	丙氯拉嗪	$DRD2,DRD3,DRD4,ADRA2B,S100A4,ADRA1D,HRH11,HTR2A,ADRA1B,HTR2C$
16	普罗替林	$SLC6A2,SLC6A4,ADORA3,BACE1$
17	嘌呤霉素	$RPL10L,RPL13A,RPL23,RPL15,RPL19,RPL23A,RSL24D1,RPL26L1,RPL8,RPL37,RPL3,RPL11,FOS,RBM3,KLK4$
18	乙胺嘧啶	$DHFR,HEXB,SLC46A1,CHRM1,CYP2C9,PDF,HHEX,STAT3,TYMS,DHFRL1$
19	醌类他汀	—
20	白藜芦醇	$SIRT1,SIRT3,SIRT5,TP53,NOS3,PTGS2,AKT1,ESR1,PTGS1,PPARG,NQO2,CSNK2A1,ALOX15,ALOX5,AHR,P14K2B,ITGA5,ITGB3,APP,SNCA,MTNR1A,MTNR1B,CLEC14A,NR1I2,NR1I3,SLC2A1,CBR1,PPARA,PPARG,KHSRP,YARS$

续表

序号	药品名称	靶基因
21	利福布汀	HSP90AA1, HSP90B1, BCL6, CYP3A4, CYP3A5, AADAC, CYP3A7, ABCB11
22	组蛋白去乙酰化酶（HDAC）抑制剂	REN, AGT, CASP3, TP53, XRCC5, HDAC1, HDAC2, HDAC3, HDAC6
23	司美替尼	DPEP1, EIF2AK3, BCL2L11, FOXO3, STAT3, MAPK1, MAPK3, MAP2K1
24	西罗莫司（雷帕霉素）	MTOR, FKBP1A, FGF2, FKBP3, FKBP5, FKBP4, AKT1, RPTOR, RPS6KB1, IRS1, EIF4EBP1
25	坦内霉素	HSP90AA1, HSP90AB1, HSPA4, EGFR, ERBB2, TP53, CCND1, VEGFA, AKT1, HSPB1
26	硫利达嗪	DRD2, DRD1, ADRA1A, ADRA1B, HTR2A, KCNH2, HTR6, DRD3, HTR1A, CYP2D6, HTR2C, ADRA1A, HRH1
27	曲美替尼	MAP2K1, MAP2K2, MAPK1, MAPK3, RPS6KB1, RB1, ATK1, EIF2AK3, GNAQ, GNA11
28	曲古抑素 A	HIST4H4, HDAC9, HDAC8, HDAC10, HDAC2, HDAC1, HDAC3, HDAC4, HDAC6, HDAC7
29	丙戊酸	HDAC9, ABAT, ACADSB, OGDH, ALDH5A1, HDAC2, PPARA, PPARD, PPARG, GSK3B, SMN1, ABCB1, CYP2C9, CYP2B6, CYP2A6, TSPO, BDNF, RELN
30	伏立诺他	HDAC1, HDAC2, HDAC3, HDAC6, HDAC8, HDAC7, HSP90AA1, TP53, BCL2L1, H2AFX
31	渥曼青霉素	PIK3CG, PLK1, PIK3R1, PIK3CA, PIK3CD, PLK3, MYLK, NOS3, AKT1, PIK3C3

注：—. 无内容。

（三）Hub 基因与候选药物的分子对接研究

将 31 种药物分别与 15 个 Hub 基因对接，以研究药物-靶标复合物的相互作用和稳定性。最佳的药物-靶标复合物由达拉非尼和 MAPK1 形成，结合能为 －9.9 kcal/mol（图 2-2、表 2-4）。组蛋白去乙酰化酶（HDAC）抑制剂-AURKB 复合物也非常稳定，结合能为－9.8 kcal/mol（图 2-2）。17 个药物-靶标配合物结合能为 ≤－9.0 kcal/mol，429 个药物-靶标复合物结合能＜－5.0 kcal/mol。

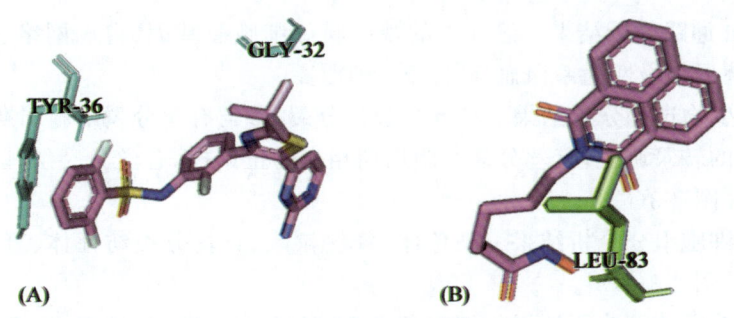

图 2-2 优选受体-药物复合物

注：(A)达拉非尼-MAPK1 复合物；(B) HDAC 抑制剂-AURKB 复合物。

表 2-4 优选受体-药物复合物

配位体	靶基因	结合能/kcal·mol^{-1}
达拉非尼	MAPK1	−9.9
HDAC 抑制剂	AURKB	−9.8
甲麦角林	MAPK1	−9.8
多韦替尼	AURKB	−9.5
甲麦角林	AURKB	−9.5
HDAC 抑制剂	SKP2	−9.5
达拉非尼	AURKB	−9.3
吐根碱	AURKB	−9.3
恩替诺司他	AURKB	−9.3
LY-294002	AURKA	−9.3
达拉非尼	CCND1	−9.3
拉氧头孢	AURKB	−9.2
芬地林	SKP2	−9.1
哌柏西利	MAPK1	−9.1
甲麦角林	AURKA	−9
达拉非尼	PNMT	−9
醌类他汀	PNMT	−9

注：HDAC. 组蛋白去乙酰化酶。

(四)通路与本体分析

笔者利用 KEGG 和 WikiPathways 数据库对 1075 个 DEG 进行了通路分析。对基因本体论(gene ontology,GO)富集分析的所有术语，即生物过程、细胞组分和分子功能进行分析。根据 P 值，发现以下结果具有显著性。

1. KEGG 通路分析结果 小细胞肺癌、急性髓系白血病、膀胱癌和子宫内膜癌[图 2-3(A)]。

2. Wiki 通路分析结果　癌症中的视网膜母细胞瘤基因、胃癌网络、转移性脑肿瘤、伊马替尼和慢性髓系白血病[图 2-3(B)]。

3. GO 生物过程分析结果　有丝分裂核分裂，参与有丝分裂细胞周期 G1/S 期转变过程中的转录调控，有丝分裂细胞周期相变的正调控，有丝分裂纺锤体微管附着于着丝点[图 2-3(C)]。

4. GO 细胞组分分析结果　染色体、着丝粒区、有丝分裂纺锤体、凝聚染色体和着丝粒区[图 2-3(D)]。

5. GO 分子功能分析结果　细胞色素 b5 还原酶活性，作用于 NAD(P)H，组蛋白丝氨酸激酶活性，MAP 激酶酪氨酸/丝氨酸/苏氨酸磷酸酶活性，以及组蛋白激酶活性[图 2-3(E)]。

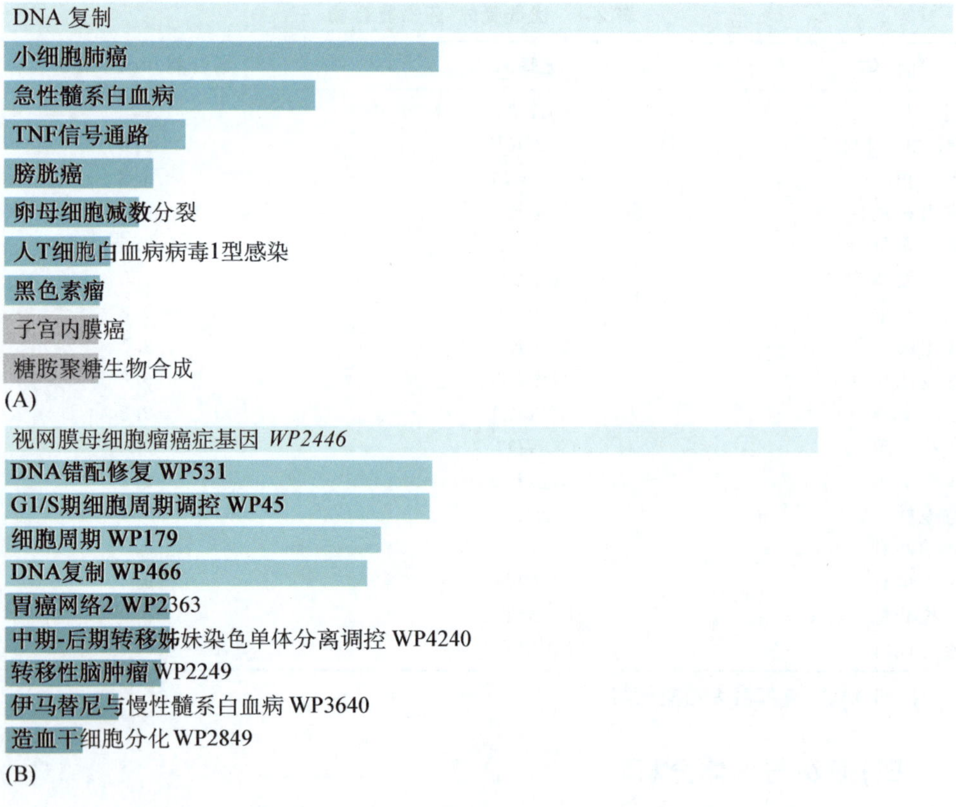

DNA 复制
小细胞肺癌
急性髓系白血病
TNF信号通路
膀胱癌
卵母细胞减数分裂
人T细胞白血病病毒1型感染
黑色素瘤
子宫内膜癌
糖胺聚糖生物合成
(A)

视网膜母细胞瘤癌症基因 WP2446
DNA错配修复 WP531
G1/S期细胞周期调控 WP45
细胞周期 WP179
DNA复制 WP466
胃癌网络2 WP2363
中期-后期转移姊妹染色单体分离调控 WP4240
转移性脑肿瘤 WP2249
伊马替尼与慢性髓系白血病 WP3640
造血干细胞分化 WP2849
(B)

图 2-3*

注：(A)KEGG 通路分析柱状图；(B)Wiki 通路分析柱状图。

---

*译者注：原著无图题。

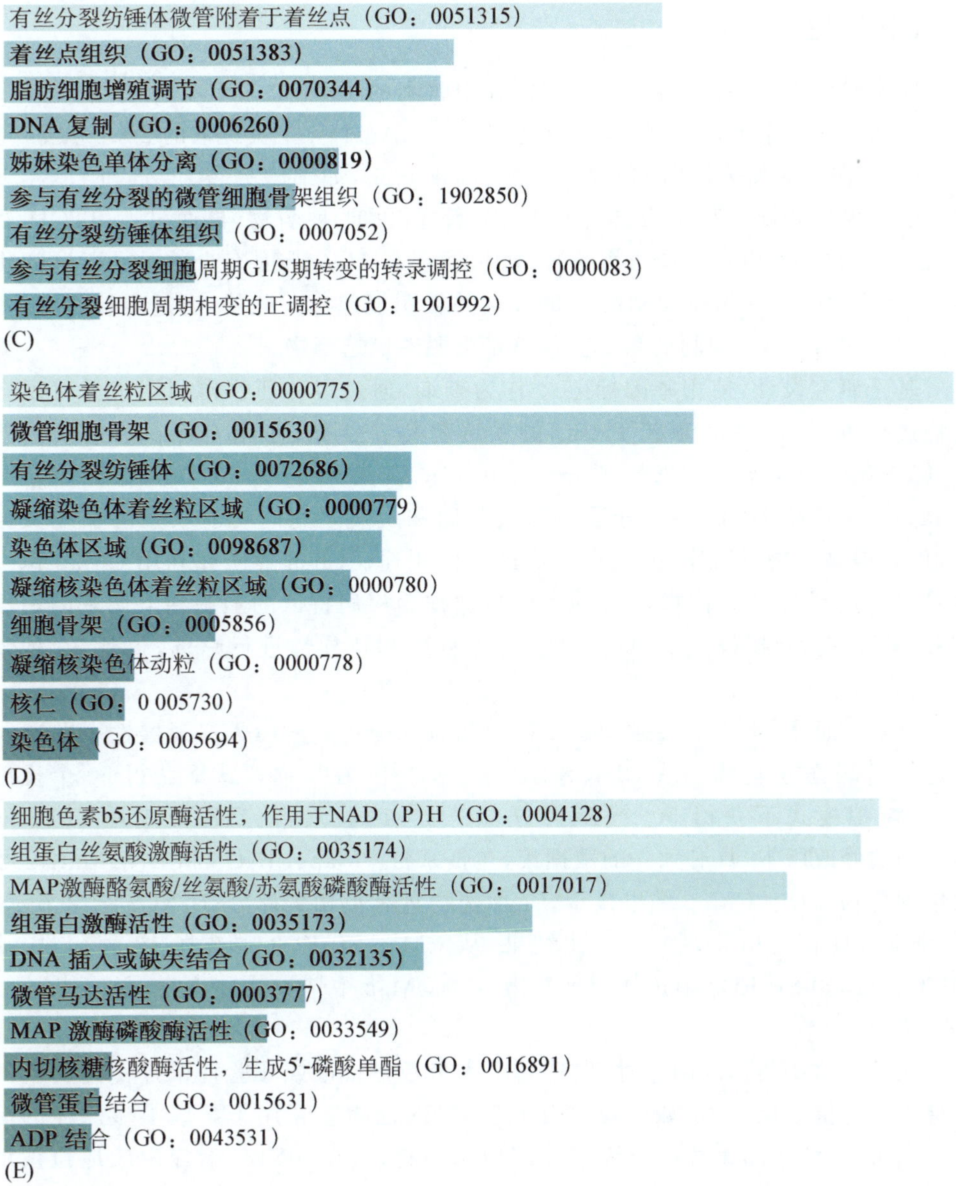

第 2 章 筛选三阴性乳腺癌的潜在治疗药物 | 43

有丝分裂纺锤体微管附着于着丝点（GO：0051315）
着丝点组织（GO：0051383）
脂肪细胞增殖调节（GO：0070344）
DNA 复制（GO：0006260）
姊妹染色单体分离（GO：0000819）
参与有丝分裂的微管细胞骨架组织（GO：1902850）
有丝分裂纺锤体组织（GO：0007052）
参与有丝分裂细胞周期G1/S期转变的转录调控（GO：0000083）
有丝分裂细胞周期相变的正调控（GO：1901992）
(C)

染色体着丝粒区域（GO：0000775）
微管细胞骨架（GO：0015630）
有丝分裂纺锤体（GO：0072686）
凝缩染色体着丝粒区域（GO：0000779）
染色体区域（GO：0098687）
凝缩核染色体着丝粒区域（GO：0000780）
细胞骨架（GO：0005856）
凝缩核染色体动粒（GO：0000778）
核仁（GO：0 005730）
染色体（GO：0005694）
(D)

细胞色素b5还原酶活性，作用于NAD（P)H（GO：0004128）
组蛋白丝氨酸激酶活性（GO：0035174）
MAP激酶酪氨酸/丝氨酸/苏氨酸磷酸酶活性（GO：0017017）
组蛋白激酶活性（GO：0035173）
DNA 插入或缺失结合（GO：0032135）
微管马达活性（GO：0003777）
MAP 激酶磷酸酶活性（GO：0033549）
内切核糖核酸酶活性，生成5'-磷酸单酯（GO：0016891）
微管蛋白结合（GO：0015631）
ADP 结合（GO：0043531）
(E)

图 2-3 （续）

注：(C)GO 生物过程柱状图；(D)GO 细胞组分柱状图；(E)GO 分子功能柱状图。

四、讨论

在本研究中,笔者甄选了从前期研究中收集的 1075 个 TNBC DEG 中 589 个上调基因和 486 个下调基因,以及通过 NetworkAnalyst 工具提取的 20 个 Hub 基因。DEG 在癌症相关通路和生物过程中高度富集,如细胞分裂、增殖和 DNA 复制。通过多种药物再利用工具搜索 DEG,筛选出 31 种药物;再通过 STITCH 和 DrugBank 数据库检索候选药物的靶基因,发现与 Hub 基因有少数重叠。这初步表明,药物相关靶基因在 TNBC 中的表达并无明显差异。此外,通过对接研究,考虑达拉非尼、HDAC 抑制剂和甲麦角林是重要的候选药物。

基于研究设计,使用基因标记[35]作为查询,通过多种药物再利用工具对现有药物进行再利用,逐步确定 TNBC 的候选药物。首先,使用 CMap 筛选候选药物,筛选条件为负平均连通性评分＜－0.199,富集评分＜－0.700,特异性＞0。CMap 是一个可以推断出小分子/药物、基因和疾病之间的功能联系的在线数据库,可以提高药物发现率,并检测现有药物的用途。Chen 等研究利用 CMap 识别食管癌候选新药[36]。同样,在该研究中,被称为疾病特征的上调和下调基因用作 CMap 的查询,并根据负平均连通性、富集分数和特异性进行筛选,得到 50 种候选药物。

进一步通过 sscMap,根据 setsize(＞5)和 setscore(＜－0.085),显著性水平为 1,筛选出 10 个候选药物。从 LINCS-L1000CDS2 中,在反向模式下获得 50 个扰动源,在模拟模式下获得 50 个 Z 得分＜－2.000 扰动源。SPIED3 是 SPIEDw (v2.0)的修改版本,具有独立的数据集,包括来自 CMap、LINCS 和 DrugMatrix 数据集的药物治疗。CMap 结果显示,51 种药物具有负相关评分;LINCS 结果显示,50 种药物具有负相关评分。对比结果,从 CMap-SPIED3 中选择 17 种药物,从 LINCS-L1000-SPIED3 中选择 8 种药物,从 sscMap 中选择 9 种药物,合计选定 31 种药物。

在验证这些药物的用途时,发现其中大多数是批准或实验性治疗不同类型的癌症。一些抗疟疾药物,如甲氟喹和乙胺嘧啶,已被重新用于某些类型癌症的治疗。据报道,药物曲美替尼成为潜在的候选药物,其在 TNBC 治疗中的地位被重新确定。

使用 DrugBank、STITCH 和文献检索进一步对药物进行分析。研究发现,曲美替尼已经通过不同的方案被重新用于 TNBC[33]。部分药物已经被用于癌症治疗,如达拉非尼、米托蒽醌、哌柏西利、达沙替尼、伏立诺他和氟维司群。多维替尼、司美替尼和坦内霉素等药物正在临床试验中,用于治疗淋巴瘤、乳腺癌和其他类型癌症。目前正在研究中的曲古霉素 A[37]和白藜芦醇[38]是具有潜在抗癌作用的天然衍生物。曲古霉素 A 是从链霉菌属细菌中分离出来的二烯羟肟酸天然衍生物。白藜芦醇是从葡萄和其他食品中提取的植物抗生素,具有抗氧化和潜在的化学预防活性。抗疟疾药物(如乙胺嘧啶和甲氟喹)已分别成功用于治疗肝细胞癌和结直肠癌。

此外,笔者对之前研究中发现的 TNBC 相关 *Hub* 基因进行了进一步分析。除生物信息学数据库分析外,还通过结构进一步探索药物再利用。使用 AutoDock Vina 对 *Hub* 基因与 31 个潜在候选药物进行对接研究。在这项研究中,确定了药物分子与蛋白质之间的结合亲和力。结果表明,达拉非尼和 *MAPK1* 的结合能最佳,为 -9.9 kcal/mol,其次是 HDAC 抑制剂和甲麦角林。负结合能越大,药物-靶标复合物的稳定性越大。因此,通过药物重新利用和对接研究,考虑达拉非尼、HDAC 抑制剂和甲麦角林为潜在的候选药物,可能针对影响发病机制的 *Hub* 基因。因此,这些药物是治疗 TNBC 的潜在候选药物。

五、结论

由于 TNBC 的治疗选择有限,对有效治疗的需求日益增加,药物再利用比新药发现更节省时间,因此成为最佳选择之一。这项工作根据已知的靶基因、药理学用法和基因特征确定可能的候选药物,这些候选药物可以重复用于治疗高度侵袭性乳腺癌亚型。笔者筛选了 31 种药物并提取了它们现有的靶点,观察到这些药物的使用主要与抗癌活性有关。预测达拉非尼、HDAC 抑制剂和甲麦角林可能是针对 TNBC 相关 *Hub* 基因的潜在候选药物。这些候选药物,可用于治疗 TNBC。在对接研究的帮助下,可为这些药物确定更多的新靶点。

致谢

感谢本地治里大学生物信息学中心为开展这项工作提供了计算机设备。Leimarembi Devi Naorem 感谢科学与工业研究理事会(Council Of Scientific & Industrial Research,CSIR)的高级研究奖学金。Mathavan Muthaiyan 感谢拉吉夫·甘地国家奖学金(Rajiv Gandhi National Fellowship,RGNF)的高级研究奖学金。

参考文献

[1] Shao F, Sun H, Deng CX. Potential therapeutic targets of triple-negative breast cancer based on its intrinsic subtype. Oncotarget 2017;8(42):73329.

[2] Wahba HA, El-Hadaad HA. Current approaches in treatment of triple-negative breast

cancer. Cancer Biol Med 2015;12(2):106.

[3] Jia H, Truica CI, Wang B, Wang Y, Ren X, Harvey HA, Song J, Yang JM. Immunotherapy for triplenegative breast cancer: existing challenges and exciting prospects. Drug Resist Updat 2017;32:1-15.

[4] Cyprian FS, Akhtar S, Gatalica Z, Vranic S. Targeted immunotherapy with a checkpoint inhibitor in combination with chemotherapy: a new clinical paradigm in the treatment of triple-negative breast cancer. Bosn J Basic Med Sci 2019;19(3):227.

[5] Gns HS, Saraswathy GR, Murahari M, Krishnamurthy M. An update on drug repurposing: re-written saga of the drug's fate. Biomed Pharmacother 2019;110:700-16.

[6] Mirza N, Sills GJ, Pirmohamed M, Marson AG. Identifying new antiepileptic drugs through genomicsbased drug repurposing. Hum Mol Genet 2017;26(3):527-37.

[7] Luo B, Gu YY, Wang XD, Chen G, Peng ZG. Identification of potential drugs for diffuse large b-cell lymphoma based on bioinformatics and Connectivity Map database. Pathol Res Pract 2018;214(11):1854-67.

[8] Siavelis JC, Bourdakou MM, Athanasiadis EI, Spyrou GM, Nikita KS. Bioinformatics methods in drug repurposing for Alzheimer's disease. Brief Bioinform 2016;17(2):322-35.

[9] Zhang SD, Gant TW. sscMap: an extensible Java application for connecting small-molecule drugs using gene-expression signatures. BMC Bioinform 2009;10(1):236.

[10] Williams G. SPIEDw: a searchable platform-independent expression database web tool. BMC Genomics 2013;14(1):765.

[11] Duan Q, Reid SP, Clark NR, Wang Z, Fernandez NF, Rouillard AD, Readhead B, Tritsch SR, Hodos R, Hafner M, Niepel M. L1000CDS 2: LINCS L1000 characteristic direction signatures search engine. NPJ Syst Biol Appl 2016;2(1):1-12.

[12] Wishart DS, Knox C, Guo AC, Shrivastava S, Hassanali M, Stothard P, Chang Z, Woolsey J. Drug-Bank: a comprehensive resource for in silico drug discovery and exploration. Nucleic Acids Res 2006;34(Suppl_1):D668-72.

[13] Kuhn M, von Mering C, Campillos M, Jensen LJ, Bork P. STITCH: interaction networks of chemicals and proteins. Nucleic Acids Res 2007;36(Suppl_1):D684-8.

[14] Naorem LD, Muthaiyan M, Venkatesan A. Integrated network analysis and machine learning approach for the identification of key genes of triple-negative breast cancer. J Cell Biochem 2019;120(4):6154-67.

[15] Lamb J, Crawford ED, Peck D, Modell JW, Blat IC, Wrobel MJ, Lerner J, Brunet JP, Subramanian A, Ross KN, Reich M. The Connectivity Map: using gene-expression signatures to connect small molecules, genes, and disease. Science 2006;313(5795):1929-35.

[16] Rashidieh B, Madani Z, Azam M, Maklavani SK, Akbari NR, Tavakoli S, Rashidieh G, Madani B, Azam Z, Maklavani MK, Akbari SK, Tavakoli NR, Rigi G. Molecular docking based virtual screening of compounds for inhibiting sortase A in *L. monocytogenes*. Bioin-

formation 2015;11(11):501.

[17] Trott O, Olson AJ. AutoDock Vina: improving the speed and accuracy of docking with a new scoring function, efficient optimization, and multithreading. J Comput Chem 2010;31(2):455-61.

[18] Yuan S, Chan HS, Hu Z. Using PyMOL as a platform for computational drug design. Wiley Interdiscip Rev Comput Mol Sci 2017;7(2):e1298.

[19] Kuleshov MV, Jones MR, Rouillard AD, Fernandez NF, Duan Q, Wang Z, Koplev S, Jenkins SL, Jagodnik KM, Lachmann A, McDermott MG. Enrichr: a comprehensive gene set enrichment analysis web server 2016 update. Nucleic Acids Res 2016;44(W1):W90-7.

[20] Long GV, Flaherty KT, Stroyakovskiy D, Gogas H, Levchenko E, De Braud F, Larkin J, Garbe C, Jouary T, Hauschild A, Chiarion-Sileni V. Dabrafenib plus trametinib versus dabrafenib monotherapy in patients with metastatic BRAF V600E/K-mutant melanoma: long-term survival and safety analysis of a phase 3 study. Ann Oncol 2017;28(7):1631-9.

[21] Ongoren S, Eskazan AE, Suzan V, Savci S, Erdogan Ozunal I, Berk S, Yalniz FF, Elverdi T, Salihoglu A, Erbilgin Y, Iseri SA. Third-line treatment with second-generation tyrosine kinase inhibitors (dasatinib or nilotinib) in patients with chronic myeloid leukemia after two prior TKIs: real-life data on a single center experience along with the review of the literature. Hematology 2018;23(4):212-20.

[22] Connolly RM, Rudek MA, Piekarz R. Entinostat: a promising treatment option for patients with advanced breast cancer. Future Oncol 2017;13(13):1137-48.

[23] Lagast H, Meunier-Carpentier F, Klastersky J. Moxalactam treatment of anaerobic infections in cancer patients. Antimicrob Agents Chemother 1982;22(4):604-10.

[24] Liu J, Fu XQ, Zhou W, Yu HG, Yu JP, Luo HS. LY294002 potentiates the anti-cancer effect of oxaliplatin for gastric cancer via death receptor pathway. World J Gastroenterol 2011;17(2):181.

[25] Ahmedzai S, Carlyle DL, Calder IT, Moran F. Anti-emetic efficacy and toxicity of nabilone, a synthetic cannabinoid, in lung cancer chemotherapy. Br J Cancer 1983;48(5):657-63.

[26] Kong L, Zhang X, Li C, Zhou L. Potential therapeutic targets and small molecular drugs for pediatric B-precursor acute lymphoblastic leukemia treatment based on microarray data. Oncol Lett 2017;14(2):1543-9.

[27] Liu L, Sun X, Xie Y, Zhuang Y, Yao R, Xu K. Anticancer effect of histone deacetylase inhibitor scriptaid as a single agent for hepatocellular carcinoma. Biosci Rep 2018;38(4):1-9.

[28] Woo HN, Chung HK, Ju EJ, Jung J, Kang HW, Lee SW, Seo MH, Lee JS, Lee JS, Park HJ, Song SY. Preclinical evaluation of injectable sirolimus formulated with polymeric nanoparticle for cancer therapy. Int J Nanomedicine 2012;7:2197.

[29] Knispel S, Zimmer L, Kanaki T, Ugurel S, Schadendorf D, Livingstone E. The safety and efficacy of dabrafenib and trametinib for the treatment of melanoma. Expert Opin Drug

Saf 2018;17(1):73-87.

[30] Kim S, Thiessen PA, Bolton EE, Chen J, Fu G, Gindulyte A, Han L, He J, He S, Shoemaker BA, Wang J. BS The PubChem Project. Nucleic Acids Res 2016;44(D1): D1202-13.

[31] Gaulton A, Hersey A, Nowotka M, Bento AP, Chambers J, Mendez D, Mutowo P, Atkinson F, Bellis LJ, Cibrián-Uhalte E, Davies M. The ChEMBL database in 2017. Nucleic Acids Res 2017;45(D1):D945-54.

[32] Mendez D, Gaulton A, Bento AP, Chambers J, De Veij M, Félix E, Magariños MP, Mosquera JF, Mutowo P, Nowotka M, Gordillo-Marañón M. ChEMBL: towards direct deposition of bioassay data. Nucleic Acids Res 2019;47(D1):D930-40.

[33] Vitali F, Cohen LD, Demartini A, Amato A, Eterno V, Zambelli A, Bellazzi R. A network-based data integration approach to support drug repurposing and multi-target therapies in triple negative breast cancer. PLoS One 2016;11(9), e0170363.

[34] Xu X, Wang J, Han K, Li S, Xu F, Yang Y. Antimalarial drug mefloquine inhibits nuclear factor kappa B signaling and induces apoptosis in colorectal cancer cells. Cancer Sci 2018;109(4):1220-9.

[35] Malcomson B, Wilson H, Veglia E, Thillaiyampalam G, Barsden R, Donegan S, El Banna A, Elborn JS, Ennis M, Kelly C, Zhang SD. Connectivity mapping (ssCMap) to predict A20-inducing drugs and their antiinflammatory action in cystic fibrosis. Proc Natl Acad Sci 2016;113(26):E3725-34.

[36] Chen YT, Xie JY, Sun Q, Mo WJ. Novel drug candidates for treating esophageal carcinoma: a study on differentially expressed genes, using connectivity mapping and molecular docking. Int J Oncol 2019;54(1):152-66.

[37] Zhang XF, Yan Q, Shen W, Gurunathan S. Trichostatin A enhances the apoptotic potential of palladium nanoparticles in human cervical cancer cells. Int J Mol Sci 2016;17(8):1354.

[38] Ko JH, Sethi G, Um JY, Shanmugam MK, Arfuso F, Kumar AP, Bishayee A, Ahn KS. The role of resveratrol in cancer therapy. Int J Mol Sci 2017;18(12):2589.

第 3 章
女性特异性癌症的化疗耐药性及相关处理

S. Sumathi, K. Santhiya, J. Sivaprabha

Department of Biochemistry, Biotechnology and Bioinformatics, Avinashilingam Institute for Home Science and Higher Education for Women, Coimbatore, Tamil Nadu, India

摘要

癌症是一种细胞不受控制的异常增殖,侵袭并扩散到身体其他部位的疾病。各种类型的癌症以其稳定的行为和不同的治疗反应而著称。女性更容易罹患乳腺癌、卵巢癌、宫颈癌、子宫内膜癌、外阴癌和阴道癌。最常采用的治疗方法包括化学治疗(简称"化疗")和放射治疗(简称"放疗")。化疗耐药性是肿瘤细胞对化疗药物的作用表现出耐药性的现象。本综述将重点介绍女性特异性癌症化疗耐药的不同机制及其治疗方式。

关键词

雌激素,耐药性,癌症,孕酮,转移性乳腺癌,化疗药物,蒽环类药物耐药性

缩略词

ABC receptor	ATP 结合受体
ABC	晚期乳腺癌共识
Akt	蛋白激酶 B
ARID1A	AT 丰富结构域 1A
ATF6	活化转录因子 6
BAX	Bcl-2 样蛋白 4
Bcl-2	B 细胞淋巴瘤 2
BIM	Bcl-2 样蛋白 11
BRAF	B-Raf 原癌基因
BRCA gene	乳腺癌基因
BUBR1	有丝分裂检查点相关蛋白
CD	分化抗原簇
C-erbB-2/ErbB2	表皮生长因子受体家族

COX2	环氧合酶-2
CTLA4	细胞毒性 T 淋巴细胞相关蛋白 4
CTNNB1	连环蛋白 β1
DDP	顺铂
EMA	欧洲药品管理局
EMT	上皮间充质转化
ER	内质网
ER	雌激素
ERK	胞外信号调节激酶
FDA	美国食品药品管理局
GLOBOCAN	全球癌症发病率、死亡率和患病率
GST	谷胱甘肽转移酶 S
HER2/neu	人表皮生长因子受体-2
HIF	缺氧诱导因子
HIPEC	腹腔内热灌注化疗
ICI	免疫检查点抑制剂
IL	白介素
IRE1α	肌醇依赖性激酶 1α
ITH	肿瘤内异质性
KRAS	Ki-ras2 Kirsten 大鼠肉瘤病毒癌基因同源物
MAD2	有丝分裂阻滞缺陷蛋白 2
MAP	微管相关蛋白
MDR1	多药耐药蛋白 1
MEK	丝裂原活化蛋白激酶
MRP1	多药耐药相关蛋白 1
OS	总生存期
P21$^{cip/waf}$	细胞周期蛋白依赖性激酶抑制剂 1
P34$^{cdc\,2}$	蛋白激酶细胞分裂周期 2
PAMAM	聚酰胺-胺
PARP	多聚 ADP 核糖聚合酶
PD-1	程序性细胞死亡蛋白-1
PFS	无进展生存期
P-gp	P 糖蛋白
PgR	孕激素

PI3K	磷脂酰肌醇-3-激酶
PIK3CA	磷脂酰肌醇-4,5-二磷酸 3-激酶催化亚基 α
PLD	聚乙二醇脂质体多柔比星
PPP2R1A	蛋白磷酸酶 2 支架亚基 α
Prosigna	乳腺癌预后基因特征分析
PTB	多聚嘧啶区结合蛋白
PTEN	磷酸酶-张力蛋白基因
RAF	快速进展纤维肉瘤
SAC	纺锤体组装检查点
SIOG	国际老年肿瘤学会
SRp20	富丝氨酸/精氨酸蛋白 20
Topo Ⅰ	拓扑异构酶Ⅰ
Topo Ⅱ	拓扑异构酶Ⅱ
TOR	托瑞米芬
TP53	肿瘤蛋白 53
VEGF	血管内皮生长因子
XiaP	X 染色体连锁凋亡抑制因子

一、乳腺癌

(一)流行病学

乳腺癌是女性最常见的恶性肿瘤,在全球肿瘤负担数据中排名第二,仅次于肺癌。2020 年,全球有 170 万人被确诊乳腺癌,约 50 万人死于乳腺癌[1]。根据全球癌症数据库(GLOBOCAN)2018 报告,乳腺癌的发病率为 1.6%,病死率为 6.6%[2]。现代化的生活方式,以及先进诊断和治疗手段的缺乏导致其发病率和死亡率的快速上升。

(二)乳腺癌分子分型

既往乳腺癌分为 4 种临床亚型,包括 Luminal A 型、Luminal B 型、HER2 过表达型和三阴性乳腺癌。目前,基因拷贝数和表达分析技术已预测出 10 种不同的分子亚型[3]。传统的 4 种乳腺肿瘤亚型可直接使用 prosigna(NanoString Technologies)和 BluePrint(Agendia)技术的多基因检测分析来进行评估;还可间接通过免疫组化手段对雌激素(estrogen,ER)、孕激素(progesterone,PgR)和 HER2 等类固醇激素受体,以及揭示肿瘤生物学特性的肿瘤增殖标志物 Ki67 进行分析。Luminal A 型为 ER 或 PgR 阳性或两者均阳性、HER2 阴性,且增殖能力低。Luminal B 型与 Luminal A 型的区别在于其增殖率较高。HER2 亚型(非 Luminal 型)为 HER2 阳性,不表达 ER 和 PgR。3 种受体表达均阴性是基底细胞样或三阴性乳腺癌(HER2、ER、PgR 阴性)的特征性表现。对患者的治疗决策取决于分子亚型、局部肿瘤负荷和患者的个人意愿[4,5]。

(三)早期乳腺癌的治疗方法

未转移的早期乳腺癌可以治愈。治疗方式需要结合活检和乳腺的影像学检查(如 X 线和超声检查)[6]。局部治疗包括手术和放疗,全身治疗包括内分泌治疗和化疗。

(四)早期乳腺癌局部治疗

1. 手术治疗 通过肿瘤整形外科技术和系统性治疗的建立,提高了其他器官保留手术的可行性[7]。保乳手术已成为一种不可或缺的治疗措施,通过肿瘤整形技术和新辅助化疗使肿瘤缩小后行保乳手术是取代乳房切除术的主要选择[8]。在新辅助化疗或系统治疗后,进行保乳手术,应满足"切缘染色处没有肿瘤细胞"(no ink on tumor rule)原则,即确保切缘无肿瘤累及,以预防复发[9]。前哨淋巴结活检减轻了腋窝淋巴结清扫的严重不良反应[10]。在某些情况下,腋窝淋巴结清扫对治疗结局没有影响[11]。

2. 放射治疗 侵入性较小的放射治疗方法包括局部乳房照射或低分割放射治疗,以减轻肿瘤负荷[12]。术中放疗或独立放疗往往能减轻长期毒性反应,这种治疗通常在腋窝和锁骨上区域进行。众所周知,现代放射疗法通过优化增强来解决剂量相关问题[13]。即使不进行腋窝手术处理,淋巴结照射对阳性肿瘤淋巴结仍有作用,但会产生一定的毒副作用[14]。

3. 早期乳腺癌的系统治疗 HER2 阴性 Luminal 肿瘤根据肿瘤增殖程度、肿瘤分级、淋巴结受累情况等因素进行新辅助或辅助化疗。这些都是通过多基因表达检测确定的,同时也可追踪早期和晚期复发的风险[15]。

4. 内分泌治疗 对绝经前女性的早期 Luminal 型乳腺癌患者进行为期 5~10 年的辅助内分泌治疗,标准剂量为他莫昔芬每天 20 mg,这种治疗已被证明可减少 ER 阳性肿瘤的复发[16]。持续服用他莫昔芬治疗 10 年可使受益患者的乳腺癌相关病死率减半,但在治疗后期生活中具有明显的不良反应[17]。内分泌治疗作为 HER2 阴性的 Luminal 型转移性乳腺癌患者的一线治疗选择非常有效,因为仅器官损伤等不良反应就会影响化疗发挥作用[18]。芳香化酶抑制剂是绝经后女性的首选药物。参与内分泌治疗方案的其他药物包括氟维司群、孕激素和他莫昔芬。内分泌单药治疗或内分泌与靶向药物联合治疗可能适用于进展缓慢的肿瘤[15]。

5. 转移性乳腺癌的治疗特点 由不到5%的长期幸存者证实[19],临床并无治愈转移性乳腺癌患者的潜在方法,而是以延长生存期并减轻症状为目标。根据每2年一度的晚期乳腺癌国际共识(Advanced Breast Cancer conference,ABC)会议报告,系统治疗是转移性乳腺癌的首选治疗方案,而局部治疗在某些情况下可以采用,如原发转移性肿瘤。由于肿瘤的异质性,从原发性肿瘤部位到转移部位的组织学都不尽相同,这有助于确定潜在的治疗靶点。在首次骨转移期间,可使用双膦酸盐或地舒单抗等骨稳定药物维持治疗[20]。

6. 化疗药物的大型临床试验 对早期乳腺癌患者进行术前和术后化疗试验,通常可延长总的无病生存期[21]。三阴性和HER2阳性乳腺癌的患者通过化疗可获得良好的病理学完全缓解和更好的预后[22]。研究发现,将蒽环类药物与其他紫杉烷类药物协同应用,即标准化疗方案在18~24周期间给药时,通过4周一次的蒽环类药物、每周一次的紫杉醇单药治疗和每3周一次的多西他赛治疗,能够降低乳腺癌的10年死亡率[23]。4~6个周期的多西他赛-环磷酰胺(docetaxel-cyclophosphamide,TC)可有效替代蒽环类药物,但其并非标准治疗方案[24]。GIM试验发现,与其他标准化疗方案相比,大剂量含蒽环和/或紫杉类的化疗方案可提高患者的5年无病生存率[25]。在化疗过程中,患者的生理年龄被认为是比实际年龄更重要的因素,因此,对于身体健康的老年人来说,最好遵循标准的用药方案。国际老年肿瘤学会(International Society of Geriatric Oncology,SIOG)记录了符合老年人需求的药物剂型[26]。在基于 *BRCA*1/2 突变和野生型 *BRCA* 的三阴性乳腺癌中,通过在标准化疗方案基础上联合铂类药物治疗可获得病理学完全缓解[27]。在转移性乳腺癌中,抗血管内皮生长因子(vascular endothelial growth factor,VEGF)抗体贝伐珠单抗可以延长无进展生存期(progression-free survival,PFS),然而,与紫杉醇或卡培他滨等联合用药不能保证总生存期。贝伐珠单抗已获得欧洲药品管理局(European Medicines Agency,EMA)的批准,但尚未获得美国食品药品管理局(Food and Drug Administration,FDA)的批准,因此,仅在限定国家作为一种治疗措施使用[28]。

7. 乳腺癌的化疗耐药 细胞化疗耐药性是导致总生存率下降的主要原因,它在分子水平上通过多种机制导致不良预后。

8. CD73在蒽环类耐药性中的作用 通过对6000例患者基因表达谱分析的结果显示,分化抗原簇73(cluster of differentiation73,CD73)的高表达与蒽环类化疗药物疗效的抑制作用相关。CD73的高表达显著降低了新辅助化疗后的病理学完全缓解率,导致侵袭性肿瘤在手术中消失(译者注:此处应勘误,CD73的高表达显著降低了新辅助化疗后的病理学完全缓解率,影响侵袭性肿瘤在手术中消失)。腺苷受体的激活导致多柔比星的化疗耐药,从而降低了抗肿瘤效果[29]。

9. 微管稳定剂 某些紫杉烷类药物如紫杉醇和多西他赛作为微管稳定剂,破坏纺锤体微管动力学,导致细胞死亡和凋亡。对紫杉醇类的化疗耐药性研究涉及纺锤体组装检查点(spindle assembly checkpoint,SAC)和细胞凋亡信号调节失调。有丝分裂阻滞缺陷蛋白2(mitotic arrest deficient 2,MAD2)、有丝分裂检查点相关蛋白1(budding uninhibited by benzimidazole-related 1,BUBR1)、γ-突触核蛋白和Aurora A 等 SAC 蛋白是紫杉醇耐药性的重要标志物。药物外排泵:多药耐药蛋白1(multidrug resistance protein 1,MDR-1)/P糖蛋白(P-glycoprotein,P-gp)的过表达改变了微管相关蛋白(microtubule-associated protein,MAP)如 Tau、stathmin 和 MAP4 的表达,决定了肿瘤复发的概率,同时也检查了紫杉类药物治疗的有效性[30]。

10. β微管蛋白突变 这些突变改变了微管的动力学和稳定性[31],进而阻碍了紫杉醇等抗有丝分裂药物与β微管蛋白亚基的结合[32]。由于高度耐药的微管蛋白等位基因的杂合性丢失,癌细胞反复暴露于抗有丝分裂药物可能会产生高度耐药的表型[33]。人体中存在7种β微管蛋白异型。由βⅢ和βⅣ微管蛋白异型组成的微管可能需要与紫杉醇结合才能诱导微管的稳定性[34]。βⅢ微管蛋白第277位的丝氨酸/精氨酸置换改变了结合位点,从而促进了药物耐药[35]。

11. 微管相关蛋白(MAP) 参与微管动力学的MAP有助于调节微管蛋白聚合物和微管之间的相互作用。它们还调节细胞对有丝分裂抑制剂药物的反应[36]。Tau 是一种神经元相关 MAP,在低表达水平下会对紫杉醇的结合产生抵抗。微管稳定剂癌蛋白18(stathmin)的功能紊乱会导致紫杉类药物的耐药性[37]。MAP4的下调可提高微管的动态性,并影响紫杉醇的耐药性[36]。

12. 多药耐药蛋白(MDR) MDR1 基因编码的 P-gp 是一种能量依赖性药物外排泵,它与多种疏水药物如紫杉醇、多柔比星、长春新碱和长春碱结合,并随后诱导耐药性[38]。

13. 表皮生长因子受体家族/人表皮生长因子受体-2(C-erbB-2/HER 2-neu) 由于相应的人表皮生长因子受体-2(*HER2/neu*)原癌基因过度表达,细胞对紫杉醇的耐药性有2种机制。P21$^{waf1/cip-1}$ 与激酶 P34^{cdc2} 的协同或结合抑制了激酶 P34^{cdc2} 在紫杉醇诱导下的活化,导致 G2/M 期细胞凋亡,进而导致 HER2/neu 的高表达[39]。ErbB2受体酪氨酸激酶的过度表达会抑制原发性乳腺肿瘤中 P34^{cdc2} 的活化,从而对紫杉醇诱导的细胞凋亡产生抵抗作用[40]。HER2/PI3K/Akt 信号通路促进了肿瘤对紫杉醇、多柔比星和氟尿嘧啶的高耐药性[41]。

14. 抗凋亡信号转导 Raf/MEK/ERK 是一种细胞存活途径,涉及各种促凋亡和抗凋亡蛋白。Bcl-2样蛋白11(Bcl-2-like Protein 11,BIM)是一种由胞外信号调节激酶(extracellular signal-regulated kinase,ERK)引起的促凋亡蛋白,BIM的磷酸化阻止了Bcl-2诱导的Bax-Bax同源二聚体化,并激发了显著的抗凋亡活性[42]。蛋白酪氨酸激酶(protein tyrosine kinases,PTK)通过调节抗凋亡信号通路磷脂酰肌醇3-激酶/蛋白激酶B(phosphotidyl inositol-3-kinase/protein kinase B,PI3K/Akt)诱导耐药性[43]。

(五)改善乳腺癌的化疗耐药性

1. 抗化疗耐药的生物标志物 缺氧诱导因子(hypoxia inducible factors,HIF)及其基因产物在三阴性乳腺癌中普遍存在。化疗诱导的HIF活性通过白介素(interleukin,IL)-6和IL-8信号影响乳腺癌干细胞的增殖,从而导致MDR效应增强。HIF抑制剂地高辛与紫杉醇或吉西他滨联合使用可通过消除耐药性控制肿瘤[44]。

2. 抗肿瘤候选药物 塞来昔布作为一种特异性环氧合酶2(cyclooxygenase 2,COX-2)抑制剂,作用于P-gp药物外排泵[45]。LY294002是PI3K的特异性抑制剂,能使P-gp失活并降低存活蛋白的浓度[46]。托瑞米芬(toremifene,TOR)可增加多柔比星在细胞中的积累[47],洛贝林可逆转MDR。

3. 联合疗法 他莫昔芬与依维莫司合用可大大降低继发性耐药的发生率,抑制细胞增殖或诱导细胞凋亡。槲皮素在高热条件下可增加肿瘤细胞凋亡,并可逆转MDR[48]。

4. 新型药物递送系统 药物递送系统用于靶向药物释放、维持血药浓度和优化生物相容性,该系统通常以纳米尺度制备。聚酰胺-胺(polyamidoamine,PAM-AM)通过调节细胞内耐药性来克服多药耐药性,促进了主要拱顶蛋白靶向小干扰RNA和多柔比星的同时递送[49]。脂质体青蒿内酯和长春瑞滨可以消除乳腺癌干细胞[50]。

5. 免疫治疗 免疫检查点抑制剂(immune checkpoint inhibitor,ICI)利用免疫系统的漏洞选择性地杀死癌细胞[51]。纳武利尤单抗的作用靶点是程序性死亡受体-1(programmed cell death protein-1,PD-1)。环孢素等免疫调节剂对P-gp的抑制可减小MDR[52]。ICI、免疫增强剂、靶向药物,以及表观遗传修饰剂如组蛋白去乙酰化酶抑制剂可以逆转乳腺肿瘤的MDR[51]。

二、卵巢癌

(一)全球卵巢癌概况

卵巢癌是一种常见的妇科肿瘤,发病率仅次于宫颈癌和子宫内膜癌,居第三位。预后不良、死亡率高而发病率低、肿瘤生长隐匿和症状出现较晚等特点使其被称为"沉默杀手"[53,54]。卵巢癌的致死率是乳腺癌的3倍,预计到2040年,死亡率还将上升[55]。卵巢癌是一组具有不同生物学特性和分子特征的恶性肿瘤。超过90%的卵巢肿瘤为上皮源性,在非西班牙裔白人中,浆液性癌的发病率最高(每10万人中有5.2例),而非西班牙裔黑人和亚太岛民中其发病率最低(每10万人中有3.4例)。然而,后者发生子宫内膜样癌和透明细胞癌的风险较高。在Ⅲ期或Ⅳ期,延迟诊断会促进肿瘤的进展,特别是浆液性癌[56]。

(二)独特亚型

卵巢癌在女性肿瘤中发病率排第七位,可分为上皮性和非上皮性两种。上皮源性卵巢癌是最主要的类型,因为它有5个亚型,分别具有不同的发育、组织学、分子和预后模式及特征[57]。这些亚型包括70%的高级别浆液性癌、<5%的低级别浆液性癌、10%的子宫内膜样癌,10%的透明细胞癌和3%的黏液性癌。上皮性卵巢癌与子宫体癌,以及起源于输卵管或子宫内膜的癌症的肿瘤形态相似,并且最初常被误诊为上皮源性癌症[58]。根据上皮性癌的肿瘤基因特征,可将其分为两类:Ⅰ型包括低级别浆液性癌、黏液性癌、子宫内膜样癌、透明细胞癌和Brenner瘤,其特征是 *KRAS*、*BRAF*、*PTEN*、*PIK3CA*、*CTNNB1*、*ARID1A* 和 *PPP2R1A* 等特异基因的高度突变;Ⅱ型包括高级别浆液性和子宫内膜样癌,具有高度遗传不稳定性[59]。高级别浆液性和子宫内膜样癌是由肿瘤蛋白53(tumor protein 53,*TP53*)突变和 *BRCA1* 和/或 *BRCA2* 功能异常引起的[60]。

(三)诱发卵巢癌的因素

绝经后女性的上皮性卵巢癌发病率通常更高,其5年生存率为22%,而绝经前年轻女性的5年生存率为48%。年轻女性在癌症进展的各阶段都显示出更高的生存优势,这由独立预后因素决定,如年龄、活性和细胞减灭术的范围[61]。导致侵袭性肿瘤的另一个机会因素是早产,生育男婴会使风险加倍[62]。盆腔炎性疾病的复发与卵巢癌的风险相关[63]。乳腺肿瘤家族史是一个重要的遗传易感因素[64]。生活习惯,如缺乏运动和伴随的肥胖是这种危及生命的癌症的关键因素,会降低患者的生存率[65]。

(四)治疗方法

1. 手术治疗 诊断和治疗策略包括减瘤术或肿瘤细胞减灭术[66],旨在切除所有可见的肿瘤组织,以降低复发的风险[67]。二次减瘤术后PFS增加5.6个月,这一点证实了铂类敏感患者可以从中获益[68]。腹腔内热灌注化疗(hyperthermic intraperitoneal chemotherapy,HIPEC)的最佳效果也是在肿瘤细胞减灭术后得以保证和正常进行的[69]。手术获益较小的个体可以进行新辅助化疗[70]。

2. 靶向治疗

(1)抗血管生成素：贝伐珠单抗可与一线化疗联合使用，也可用于铂类敏感或铂类耐药的复发患者[71]。这种使用贝伐珠单抗等抗血管生成药物的给药模式可延长Ⅲ期或Ⅳ期上皮性卵巢癌患者的PFS，并改善患者的生活质量[72]。化疗结束后，贝伐珠单抗的长周期序贯方案对于维持PFS期至关重要。在贝伐珠单抗的使用过程中也会发生高血压和胃肠道毒性等不良反应，这些不良反应的发生率可能仅占观察到有不良反应病例的3%。当贝伐珠单抗与标准化疗方案卡铂-吉西他滨联合使用时，铂敏感复发上皮性癌患者的平均PFS为12.4个月，而单独化疗的平均PFS为8.4个月。然而，两组之间的总生存期(overall survival,OS)保持不变[73]。意大利肿瘤内科协会[67]建议，对高级别肿瘤患者进行减瘤术后，应接受贝伐珠单抗与卡铂-紫杉醇联合治疗6个周期的治疗方案。

(2)PARP抑制剂：在 *BRCA* 基因突变的癌细胞中，化疗驱动的DNA损伤通过单链或替代的DNA修复途径来克服，这需要多聚ADP核糖聚合酶(poly ADP ribose polymerase,PARP)的功能，抑制PARP可以促进合成致死过程[74]。有 *BRCA* 基因突变的高级别卵巢癌患者通过使用奥拉帕利(400 mg，每天2次)进行单药维持治疗可获得较长的PFS。用药后也会出现恶心、贫血和疲劳等不良反应[75]。2种新型PARP抑制剂，即尼拉帕利(于2017年11月获得EMA批准)和鲁卡帕利目前尚未上市。据了解，尼拉帕利和卢卡帕利能为铂敏感复发性卵巢癌患者带来明显较长的PFS，无论其是否存在 *BRCA* 突变和同源重组缺陷状态[76,77]。

(3)一线化疗：铂类药物在卵巢癌的早期治疗中应用最为广泛，顺铂是首个用于治疗卵巢癌的铂类药物。然而，它具有与剂量相关的毒性作用，如恶心、周围神经病变和肾毒性。因此，以卡铂为代表的顺铂有机类似物成为主要的化疗药物[78]。紫杉醇联合卡铂的标准化疗方案被认为是一线治疗策略，尽管这种方案在最初2年内的复发率高达70%～80%，但并无其他药物能达到相同的卓越疗效[67]。可耐受剂量下每3周一次卡铂联合每周一次紫杉醇的治疗方案，以及贝伐珠单抗联合卡铂-紫杉醇3周方案也能取得良好疗效[79,80]。

(4)二线化疗：在复发性卵巢癌患者中，二线治疗旨在确保延长生存期，并通过延缓症状进展以提高生活质量。预后因素包括肿瘤大小、组织学类型、*BRCA* 突变及转移灶数量[81]。治疗决策基于患者对于铂类药物治疗的反应性。部分或完全铂敏感复发性卵巢癌患者接受以铂为基础的联合化疗，必须具有>12个月或6~12个月的无铂间期[67]。对于铂耐药复发性卵巢癌患者，靶向治疗可提供良好的效果。据了解,曲贝替定联合聚乙二醇脂质体多柔比星(pegylated liposomal doxorubicin,PLD)能更好的改善 PFS 和 OS 率[82]。

(5)化疗耐药性:化疗耐药原因众多,如肿瘤干细胞、低效的药物转运、药物靶点的修饰、参与解毒的细胞蛋白改变、与 DNA 修复机制相关的改变,以及对药物损伤的高度耐受[83]。50%~70%的卵巢癌复发可能是由于化疗耐药和肿瘤内异质性(intratumor heterogeneity,ITH)所致[84]。

(6)药物转运蛋白问题:MDR 是肿瘤细胞在化疗过程中逐渐获得的一种交叉耐药性。它通常涉及 P-gp 和 MDR 相关蛋白 1(MDR-associated protein 1,MRP1)等三磷酸腺苷(adenosine triphosphate,ATP)结合盒转运蛋白的过表达[85]。*MRP1* 基因的高可变剪接率产生了许多剪接变体,如多聚嘧啶区结合蛋白(polypyrimidine tract binding protein,PTB)和丝氨酸/精氨酸丰富蛋白 20(serine/arginine-rich protein 20,SRp20),这些变体对多柔比星表现出耐药性[86]。

(7)解毒过程中细胞蛋白质的变化:谷胱甘肽和谷胱甘肽 S-转移酶(glutathione S transferase,GST)参与了一些化疗烷化剂的解毒过程。通过在酵母中进行转染实验,已经证明 GST π 1 对多柔比星、苯丁酸氮芥产生耐药性[87]。金属硫蛋白是一类低分子量蛋白质,可抵抗细胞 DNA 损伤、氧化应激及相关的凋亡,其过表达是一个重要因素,并且在卵巢癌中已有相关报道[88]。

(8)药物靶点的修饰:拓扑异构酶Ⅰ(TopoⅠ)和拓扑异构酶Ⅱ(TopoⅡ)在 DNA 修复代谢中具有重要作用。因此,它们在恶性肿瘤中的表达增加,并且是许多化疗药物[如喜树碱、依托泊苷、替尼泊苷、新生霉素、蒽环类药物(多柔比星)和米托蒽醌]的药物靶点[89]。

(9)强大的 DNA 修复活性:研究发现,卵巢癌细胞系 A2780 对顺铂(Ⅱ)(cis diamminedichloroplatinum Ⅱ,DDP)具有耐药性,这是由于去除铂-DNA 加合物所致[90]。同样,顺铂相关的耐药性也会诱导有效的 DNA 修复,特别是在链内交联处[91]。铂-DNA 损伤可以通过核苷酸切除修复过程去除[92]。

(10)药物性损伤的耐受性:增加化疗损伤的耐受性有助于降低细胞凋亡的反应性,这需要促凋亡因子或抑癌基因的表达,以及细胞存活因子的调节[92]。X 连锁凋亡抑制因子(X-linked inhibitor of apoptosis,Xiap)的表达和 Fas 配体的下调导致卵巢癌的化疗耐药性[93]。Fas/Fas 配体的功能失调促进顺铂耐药[94]。

(五)改善化疗耐药性

1. 外排泵抑制剂 与第一代和第二代抑制剂相比,P-gp 和 MDR 等药物外排泵的第三代抑制剂对细胞色素 P450 酶的抑制作用极小[95]。这些药物,如阿帕替尼和他利奎达,具有更强的特异性和疗效,并能在体外和体内系统中逆转对紫杉醇的耐药性[96,97]。在卵巢癌小鼠模型中，选择了以 CD44 为靶点的纳米制剂来递送针对 MDR1 的 siRNA，并与紫杉醇联合使用，以确保对癌细胞的特异性[98]。

2. 内皮素受体与 EMT　化疗后获得的上皮间充质转化（epithelial-mesenchymal transition，EMT）状态会导致卵巢癌的化疗耐药性。内皮素受体是 EMT 变化的前体，因此，使用齐泊腾坦（zibotentan）等拮抗剂阻断内皮素受体，被认为可以逆转耐药性和影响随后的 EMT 表型。目前，这种药物正在进行临床试验研究[99,100]。

3. 逆转 DNA 损伤耐受性和增强修复　具有 *TP53* 突变的卵巢癌细胞通过 G1 期阻滞和 G2 期延迟，显示出对铂类诱导的 DNA 损伤和抗凋亡作用的耐药性，因修复途径的增强而不再受遗传损伤的影响[101]。参与 CDC2 磷酸化的 Wee1 激酶是 *TP53* 突变体中逆转铂类耐药性的潜在药物靶点，并受到 Wee1 特异性抑制剂 MK1775 和 PD0166285 的抑制作用[102]。

4. PARP 和血管生成抑制剂　越过 VEGF 的阻断作用，通过血管生成素形成新的血管是癌细胞的常用方法。在铂类耐药性高级别卵巢浆液性癌患者中联合使用贝伐珠单抗和 trebananib 等抗血管生成药物，有助于延长患者的生存期[103,104]。对 PARP 抑制剂的耐药性是由于 MDR1 外排泵的表达，而特定药物如 6-硫鸟嘌呤可以逆转后者的拮抗作用[105]。

5. 检查点抑制剂　在高级别卵巢浆液性癌中观察到 PD-1 受体表达增加，PD-1 抑制剂如帕博利珠单抗和纳武利尤单抗正处于 FDA 试验阶段。细胞毒性 T 淋巴细胞相关蛋白 4（cytotoxic T-lymphocyte-associated protein 4，CTLA4）也是一种检查点抑制剂，与之相关的伊匹木单抗（ipilumab）目前正在研究中[106]。为躲避免疫系统的攻击，一些癌细胞会删除主要组织相容性复合体 I 类分子，并产生耐药性，而这种耐药性可以通过对检查点抑制剂的进一步预测而找到合适的靶点[107]。

三、宫颈癌

宫颈癌是由女性下生殖系统（子宫）中的细胞异常生长引发的癌症。承载胎儿的子宫上部通过宫颈与下面的阴道相连。子宫颈分为 2 个区域：上部区域称为宫颈内口，由腺细胞组成；下部靠近阴道区域称为宫颈外口，由鳞状细胞组成。这 2 种细胞在转化区交汇，转化区的位置受女性年龄和分娩情况影响。

宫颈癌通常发展在转化区的细胞中。这些正常细胞表现出一定的癌前行为，之后是否会转变为癌症并不确定。这些癌前病变以不同术语来指称，包括宫颈上皮内瘤变、鳞状上皮病变和不典型增生。宫颈癌好发于 35～44 岁的女性，20 岁之前少见，65 岁以上的病例数仅占 15%[108,109]。

(一) 诊断

年龄在 30～49 岁的女性应定期检查是否出现癌前病变,以及与宫颈癌相关的症状。通常采用巴氏涂片对患者进行检查,如结果异常,医师会建议进行进一步检查,如阴道镜检查、宫颈活检、阴道镜活检、宫颈管搔刮和锥切活检[110]。

(二) 治疗方法

传统的治疗措施包括手术、放疗、化疗和使用单克隆抗体的靶向治疗。手术包括冷冻疗法、激光疗法、环形电切术、锥切术、广泛性子宫颈切除术、单纯/根治性子宫切除术。

(三) 化疗药物及其作用方式

化疗是指使用化学物质/药物治疗宫颈癌。表 3-1 列出了用于治疗宫颈癌的化疗药物。

表 3-1　化疗药物及其对癌细胞的作用模式[111]

药物	作用方式
20 世纪 70 年代以前	
环磷酰胺	干扰 DNA 的复制和 RNA 的转录
苯丁酸氮芥	细胞周期停滞并诱导癌细胞凋亡
美法仑	烷基化鸟嘌呤并抑制 DNA 和 RNA 的合成
氟尿嘧啶	抑制核苷酸胸苷嘧啶的形成并干扰 DNA 复制
甲氨蝶呤	阻断核苷酸胸苷嘧啶的从头合成
长春新碱	抑制细胞分裂
博来霉素	诱导癌细胞 DNA 链断裂
多柔比星	干扰癌细胞的生长和扩散
丝裂霉素	抑制癌细胞生长
20 世纪 70 年代年以后	
顺铂	与 DNA 相互作用,形成 DNA 加合物
卡铂	修饰 DNA 结构,抑制 DNA 合成
异环磷酰胺	抑制 DNA 合成
紫杉醇	有丝分裂纺锤体组装缺陷,影响染色体分离和细胞分裂
伊立替康	抑制拓扑异构酶,从而阻止 DNA 合成

续表

药物	作用方式
托泊替康	诱导癌细胞 DNA 损伤
吉西他滨	抑制癌细胞 DNA 复制
长春瑞滨	阻止有丝分裂纺锤体的形成,导致肿瘤细胞在中期生长停滞
多西他赛	破坏微管的正常形成,阻止细胞分裂
多柔比星	作为嵌入剂,抑制 DNA 合成和 RNA 转录
二溴卫矛醇	干扰细胞分裂

(四)癌细胞对化疗的耐药性

在癌症治疗中使用化疗时,通常会观察到一个持续存在的问题,即癌细胞对用于治疗的化疗药物产生的耐药性逐渐增强。

内质网(endoplasmic reticulum,ER)是参与蛋白质折叠不可缺少的细胞器。任何对其正常功能的干扰都会导致内质网腔中未折叠或错误折叠蛋白质的积累。这导致 ER 应激并最终引起未折叠蛋白质反应,激活细胞死亡。多种化疗药物都采用以上策略来阻止癌细胞的生长[112]。但在某些情况下,癌细胞会通过一些分子机制对化疗药物产生耐药性,这些机制包括膜转运改变[例如,癌细胞中 ATP 结合受体(ATP-binding cassette,ABC receptor)的过度表达会促进耐药性的产生][113]、药物靶点的改变(例如,MRP-1 通过诱导拓扑异构酶 II 基因突变导致药物在癌细胞中的积累减少,从而对依托泊苷和多柔比星产生耐药性)[114,115]、抗氧化剂和解毒系统的激活(例如,谷胱甘肽 S-转移酶的增加会导致癌细胞对凋亡产生耐药性)[116],以及 ER 应激反应(例如,ATF6、IRE1 和 PERK 通常在肿瘤细胞中失调,从而导致癌基因的激活和抑癌基因的抑制)[113,117,118]。

顺铂(单药治疗或与紫杉醇联合治疗)被广泛用于宫颈癌的治疗。癌细胞会对顺铂产生耐药性,从而降低药物杀死肿瘤细胞的效果。对顺铂产生耐药性的机制包括肿瘤细胞内的铂类积累减少、DNA 损伤修复增加、抗细胞凋亡、EMT 的激活、DNA 甲基化的改变、肿瘤干细胞的特征和患者的应激反应等[119]。

(五)改善化疗耐药性

为改善 MDR 已采用多种策略。一些癌细胞的 MDR 通常是由于 ABC 转运蛋白和化疗增敏剂的过表达所致,已开发出用于阻断 ABC 转运蛋白的功能以逆转耐药性(如儿茶酚、类胡萝卜素)的化疗增敏剂[120]。缩短每次化疗的间隔时间可抑制癌细胞的 MDR[121]。

四、结论

化疗是治疗女性特异性癌症最广泛使用的治疗方式之一。然而,正如本章所述,肿瘤细胞通过各种分子机制表现出耐药性。也正因如此,一个新的研究领域应运而生,即关注更有效的低耐药性化疗药物,或者改变治疗方法以适应患者需求,给患者带来福祉。

参 考 文 献

[1] Ferlay J, Soerjomataram I, Dikshi R, et al. Cancer incidence and mortality worldwide: sources, methods and major patterns in GLOBOCAN 2012. Int J Cancer 2015;136: E359-86.

[2] Bray F, Ferlay J, Soerjomataram I, Siegel RL, Torre LA, Jemal A. Global Cancer Statistics 2018: GLOBOCAN estimates of incidence and mortality worldwide for 36 cancers in 185 countries. CA Cancer J Clin 2018;68:394-424.

[3] Curtis C, Shah SP, Cgin SF, et al. The genomic and transcriptomic architecture of 2000 breast tumours reveals novel subgroups. Nature 2012;486:346-52.

[4] Goldhirsch A, Winer EP, Coats AS, et al. Personalizing the treatment of women with early breast cancer: highlights of St. Gallen International Expert Consensus on the primary therapy of early breast cancer 2013. Ann Oncol 2013;24:206-23.

[5] Coats AS, Winer EP, Goldhirsch A, et al. Tailoring therapies-improving the management of early breast cancer, St. Gallen International Expert Consensus on the primary therapy of early breast cancer 2015. Ann Oncol 2015;26:1533-46.

[6] AGO Breast Commission Recommendations. Diagnosis and therapy of primary and metastatic breast cancer, 2016. Available from: http://www.ago-online.de/en/guidelines-mamma/. (Accessed 15 September 2019).

[7] McLaughlin SA. Surgical management of the breast: breast conservation therapy and mastectomy. Surg Clin North Am 2013;93:411-28.

[8] Haloua MH, Krekel NM, Winters HA, et al. A systematic review of oncoplastic breast-conserving surgery: current weaknesses and future prospects. Ann Surg 2013;257:609-20.

[9] Kümmel S, Holtschmidt J, Loibl S. Surgical treatment of primary breast cancer in the neoadjuvant setting. Br J Surg 2014;101:912-24.

[10] Krag DN, Julian TB, Harlow SP, et al. NSABP-32: phase Ⅲ, randomized trial comparing axillary resection with sentinel lymph node dissection: a description of the trial. Ann Surg Oncol 2004;11:208S-10.

[11] Giuliano AE, Hunt KK, Ballman KV, et al. Axillary dissection vs no axillary dissection in

women with invasive breast cancer and sentinel node metastasis: a randomized clinical trial. JAMA 2011;305:589.

[12] Haviland JS, Owen JR, Dewar JA, et al. The UK Standardisation of Breast Radiotherapy (START) trials of radiotherapy hypofractionation for treatment of early breast cancer: 10-year follow-up results of two randomised controlled trials. Lancet Oncol 2013;14:1086-94.

[13] Franco P, Cante D, Sciacero P, Girelli G, La Porta MR, Ricardi U. Tumor bed boost integration during whole breast radiotherapy: a review of the current evidence. Breast Care (Basel) 2015;10:44-9.

[14] Brown LC, Mutter RW, Halyard MY. Benefits, risks, and safety of external beam radiation therapy for breast cancer. Int J Womens Health 2015;7:449-58.

[15] Harbeck N, Gnant M. Breast cancer. Lancet 2017;389:1134-50.

[16] Early Breast Cancer Trialists' Collaborative Group (EBCTCG). Relevance of breast cancer hormone receptors and other factors to the efficacy of adjuvant tamoxifen: patient-level meta-analysis of randomised trials. Lancet 2011;378:771-84.

[17] Fisher B, Costantino JP, Wickerham DL, et al. Tamoxifen for prevention of breast cancer: report of the National Surgical Adjuvant Breast and Bowel Project P-1 study. J Natl Cancer Inst 1998;90:1371-88.

[18] Cardoso F, Costa A, Norton L, et al. ESO-ESMO 2nd international consensus guidelines for advanced breast cancer (ABC2). Breast 2014;23:489-502.

[19] Greenberg PA, Hortobagyi GN, Smith TL, Ziegler LD, Frye DK, Buzdar AU. Long-term follow-up of patients with complete remission following combination chemotherapy for metastatic breast cancer. J Clin Oncol 1996;14:2197-205.

[20] Wang X, Yang KH, Wanyan P, Tian JH. Comparison of the efficacy and safety of denosumab versus bisphosphonates in breast cancer and bone metastases treatment: a meta-analysis of randomized controlled trials. Oncol Lett 2014;7:1997-2002.

[21] Rastogi P, Anderson SJ, Bear HD, et al. Preoperative chemotherapy: updates of National Surgical Adjuvant Breast and Bowel Project Protocols B-18 and B-27. J Clin Oncol 2008;26:778-85.

[22] Cortazar P, Zhang L, Untch M, et al. Pathological complete response and long-term clinical benefit in breast cancer: the CTNeoBC pooled analysis. Lancet 2014;384:164-72.

[23] Sparano JA, Zhao F, Martino S, et al. Long-term follow-up of the E1199 phase iii trial evaluating the role of taxane and schedule in operable breast cancer. J Clin Oncol 2015;33:2353-60.

[24] Joensuu H, Kellokumpu-Lehtinen PL, Huovinen R, et al. Adjuvant capecitabine, docetaxel, cyclophosphamide, and epirubicin for early breast cancer: final analysis of the randomized FinXX trial. J Clin Oncol 2012;30:11-8.

[25] Del Mastro L, De Placido S, Bruzzi P, et al. Fluorouracil and dose-dense chemotherapy in adjuvant treatment of patients with early-stage breast cancer: an open-label, 2×2 factorial,

randomised phase 3 trial. Lancet 2015;385:1863-72.

[26] Biganzoli L, Aapro M, Loibl S, Wildiers H, Brain E. Taxanes in the treatment of breast cancer: have we better defined their role in older patients? A position paper from a SIOG Task Force. Cancer Treat Rev 2016;43:19-26.

[27] Alba E, Chacon JI, Lluch A, et al. A randomized phase II trial of platinum salts in basal-like breast cancer patients in the neoadjuvant setting. Results from the GEICAM/2006-03, multicenter study. Breast Cancer Res Treat 2012;136:487-93.

[28] Miles DW, Diéras V, Cortes J, Duenne AA, Yi J, O'Shaughnessy J. First-line breast cancer: pooled and subgroup analyses of data from 2447 patients. Ann Oncol 2013;24:2773-80.

[29] Loi S, Pommey S, Haibe-Kains B, Beavis PA, Darcy PK, Smyth MJ, Stagg J. CD73 promotes anthracycline resistance and poor prognosis in triple negative breast cancer. PNAS 2013;110:11091-6.

[30] McGrogan BT, Gilmartin B, Carney DN, McCann A. Taxanes, microtubules and chemoresistant breast cancer. Biochimica et Biophysica Acta 2008;1785:96-132.

[31] Gonzalez-Garay ML, Chang L, Blade K, Menick DR, Cabral F. A beta-tubulin leucine cluster involved in microtubule assembly and paclitaxel resistance. J Biol Chem 1999;274:23875-82.

[32] Berrieman HK, Lind MJ, Cawkwell L. Do beta-tubulin mutations have a role in resistance to chemotherapy? Lancet Oncol 2004;5:158-64.

[33] Wang Y, O'Brate A, Zhou W, Giannakakou P. Resistance to microtubule-stabilizing drugs involves two events, beta-tubulin mutation in one allele followed by loss of the second allele. Cell Cycle 2005;4:1847-53.

[34] Derry W, Wilson L, Khan IA, Ludena RF, Jordan MA. Taxol differentially modulates the dynamics of microtubules assembled from unfractionated and purified beta-tubulin isotypes. Biochemistry 1997;36:3554-62.

[35] Ferlini C, Raspaglio G, Mozzetti S, Cicchillitti L, Filippetti F, Gallo D, Fattorusso C, Campiani G, Scambia G. The seco-taxane IDN5390 is able to target class III beta-tubulin and to overcome paclitaxel resistance. Cancer Res 2005;65:2397-405.

[36] Orr G, Verdier-Pinard P. Mechanisms of taxol resistance related to microtubules. Oncogene 2003;22:7280-95.

[37] Honore S, Pasquier E, Braguer D. Understanding microtubule dynamics for improved cancer therapy. Cell Mol Life Sci 2005;62:3039-56.

[38] Schinkel AH, Mayer U, Wagenaar E, Mol CA, Van Deemter L, Smit JJ, Van Der Valk MA, Voordouw AC, Spits H, Van Tellingen O, Zijlmans JM, Fibbe WE, Borst P. Normal viability and altered pharmacokinetics in mice lacking Mdr1-Type (drug-transporting) P-glycoproteins. Proc Natl Acad Sci U S A 1997;94:4028-33.

[39] Yu D, Jing T, Liu B, Yao J, Tan M, Mc Donnell TJ, Hung MC. Overexpression of

ErbB2 blocks taxol-induced apoptosis by upregulation of p21cip1, which inhibits p34Cdc2 kinase. Mol Cell 1998;2:581-91.

[40] Tan M, Jing T, Lan K-H, Neal CL, Li P, Lee S, Fang D, Nagata Y, Liu J, Arlinghaus R, Hung M-C, Yu D. Phosphorylation on tyrosine-15 of p34Cdc2 activation and is involved in resistance to taxolinduced Apoptosis. Mol Cell 2002;9:993-1004.

[41] Knuefermann C, Lu Y, Liu B, Jin W, Liang K, Wu L, Schmidt M, Mills GB, Mendelsohn J, Fan Z. HER2/PI-3K/Akt activation leads to a multidrug resistance in human breast adenocarcinoma cells. Oncogene 2003;22:3205-12.

[42] Harada H, Quearry B, Ruiz-Vela A, Korsmeyer SJ. Survival factor induced extracellular signalregulated kinase phosphorylates BIM, inhibiting its association with BAX and pro-apoptotic activity. Proc Natl Acad Sci U S A 2004;101:15313-7.

[43] Fresno Vara JA, Casado E, De Castro J, Cejas P, Belda-Iniesta C, Gonzalez-Baron M. PI3K/Akt signaling pathway and cancer. Cancer Treat Rev 2004;30:193-204.

[44] Samanta D, Gilkes DM, Chaturvedi P, Xiang L, Semenza GL. Hypoxia-inducible factors are required for chemotherapy resistance of breast cancer stem cells. Proc Natl Acad Sci U S A 2014;111(50):E5429-38. https://doi.org/10.1073/pnas.1421438111.

[45] Kang HK. Cyclooxygenase-independent down-regulation of multidrug resistance associated protein-1 expression by celecoxib in human lung cancer cells. Mol Cancer Ther 2005;4:1358-63.

[46] Zhang W, Ding W, Chen Y, Feng M, Ouyang Y, Yu Y, He Z. Up-regulation of breast cancer resistance protein plays a role in HER2-mediated chemoresistance through PI3K/Akt and nuclear factorkappa B signaling pathways in MCF7 breast cancer cells. Acta Biochim Biophys Sin (Shangai) 2011;43:647-53.

[47] Mubashar M, Harrington KJ, Chaudhary KS, El Lalani N, Stamp GW, Peters AM. P-glycoprotein expressing breast and head and neck cancer cell lines. Acta Oncol 2004;43:443-52.

[48] Bachelot T, Bourgier C, Cropet C, Ray-Coquard I, Ferrero J, Freyer GM, Abadie-Lacourtoisie S, Eymard JC, Debled M, Spaëth D, Legouffe E, Allouache D, El Kouri C, Pujade-Lauraine E. Randomized phase II trial of everolimus in combination with tamoxifen in patients with hormone receptor-positive, human epidermal growth factor receptor 2-negative metastatic breast cancer with prior exposure to aromatase inhibitors: a GINECO study. J Clin Oncol 2012;30:2718-24.

[49] Han M, Lv Q, Tang X, Hu YL, Xu DH, Li FZ, Liang WQ, Gao JQ. Overcoming drug resistance of MCF-7/ADR cells by altering intracellular distribution of doxorubicin via MVP knockdown with a novel siRNA polyamidoamine-hyaluronic acid complex. J Control Release 2012;163:136-44.

[50] Liu Y, Lu WL, Guo J, Du J, Li T, Wu JW, Wang GL, Wang JC, Zhang X, Zhang Q. A potential target associated with both cancer and cancer stem cells: a combination therapy

for eradication of breast cancer using vinorelbine stealthy liposomes plus parthenolide stealthy liposomes. J Control Release 2008;129:18-25.

[51] Sharma P, Hu-Lieskovan S, Wargo JA, Ribas A. Primary, adaptive, and acquired resistance to cancer immunotherapy. Cell 2017;168:707-23.

[52] Muraro E, Furlan C, Avanzo M, Martorelli D, Comaro E, Rizzo A, Fae' DA, Berretta M, Militello L, Del Conte A, Spazzapan S, Dolcetti R, Trovo' M. Local high-dose radiotherapy induces systemic immunomodulating effects of potential therapeutic relevance in oligometastatic breast cancer. Front Immunol 2017;8:1476. https://doi.org/10.3389/fimmu.2017.01476.

[53] Coburn S, Bray F, Sherman M, Trabert B. International patterns and trends in ovarian cancer incidence, overall and by histologic subtype. Int J Cancer 2017;140(11):2451-60.

[54] Jacobs IJ, Menon U. Progress and challenges in screening for early detection of ovarian cancer. Mol Cell Proteomics 2004;3(4):355-66.

[55] Momenimovahed Z, Tiznobaik A, Taheri S, Salehiniya H. Ovarian cancer in the world: epidemiology and risk factors. Int J Womens Health 2019;11:287-99.

[56] Lindsey AT, Trabert B, DeSantis CE, Miller KD, Samimi G, Runowicz CD, Gaudet MM, Ahmedin Jemal DVM, Siegel RL. Ovarian cancer statistics, 2018. CA Cancer J Clin 2018;68:284-96.

[57] Reid BM, Permuth JB, Sellers TA. Epidemiology of ovarian cancer: a review. Cancer Biol Med 2017;14(1). https://doi.org/10.20892/j.issn.2095-3941.2016.0084.

[58] Prat J. Ovarian carcinomas: five distinct diseases with different origins, genetic alterations, and clinicopathological features. Virchows Arch 2012;460(3):237-49.

[59] Gadducci A, Guarneri V, Alessandro Peccatori F, Ronzino G, Scandurra G, Zamagni C, Zola P, Salutari V. Current strategies for the targeted treatment of high-grade serous epithelial ovarian cancer and relevance of BRCA mutational status. J Ovarian Res 2019;12:9. https://doi.org/10.1186/s13048-019-0484-6.

[60] Bell DA. Origins and molecular pathology of ovarian cancer. Mod Pathol 2005;18(S2):S19. https://doi.org/10.1038/modpathol.3800306.

[61] Chan JK, Loizzi V, Lin YG, et al. IV invasive epithelial ovarian carcinoma in younger versus older women: what prognostic factors are important? Obstet Gynecol 2003;102(1):156-61.

[62] Jordan SJ, Green AC, Nagle CM, et al. Beyond parity: association of ovarian cancer with length of gestation and offspring characteristics. Am J Epidemiol 2009;170(5):607-14.

[63] Risch HA, Howe GR. Pelvic inflammatory disease and the risk of epithelial ovarian cancer. Cancer Epidemiol Biomarkers Prev 1995;4(5):447-51.

[64] Kazerouni N, Greene MH, Lacey Jr. JV, Mink PJ, Schairer C. Family history of breast cancer as a risk factor for ovarian cancer in a prospective study. Cancer 2006;107(5):1075-83.

[65] Bandera EV, Lee VS, Qin B, Rodriguez-Rodriguez L, Powell CB, Kushi LH. Impact of body mass index on ovarian cancer survival varies by stage. Br J Cancer 2017;117(2):282-9.

[66] Jelovac D, Armstrong DK. Recent progress in the diagnosis and treatment of ovarian cancer. CA Cancer J Clin 2011;61(3):183-203.

[67] Associazione Italiana di Oncologia Medica (AIOM). Linee guida AIOM: tumoridell'ovaio. Edizione(2017) Available from: http://www.aiom.it/[Accessed 22 September 2019].

[68] Du Bois A, Vergote I, Ferron G, Reuss A, Meier W, Greggi S, et al. Randomized controlled phase III study evaluating the impact of secondary cytoreductive surgery in recurrent ovarian cancer: AGO DESKTOP III/ENGOT ov20. J Clin Oncol 2017;35(suppl) Abstract 5501.

[69] van Driel WJ, Koole SN, Sikorska K, Schagen van Leeuwen JH, Schreuder HWR, Hermans RHM, et al. Hyperthermic intraperitoneal chemotherapy in ovarian cancer. N Engl J Med 2018;378(3): 230-40.

[70] May T, Comeau R, Sun P, Kotsopoulos J, Narod SA, Rosen B, et al. A comparison of survival outcomes in advanced serous ovarian cancer patients treated with primary debulking surgery versus neoadjuvant chemotherapy. Int J Gynecol Cancer 2017;27(4):668-74.

[71] Perren TJ, Swart AM, Pfisterer J, Ledermann JA, Pujade-Lauraine E, Kristensen G, et al. A phase 3 trial of bevacizumab in ovarian cancer. N Engl J Med 2011;365(26): 2484-96.

[72] Burger RA, Brady MF, Bookman MA, Fleming GF, Monk BJ, Huang H, et al. Incorporation of bevacizumab in the primary treatment of ovarian cancer. N Engl J Med 2011;365(26):2473-83.

[73] Aghajanian C, Blank SV, Goff BA, Judson PL, Teneriello MG, Husain A, et al. OCEANS: a randomized, double-blind, placebo-controlled phase III trial of chemotherapy with or without bevacizumab in patients with platinumsensitive recurrent epithelial ovarian, primary peritoneal, or fallopian tube cancer. J Clin Oncol 2012;30(17):2039-45.

[74] Kaelin Jr. WG. The concept of synthetic lethality in the context of anticancer therapy. Nat Rev Can cer 2005;5(9):689-98.

[75] Ledermann J, Harter P, Gourley C, Friedlander M, Vergote I, Rustin G, et al. Olaparib maintenance therapy in patients with platinum-sensitive relapsed serous ovarian cancer: a preplanned retrospective analysis of outcomes by BRCA status in a randomised phase 2 trial. Lancet Oncol 2014; 15(8):852-61.

[76] Mirza MR, Monk BJ, Herrstedt J, Oza AM, Mahner S, Redondo A, et al. Niraparib maintenance therapy in platinum-sensitive, recurrent ovarian cancer. N Engl J Med 2016;375(22):2154-64.

[77] Coleman RL, Oza AM, Lorusso D, Aghajanian C, Oaknin A, Dean A, et al. Rucaparib maintenance treatment for recurrent ovarian carcinoma after response to platinum therapy

(ARIEL3): a randomised, double-blind, placebo-controlled, phase 3 trial. Lancet 2017; 390(10106):1949-61.

[78] Kim S, Han Y, Kim SI, Kim HS, Kim SJ, Song YS. Tumor evolution and chemoresistance in ovarian cancer. NPJ Precis Oncol 2018;2:20. https://doi.org/10.1038/s41698-018-0063-0.

[79] Chan JK, Brady MF, Penson RT, Huang H, Birrer MJ, Walker JL, et al. Weekly vs. every-3-week paclitaxel and carboplatin for ovarian cancer. N Engl J Med 2016;374(8): 738-48.

[80] Katsumata N, Yasuda M, Takahashi F, Isonishi S, Jobo T, Aoki D, et al. Dosedense paclitaxel once a week in combination with carboplatin every 3 weeks for advanced ovarian cancer: a phase 3, openlabel, randomised controlled trial. Lancet 2009; 374 (9698): 1331-8.

[81] Rustin GJ, van der Burg ME, Griffin CL, Guthrie D, Lamont A, Jayson GC, et al. Early versus delayed treatment of relapsed ovarian cancer (MRC OV05/EORTC 55955): a randomised trial. Lancet 2010;376(9747):1155-63.

[82] Poveda A, Vergote I, Tjulandin S, Kong B, Roy M, Chan S, et al. Trabectedin plus pegylated liposomal doxorubicin in relapsed ovarian cancer: outcomes in the partially platinum-sensitive (platinumfree interval 6-12 months) subpopulation of OVA-301 phase Ⅲ randomized trial. Ann Oncol 2011; 22(1):39-48.

[83] el-Deiry WS. Role of oncogenes in resistance and killing by cancer therapeutic agents. Curr Opin Oncol 1997;9:79-87.

[84] Swanton C. Intratumor heterogeneity: evolution through space and time. Cancer Res 2012;72: 4875-82.

[85] Gottesman MM, Fojo T, Bates SE. Multidrug resistance in cancer: role of ATP-dependent transporters. Nat Rev Cancer 2002;2:48-58.

[86] He X, Ee PL, Coon JS, Beck WT. Alternative splicing of the multidrug resistance protein 1/ATP binding cassette transporter subfamily gene in ovarian cancer creates functional splice variants and is associated with increased expression of the splicing factors PTB and SRp20. Clin Cancer Res 2004;10:4652-60.

[87] Black SM, Beggs JD, Hayes JD, Murarratsu M, Sakai M, Wolfe CR. Expression of human glutathione S-transferase in S. cerevisiae confers resistance to the anticancer drugs adriamycin and chlorambucil. Biochem J 1990;268:309-15.

[88] Cherian MG, Jayasurya A, Bay BH. Metallothioneins in human tumors and potential roles in carcinogenesis. Mutat Res 2003;533:201-9.

[89] Kellner U, Sehested M, Jensen P, et al. Culprit and victim-DNA topoisomerase Ⅱ. Lancet Oncol 2002;3:235-43.

[90] Masuda H, Tanaka T, Matsuda H, Kusaba I. Increased removal of DNA-bound platinum in a human ovarian cancer cell line resistant to cis-diamminedichloroplatinum (Ⅱ). Cancer

Res 1990;50:1863-6.

[91] Zhen W, Link CJ, O'Connor Jr. PM, et al. Increased gene specific repair of cisplatininterstrand crosslinks in cisplatinresistanthuman ovarian cancer cell lines. Mol Biol Cell 1992;12:3689-98.

[92] Ferry KV, Hamilton TC, Johnson SW. Increased nucleotide excision repair in cisplatin resistant ovarian cancer cells. Biochem Pharmacol 2000;60:1305-13.

[93] Mansouri A, Zhang Q, Ridgway LD, Tian L, Claret FX. Cisplatin resistance in an ovarian carcinoma is associated with a defect in programmed cell death control through XIAP regulation. Oncol Res 2003;13:399-404.

[94] Fraser M, Leung B, Jahani-Asl A, Yan X, Thompson WE, Tsang BK. Chemoresistance in human ovarian cancer: the role of apoptotic regulators. Reprod Biol Endocrinol 2003;1:66.

[95] Binkhathlan Z, Lavasanifar A. P-glycoprotein inhibition as a therapeutic approach for overcoming multidrug resistance in cancer: current status and future perspectives. Curr Cancer Drug Targets 2013;13:326-46.

[96] Mi YJ, Liang YJ, Huang HB, Zhao HY, Wu CP, Wang F, Tao LY, Zhang CZ, Dai CL, Tiwari AK, et al. Apatinib (YN968D1) reverses multidrug resistance by inhibiting the efflux function of multiple ATP-binding cassette transporters. Cancer Res 2010;70:7981-91.

[97] Chung FS, Santiago JS, De Jesus MFM, Trinidad CV, See MFE. Disrupting P-glycoprotein function in clinical settings: what can we learn from the fundamental aspects of this transporter? Am J Cancer Res 2016;6:1583-98.

[98] Yang X, Iyer AK, Singh A, Milane L, Choy E, Hornicek FJ, Amiji MM, Duan Z. Cluster of differentiation 44 targeted hyaluronic acid based nanoparticles for MDR1 siRNA delivery to overcome drug resistance in ovarian cancer. Pharm Res 2015;32:2097-109.

[99] Davidson B, Tropé CG, Reich R. Epithelial-mesenchymal transition in ovarian carcinoma. Front Oncol 2012;2:33.

[100] Tomkinson H, Kemp J, Oliver S, Swaisland H, Taboada M, Morris T. Pharmacokinetics and tolerability of zibotentan (ZD4054) in subjects with hepatic or renal impairment: two open-label comparative studies. BMC Clin Pharmacol 2011;11:3.

[101] Selvakumaran M, Pisarcik DA, Bao R, Yeung AT, Hamilton TC. Enhanced cisplatin cytotoxicity by disturbing the nucleotide excision repair pathway in ovarian cancer cell lines. Cancer Res 2003;63:1311-6.

[102] Leijen S, Beijnen JH, Schellens JHM. Abrogation of the G2 checkpoint by inhibition of Wee-1 kinase results in sensitization of p53-deficient tumor cells to DNA-damaging agents. Curr Clin Pharmacol 2010;5:186-91.

[103] Pujade-Lauraine E, Hilpert F, Weber B, Reuss A, Poveda A, Kristensen G, Sorio R, Vergote I, Witteveen P, Bamias A, et al. Bevacizumab combined with chemotherapy for platinum-resistant recurrent ovarian cancer: the AURELIA open-label randomized phase

Ⅲ trial. J Clin Oncol 2014;32:1302-8.

[104] Monk BJ, Poveda A, Vergote I, Raspagliesi F, Fujiwara K, Bae DS, Oaknin A, Ray-Coquard I, Provencher DM, Karlan BY, et al. Anti-angiopoietin therapy with trebananib for recurrent ovarian cancer (TRINOVA-1): a randomised, multicentre, double-blind, placebo-controlled phase 3 trial. Lancet Oncol 2015;15:799-808.

[105] Issaeva N, Thomas HD, Djurenovic T, Jaspers JE, Stoimenov I, Kyle S, Pedley N, Gottipati P, Zur R, Sleeth K, et al. 6-thioguanine selectively kills BRCA2-defective tumors and overcomes PARP inhib itor resistance. Cancer Res 2010;70:6268-76.

[106] Buchbinder EI, Desai A. CTLA-4 and PD-1 pathways: similarities, differences, and implications of their inhibition. Am J Clin Oncol 2016;39:98-106.

[107] Aust S, Felix S, Auer K, Bachmayr-Heyda A, Kenner L, Dekan S, Meier SM, Gerner C, Grimm C, Pils D. Absence of PD-L1 on tumor cells is associated with reduced MHC Ⅰ expression and PD-L1 expression increases in recurrent serous ovarian cancer. Sci Rep 2017;7:42929.

[108] Cancer. n. d. Available from: www. cancer. org/cancer/cancer-basics/what-is-cancer. html

[109] Cancer. n. d. Available from: www. cancer. org/cancer/cervical-cancer/causes-risks-prevention/prevention. html

[110] Cancer. n. d. Available from: www. cancer. org/cancer/cervical-cancer/prevention-and-early detection. html

[111] Kamura T, Ushijima K. Chemotherapy for advanced or recurrent cervical cancer. Taiwan J Obstet Gynecol 2013;52:161-4.

[112] Bahar E, Kim J, Yoon H. Chemotherapy resistance explained through endoplasmic reticulum stressdependent signaling. Cancer 2019; 11: https://doi. org/10. 3390/cancers11030338.

[113] Norouzi-Barough L, Sarookhani MR, Sharifi M, Moghbelinejad S, Jangjoo S, Salehi R. Molecular mechanisms of drug resistance in ovarian cancer. J Cell Physiol 2018;233:4546-62.

[114] Hait WN, Choudhury S, Srimatkandada S, Murren JR. Sensitivity of K562 human chronic myelogenous leukemia blast cells transfected with a human multidrug resistance cDNA to cytotoxic drugs and differentiating agents. J Clin Investig 1993;91:2207-15.

[115] Hoffmeyer S, Burk O, von Richter O, Arnold HP, Brockmoller J, Johne A, Cascorbi I, Gerloff T, Roots I, Eichelbaum M. Functional polymorphisms of the human multidrug-resistance gene: multiple sequence variations and correlation of one allele with P-glycoprotein expression and activity in vivo. Proc Natl Acad Sci U S A 2000;97:3473-8.

[116] Cumming RC, Lightfoot J, Beard K, Youssoufian H, O'Brien PJ, Buchwald M. Fanconianemia group C protein prevents apoptosis in hematopoietic cells through redox regulation of GSTP1. Nat Med 2001;7:814-20.

[117] Dufey E, Sepulveda D, Rojas-Rivera D, Hetz C. Cellular mechanisms of endoplasmic reticulum stress signaling in health and disease. 1. An overview. Am J Physiol Cell Physiol 2014;307:C582-94.

[118] Wang M, Kaufman RJ. The impact of the endoplasmic reticulum protein-folding environment on cancer development. Nat Rev Cancer 2014;14:581-97.

[119] Zhu H, Luo H, Zhang W, Shen Z, Hu X, Zhu X. Molecular mechanisms of cisplatin resistance in cervical cancer. Drug Des Devel Ther 2016;10:1885.

[120] Hamed AR, Abdel-Azim SN, Shams AK, Hammouda MF. Targeting multidrug resistance in cancer by natural chemosensitizers. Bull Natl Res Cent 2019;43: https://doi.org/10.1186/s42269-019-0043-8.

[121] De Sauza R, Zahedi P, Badame MR, Allen C, Piquette-Miller M. Chemotherapy dosing schedule influences drug resistance development in ovarian cancer. Mol Cancer Ther 2011;10:1289-99.

第 4 章
女性癌症的流行病学

Saritha Vara，Manoj Kumar Karnena，Bhavya Kavitha Dwarapureddi

Department of Environmental Science, GITAM Institute of Science, GITAM (Deemed to be University), Visakhapatnam, Andhra Pradesh, India

摘要

有关女性癌症流行病学的文献数量很少。本章尝试总结女性 4 种癌症（子宫体癌、卵巢癌、宫颈癌和乳腺癌）的现实负担、发展趋势和风险因素，而这 4 种癌症占女性癌症的 60% 以上。尽管低收入和中等收入国家的女性癌症发病率较低，癌症死亡人数却普遍更多。通过认识本章讨论的风险因素，可以大幅度减轻该疾病负担。

关键词

流行病学，乳腺癌，宫颈癌，卵巢癌，子宫体癌

缩略词

BMI	体重指数
DCIS	导管原位癌
ER	雌激素受体
ERT	雌激素替代疗法
HIV	人类免疫缺陷病毒
HPV	人乳头状瘤病毒
PCOS	多囊卵巢综合征

一、概述

流行病学是一门研究不同人群中疾病发生率及其病因的学科。其重要性在于流行病学信息能够帮助人们排查疾病并评估预防措施，并可指导已发病患者的治疗。与病理学和临床研究结果类似，流行病学是疾病基本描述的重要组成部分。流行病学作为一门科学学科，起源于 17 世纪，它在收集、分析和解释人口数据方面具有独特的方法。到了 18 世纪，人们开始进行人口比较学的研究，从那时起，建立并完善了人口研究组织概念和方法，并提出了多种假说。从根本上讲，流行病学涉

及多学科知识,包括社会学、生物学、统计学和其他领域[1],这构成了目前流行病学的真正核心。

癌症流行病学研究特定人群中恶性疾病的分布、决定因素和发病率[2]。其主要目的是描述致病因素,以制订有效的预防策略。临床医师可以从流行病学评估中获得癌症风险的量化数据,为高风险人群的筛查方式提供依据,并确定预防干预措施的有效性。癌症流行病学研究包括3种类型:描述性、分析性和临床性。描述性流行病学着重分析特定人群中的疾病趋势和发病率,分析性流行病学则主要涉及识别疾病发展的原因和潜在的疾病相关风险。临床流行病学则关注于制订筛查计划,评估预防策略对整体健康结果的影响[3]。本章探讨了女性数种最常见癌症的流行病学因素,包括乳腺癌、宫颈癌、卵巢癌和子宫体癌。

二、乳腺癌

乳腺癌是全球女性中最致命的恶性肿瘤之一。据美国癌症协会预测,2019年新发浸润性乳腺癌 268 600 例,新发导管原位癌(ductal carcinoma in situ,DCIS) 48 100 例。此外,预计将有 41 760 名女性死于乳腺癌。据估计,约 13% 的女性将被诊断出浸润性乳腺癌(即几乎每 8 名女性中就有 1 人),大约 3% 的女性将死于乳腺癌(即每 39 名女性中有 1 人),这些数据凸显了乳腺癌的严重威胁[4]。乳腺癌的这种重压要求人们持续关注对乳腺癌的精确理解,包括其流行病学特征。

(一)发病率

1980—1990 年,DCIS 和浸润性乳腺癌的发病率急剧上升,尤其是在 50 岁及以上的女性中。这一增长趋势主要是因为乳腺 X 线检查筛查的普及率提高,从 1987 年的 29% 到 2000 年的 70%[5]。1980—2008 年,50 岁及以上女性中 DCIS 的发病率增加了 11 倍以上。1999—2004 年,浸润性乳腺癌的发病率则出现了 13% 的显著下降,这主要归因于更年期激素摄入的减少及自 2000 年以来乳腺 X 线检查筛查率的小幅下降[6-8]。在过去十年(2012—2016 年)间,DCIS 的发病率每年下降 2.1%[9],而浸润性乳腺癌的发病率每年增加 0.3%。此外,自 20 世纪 90 年代中期以来,浸润性乳腺癌的发病率一直呈现上升趋势[10]。一些研究还指出,近期发病率的增加与体重指数(body mass index,BMI)上升和平均分娩次数减少有关[11]。

(二)年龄

乳腺癌的发病率和死亡率随年龄增长而升高,通常在 70 岁时达到峰值。这是由于随着年龄的增长,雌激素受体(estrogen receptors,ER)数量增多,因此绝经后女性更有可能罹患乳腺癌[12]。然而,80 岁及以上的女性乳腺癌发病率较低,这是因为筛查率低,以及 X 线诊断或检测不全面[12]。2012—2016 年,女性乳腺癌诊断的中位年龄是 62 岁[10]。尽管如此,年轻女性患者所患乳腺癌往往体积较大、淋巴结阳性率高、分期较晚且生存率较低[13]。

(三)种族

多种因素可能导致乳腺癌患者种族间死亡率的差异,包括乳腺 X 线检查的可及性、社会经济因素、是否及时接受治疗及生物学因素。据报道,黑人女性的乳腺癌死亡率高于白人女性,这通常归因于 ER 阴性肿瘤[14]。其他族裔/种族群体乳腺癌的发病率和死亡率通常较低[4]。在绝经前期,三阴性乳腺癌(ER 阴性、HER2 阴性和孕激素阴性)在黑人女性中比白人女性更常见。HR 阳性/HER2 阴性乳腺癌是所有种族女性中最常见的亚型。此外,最近的研究表明,社会经济地位已经取代种族/民族成为不良预后的重要预测因素[15]。

(四)诊断

浸润性乳腺癌的预后很大程度上取决于诊断时的分期。虽然大多数乳腺癌在诊断时处于局部浸润阶段,但这种趋势在不同种族间有所差异。大约 64% 的患者在初次诊断时处于原位分期,27% 患者处于局部性分期,6% 患者发生了远处转移。2012—2016 年,处于原位分期阶段乳腺癌的发病率呈现每年增长 1.1% 的趋势,早期诊断率则每年下降 0.8%[16]。

(五)母乳喂养

众多研究表明,母乳喂养与总体乳腺癌风险降低呈正相关,也就是说延长哺乳期将降低乳腺癌的风险。母乳喂养通过抑制排卵来减少女性一生中的雌激素暴露,从而降低癌症风险[17]。此外,在哺乳期间,相对于血清,乳汁中的雌激素水平较低[18]。母乳喂养可能会导致乳腺上皮细胞终止分化,使得这些细胞在分裂过程中更不容易发生基因突变,或更不容易受致癌物的影响[19]。来自 30 个国家的 47 项研究显示,母乳喂养持续 12 个月可以降低乳腺癌风险 4%[20]。特别是对于三阴性乳腺癌,这种保护作用可能更为显著,甚至可能仅限于这种类型的乳腺癌[21-23]。

(六)激素疗法

含有雌激素和孕激素的绝经后激素替代疗法会增加 HR 阳性乳腺癌的风险,这种风险与使用这些激素的时间成正比[20,24-27]。即使停止使用绝经后激素替代疗法,乳腺癌的风险也不会完全消除[28]。女性健康计划研究[29]发现,女性如果平均使用雌激素单药 6 年,乳腺癌风险会降低 25%,这与一些观察性研究报告的结果相矛盾,这些观察性研究报告认为使用雌激素治疗的女性,特别是体重较轻和绝经后早期就开始使用雌激素治疗的女性,乳腺癌风险略有增加[30,31]。自 2002 年以来,美国、欧洲和加拿大等国人群在减少使用激素后乳腺癌发病率下降了 5%~10%[32]。

(七)使用避孕激素

使用外源性激素,如雌激素和孕激素的避孕药物,与乳腺癌风险轻度增加有关。当前使用口服避孕药的女性与从未使用避孕药的女性相比,患癌风险增加高达 24%[33,34]。停止使用避孕药后,患乳腺癌风险下降,并且停药 10 年后与未服用过避孕药的女性风险相似[35]。

(八)饮食因素

多项研究检验了饮食与乳腺癌之间的关系,但结果各异。尽管近期的荟萃分析未发现乳腺癌与膳食脂肪有关,但发现大豆摄入量与降低乳腺癌风险有关,特别是在摄入大豆较多的亚洲女性中。但这种关联在西方人群中并不存在[36,37]。虽然有限,但越来越多的证据表明,摄入更多的水果和蔬菜有助于降低 HR 阴性乳腺癌的风险[38,39]。在摄入富含钙质食物的饮食情况下也发现了类似的趋势[40]。Dong 和 Qin 对前瞻性研究进行的荟萃分析显示,血浆中大豆异黄酮的浓度与乳腺癌的患癌风险呈负相关。

(九)个体体重

绝经后体重增加与 HR 阳性乳腺癌风险有关,据研究,这种风险可能高达 2 倍[41]。即使在正常 BMI 范围内,较高的体脂含量也与绝经后乳腺癌的发病风险增加有关[42]。这种风险增加归因于脂肪组织在女性绝经后成为雌激素的主要来源,以及超重女性体内往往有更高水平的胰岛素等其他相关因素[43]。一些研究表明,成年期和绝经后减肥可降低罹患乳腺癌的风险;另一些研究则发现,体重过重可防止绝经前乳腺癌的发生[44]。一项大型荟萃分析发现,与正常体重女性相比,40~49 岁的超重女性和肥胖女性的乳腺癌风险分别降低 14% 和 26%[45]。

(十)饮酒

有多项确定性研究将女性饮酒与乳腺癌风险联系起来。每天喝一杯酒的女性患癌风险增加 7%~10%,每天喝 2~3 杯酒的风险则增加 20%[46,47]。这些研究的剂量-反应关系曲线呈线性。目前还不太明确的一种假设是,饮酒可能通过提高雌激素和其他激素水平来间接增加患病风险。

(十一) 体力活动

高水平的体力活动与乳腺癌风险呈负相关[46-48]。可能的生物学机制包括体力活动对身体成分、胰岛素抵抗、激素水平、全身炎症和能量平衡的影响[51]*。

此外，遗传因素[52,53]、辐射暴露[54,55]、环境和职业致癌物[56-58]，以及倒班工作[59-61]等其他流行病学因素也表现出与乳腺癌风险呈正相关。

三、宫颈癌

宫颈癌是全球女性中第四常见的癌症，在发展中国家尤为普遍，占女性所有癌症的12%，多发现于中年女性[62,63]。如果早期诊断，5年生存率接近96%。作为病毒致癌的模型，宫颈癌也归因于持续感染致癌型人乳头状瘤病毒（human papillomavirus, HPV）亚型，以及一些其他因素，主要包括过多性伴侣数、过早性生活、长期使用口服避孕药、吸烟、生育次数多、饮食习惯和与其他性传播疾病，如沙眼衣原体和人类免疫缺陷病毒（human immunodeficiency virus, HIV）的共感染[64-67]等。宫颈癌的主要症状包括异常阴道分泌物、体重减轻、严重的盆腔疼痛和厌食[68]。

(一) 人乳头状瘤病毒

目前已有研究明确，导致癌前病变和癌性病变的主要原因是感染致癌型HPV亚型（HPV-16和HPV-18），这些亚型是宫颈癌发病机制中的重要病原体[69,70]。性接触作为感染的传播方式，会导致鳞状上皮内病变，免疫干预6~12个月后，大部分病变会消失，一小部分持续存在的病变可能会导致癌症[71]。一项荟萃分析的结果显示，25岁及以下女性中HPV的感染率最高，这主要与性行为差异有关[72,73]。HPV参与致癌的主要机制是E6和E7病毒癌蛋白活性干扰P53和视网膜母细胞瘤抑制基因的表达。此外，它也与宿主和病毒DNA的变化有关，这些变化导致DNA甲基化，从而影响调控遗传完整性、细胞凋亡、细胞黏附、细胞控制和免疫反应等主要细胞通路[74]。分子水平的流行病学研究表明，HPV感染合并吸烟的患者宫颈黏膜中存在较低剂量的亚硝胺，可能会加快致癌过程[75]。

(二) 人类免疫缺陷病毒

据报道，HIV阳性女性更容易感染HPV[76,77]。HIV阳性女性中常发现

---

*译者注：原书文献[49]和[50]在文内无标引。

HPV-16 或 HPV-18 持续感染[78,79]。此外,致癌性 HPV-16 和 HIV 感染之间的协同作用可导致免疫系统受损,使性生活活跃女性更易持续感染 HPV16[80]。

(三)沙眼衣原体

研究发现,既往感染沙眼衣原体或同时感染 HPV 与宫颈鳞状细胞癌风险增加有关[81]。7 个国家的病例对照研究发现沙眼衣原体血清抗体的存在增强宿主对 HPV 的易感性,这种影响可以使鳞状细胞癌的发病率增加 1.8 倍。沙眼衣原体的慢性感染会诱发炎症反应,该反应释放活性氧,导致 DNA 受损,增加了 HPV 相关的癌变风险。此外,感染沙眼衣原体的女性清除人乳头状瘤病毒感染的能力较弱[82]。抑制细胞凋亡可能导致癌基因 $E6/E7$ 过度表达,造成细胞畸形[83]。

(四)生殖趋势

已有流行病学提供了证据,支持宫颈浸润性癌和多次分娩之间的关联性[84,85],而母亲的初孕年龄与宫颈癌发生成反比[86]。目前,人们已发现分娩是 CIN3 的预测因子,尤其是在 HPV 感染风险较高的女性中[87]。其影响宫颈癌风险的可能生物学机制有多个假说,包括妊娠期或分娩时的免疫力、激素和营养状况的变化,以及宫颈创伤。

(五)性行为

多性伴侣性行为与宫颈癌发病风险增高有关[88,89],这归因于 HPV 感染风险增加。此外,初次性行为年龄较小也会增加宫颈癌的患病风险。使用避孕套对阴道 HPV 感染和宫颈上皮内瘤变的发生都有保护作用[90,91]。

(六)口服避孕药

近期和正在使用口服避孕药与宫颈癌患病风险升高有关[84,92],延长避孕药使用时间也会增加宫颈癌的患癌风险[93]。

(七)肥胖

宫颈腺癌的发生与超重相关的激素风险因素有关[94-96]。据报道,肥胖和超重女性患宫颈癌的概率增加了 2 倍。肥胖,尤其是绝经后的肥胖,是性激素水平升高的标志,这是因为外周脂肪组织具有将雄激素转化为雌激素的能力[94]。

(八)饮食

据了解,某些食物和营养素具有防止宫颈癌进展的潜力。研究表明,摄入视黄醇、类胡萝卜素、叶酸、维生素 C 和维生素 E、水果和蔬菜可减少宫颈癌的患病风险[97]。Tomita 等[98]的研究表明,绿色蔬菜和黄色水果的营养素摄入量越多,α-和γ-生育酚的浓度越高,宫颈癌的发病率降低 50%。Ghosh 等[99]报道了维生素 E、维生素 C、维生素 A、叶酸和番茄红素摄入量的增加与宫颈癌患病风险降低之间的显著相关性。潜在的生物机制包括维生素 C 和维生素 E 发挥重要作用,它们增强黏膜对感染的反应,从而保护黏膜免受自由基和氧化剂的侵害。这些维生素还能抑制吸烟导致的 DNA 加合物的形成。

(九)吸烟

吸烟史与宫颈癌之间的关系已经得到证实[84,100]。对于已经戒烟的女性,特别是戒烟时间超过 10 年的女性,她们的宫颈癌风险降低了 50%。吸烟女性患宫颈癌风险增加的机制之一是烟草代谢产物会诱发免疫抑制[101],而其中的尼古丁及其代谢物可导致鳞状细胞 DNA 损伤。被动吸烟,即吸入他人吸烟产生的二手烟,也会增加女性患宫颈癌的风险[102]。一些研究提出,在感染 HPV-16 的吸烟女性中,宫颈癌的风险会协同增加[75]。

四、卵巢癌

卵巢癌的发病率在宫颈癌和子宫体癌之后,排名第三[103],占所有女性癌症的 3.4%,占女性癌症死亡人数的 4.4%[103,104]。尽管其患病率低于乳腺癌,致死率却高出乳腺癌 3 倍[105],预计到 2040 年,卵巢癌的死亡率将显著增加。高死亡率通常与卵巢癌的无症状特性和隐匿性生长有关,加之缺乏有效的筛查手段和症状出现的延迟性,这些因素共同导致卵巢癌被称为"沉默杀手"。由于卵巢上皮与乳腺导管上皮含有相同的细胞膜成分,卵巢癌的风险因素在很多方面与乳腺癌的风险因素相似。

(一)年龄

上皮性卵巢癌是一种与年龄相关的绝经后疾病[106],在 60 岁以上的女性中更为多见[107]。由于与高龄相关,这种疾病更严重,生存率更低[108,109]。年龄与卵巢癌之间的关系尚不确定。

(二)遗传和家族史

卵巢癌的风险在于较强的家族史,尤其是家族中有卵巢癌、乳腺癌、子宫内膜癌或结直肠癌患者,其患病风险会增加 3~5 倍,多导致早期发病和双侧发病。大约 1/5 的卵巢癌归因于肿瘤抑制基因突变[110],而 65%～85% 是由于 BRCA 基因的胚系突变[111]。另一种导致卵巢癌的遗传性疾病是遗传性非息肉病性结直肠癌,也称为林奇综合征。

与林奇综合征相关的卵巢癌通常为非黏液性,近 84% 的病例诊断于 Ⅰ 期或 Ⅱ 期[112]。林奇综合征的发生是 4 个错配修复基因(MHL1、MSH2/6 和 PMS2)中的 1 个或多个发生遗传性突变,其中 MSH2 和 MLH1 是最常见的突变[113]。

(三) 生育药物

部分病例对照研究已经探讨了生育药物与卵巢癌之间的关系。例如,枸橼酸氯米芬等生育药物会刺激垂体分泌黄体生成素(luteinizing hormone,LH)和卵泡刺激素(follicle-stimulating hormone,FSH),从而有助于刺激排卵。然而,关于使用这些药物是否真的会增加卵巢癌风险的问题,目前仍存在争议,因为很难区分风险增加是由于使用生育药物还是其他因素(如不孕)相关潜在病理机制引起[114]。

(四) 口服避孕药

多项研究已经发现,使用口服避孕药与降低多种类型的卵巢癌风险有关[115-117]。然而,要全面理解口服避孕药的保护作用,需要结合使用时长、开始使用年龄和持续使用时间[115,118],因为一旦停止服用口服避孕药,其提供的保护作用可能会降低[119]。

(五) 激素替代疗法

据报道,使用雌激素替代疗法(estrogen replacement therapy,ERT)等外源性激素会增加 20% 的患病风险[120]。研究表明,如果使用雌激素疗法 10 年或更长时间,会进一步增加患病风险[121]。从生物学角度来看,卵巢表面上皮的细胞膜受体对雌激素产生反应。ERT 与其他细胞活动一起刺激细胞增殖,可能会通过调节 ER 导致癌变过程[122]。Mørch 等[123]认为,无论 ERT 的使用时间长短、剂量大小、制剂类型和使用方法,雌激素疗法都与卵巢癌风险的增加有关。

(六) 饮食

据报道,日间食用鱼类与卵巢癌风险之间呈正相关,每日摄入牛奶与卵巢癌风险则呈负相关[124,125]。植物雌激素的保护作用与卵巢癌风险相关,说明以植物为基础的饮食在减少与激素相关癌症方面发挥重要作用[126,127]。研究发现,血浆维生素 D 浓度增加卵巢癌患病风险降低,这与钙和乳糖摄入量对卵巢癌的影响相似[124]。

(七)肥胖

肥胖与卵巢癌风险的直接相关性主要归因于它与中央型肥胖症的关联,这种肥胖类型表明在毗邻组织中雄激素向雌激素的转化增加[128,129]。Anderson 等[130]报道了腰臀比的增加与乳腺癌风险增高的关系。Beehler 等[131]将绝经、肥胖和卵巢癌风险联系起来。流行病学的研究结果表明,长期的肥胖状态增加芳香化酶催化的雌激素生物合成,从而增加了卵巢癌的发生风险。

五、子宫体癌

子宫体癌约占所有女性特异性癌的 4.4%,其中 2.4%的患者可导致死亡[132]。在子宫体癌中,近 90%的患者属于子宫内膜癌,这种癌症起源于上皮组织;其余为间叶组织癌,起源于子宫肌层(即子宫内膜基质)。全球子宫体癌的发病模式与乳腺癌和卵巢癌存在相似性,这主要是由于共有风险因素增加了对内外源性雌激素的暴露。自 21 世纪以来,全球子宫体癌患者数急剧增加。报道显示,新发患者数和死亡人数几乎翻了 1 倍[103,133,134]。与此相关的风险因素包括缺乏母乳喂养、晚育、外源性激素摄入、高热量和高脂肪饮食、肥胖、缺乏锻炼及糖尿病等[135]。

(一)年龄

根据报道,大多数确诊患者的年龄为 50~65 岁(即绝经后年龄)[136],表明卵巢癌患病风险与年龄的增长成正比。

(二)生殖趋势

早发月经、无孕史和晚绝经等因素与内膜癌风险显著增加有关,这些因素的相反情况被认为是降低内膜癌风险的保护性因素[136]。之所以认为这些因素与内膜癌风险相关,是因为它们与较低的累积雌激素暴露有关,也符合激素机制在子宫内膜癌发生中的重要作用[137]。

(三)多囊卵巢综合征

据报道,绝经前内膜癌患者中约 30%患有多囊卵巢综合征(polycystic ovary syndrome,PCOS)[138]。患有 PCOS 的女性中,她们患内膜癌的风险是普通人群的 4 倍[139]。这种风险增加的可能机制之一是,在无排卵月经周期中,子宫内膜暴露于未受孕激素抵抗的过量雌激素[140]。

(四)卵巢颗粒细胞瘤

卵巢颗粒细胞瘤很少出现生殖道异常症状,如月经周期不规律、不孕、盆腔痛和子宫病变。尽管这些肿瘤很罕见,只占卵巢恶性肿瘤的2%~5%,但它们产生大量雌激素,增多的雌激素刺激子宫内膜及其他组织中的雌激素受体[141]。

(五)肥胖

肥胖与子宫内膜癌之间的关系已经得到了明确证实[142]。这种关系的生物学机制是肥胖女性的脂肪组织中雄烯二酮芳香化作用增强,导致内源性雌激素水平升高[143]。

(六)糖尿病

患有糖尿病的女性罹患子宫内膜癌的风险增加,2型糖尿病增加2倍,1型糖尿病增加3倍[144]。这种风险增加归因于胰岛素抵抗导致的高胰岛素血症,即血清胰岛素水平的长期升高可能通过与子宫内膜组织中的胰岛素受体结合,刺激子宫内膜上皮细胞增殖[145]。研究发现,2型糖尿病合并肥胖在增加子宫内膜癌风险方面具有协同作用[146]。

(七)激素替代疗法

流行病学研究显示,接受ERT的女性子宫内膜癌风险显著增加。已有趋势显示,患癌风险与使用时间延长直接相关。报道显示,使用雌激素1年以上的女性患子宫内膜癌的风险增加40%。这种风险还与雌激素的使用剂量有关[147]。

(八)体力活动

久坐会促进子宫内膜癌发展,体育锻炼则可能起到保护作用。据报道,体育锻炼多的女性患子宫内膜癌的风险降低了25%[148]。体育锻炼可减少中心脂肪的积累,从而有助于调整内源性雌激素和雄激素的水平,使之达到更有利的平衡状态。

林奇综合征和月经初潮过早也与子宫内膜癌风险增加有关[149,150]。

六、结论

本章目的是强调女性癌症的流行病学特征。可以得出结论,所详述的4种癌症在某些方面具有共性。外源性和内源性激素在女性癌症风险中发挥着重要作用。使用激素替代疗法似乎会增加罹患子宫内膜癌和乳腺癌的风险(表 4-1)。可依据现有的流行病学研究,提出一些可能的预防策略,包括戒烟戒酒、增加水果和蔬菜的摄入,以及接种 HPV 疫苗,这些措施都可能显著减少癌症的发生。因此,本章介绍了女性癌症的相似之处和差异,这将加深人们的认识,从而更好地理解并采取必要的预防措施。

表 4-1　4 种肿瘤常见风险因素

癌症部位	相关风险因素							非常规因素
	年龄	种族	饮食因素	体重/肥胖	生育趋势	饮酒/吸烟	体力活动	
乳腺	√	√	√	√	—	√	√	—
宫颈	—	—	√	√	√	√	—	人乳头状瘤病毒、性行为、沙眼衣原体、人类免疫缺陷病毒
卵巢	√	—	√	√	—	—	—	遗传和家族史
子宫	√	—	—	√	√	—	—	糖尿病、多囊卵巢综合征

参 考 文 献

[1] National Research Council. Epidemiologic studies. In: Analysis of cancer risks in populations near nuclear facilities: phase Ⅰ. USA: National Academies Press; 2012.

[2] Hennekens CH, Buring JE. Epidemiology in medicine. Boston: Little Brown; 198773-98.

[3] Nazario LA, Macheledt JE, Vogel VG. Epidemiology of cancer and prevention strategies. Lung 1995;169:157-400.

[4] American Cancer Society. Breast cancer facts & figures 2019-2020. Atlanta: American Cancer Society, Inc; 2019.

[5] Breen N, Gentleman JF, Schiller JS. Update on mammography trends: comparisons of rates in 2000, 2005, and 2008. Cancer 2011;117(10):2209-18.

[6] Coombs NJ, Cronin KA, Taylor RJ, Freedman AN, Boyages J. The impact of changes in hormone therapy on breast cancer incidence in the US population. Cancer Causes Control 2010;21(1):83-90.

[7] DeSantis C, Howlader N, Cronin KA, Jemal A. Breast cancer incidence rates in US women are no longer declining. Cancer 2011;20(5):733-9.

[8] Ravdin PM, Cronin KA, Howlader N, Berg CD, Chlebowski RT, Feuer EJ,… Berry DA. The decrease in breast-cancer incidence in 2003 in the United States. N Engl J Med 2007;

356(16):1670-4.
[9] SEER * Stat Databases: NAACCR Incidence Data-CiNA Analytic File, 1995-2016, for NHIAv2 Origin and for Expanded Races, Custom File With County, ACS Facts and Figures projection Project(which includes data from CDC's National Program of Cancer Registries (NPCR), CCCR's Provincial and Territorial Registries, and the NCI's Surveillance, Epidemiology and End Results(SEER) Registries), certified by the North American Association of Central Cancer Registries(NAACCR) as meeting high-quality incidence data.
[10] Howlader N, Noone AM, Krapcho M, Miller D, Brest A, Yu M,…Chen HS. SEER cancer statistics review, 1975-2016. Bethesda, MD: National Cancer Institute; 2019.
[11] Pfeiffer RM, Webb-Vargas Y, Wheeler W, Gail MH. Proportion of US trends in breast cancer incidence attributable to long-term changes in risk factor distributions. Cancer 2018; 27(10):1214-22.
[12] Yasui Y, Potter JD. The shape of age-incidence curves of female breast cancer by hormone-receptor status. Cancer Causes Control 1999;10(5):431-7.
[13] Metcalfe KA, Finch A, Poll A, Horsman D, Kim-Sing C, Scott J,… Narod SA. Breast cancer risks in women with a family history of breast or ovarian cancer who have tested negative for a BRCA1 or BRCA2 mutation. Br J Cancer 2009;100(2):421-5.
[14] Dunn BK, Agurs-Collins T, Browne D, Lubet R, Johnson KA. Health disparities in breast cancer: biology meets socioeconomic status. Breast Cancer Res Treat 2010;121(2): 281-92.
[15] Cross T, Racz G. U.S. Patent Application No. 10/025,112.
[16] DeSantis CE, Ma J, Jemal A. Trends in stage at diagnosis for young breast cancer patients in the United States. Breast Cancer Res Treat 2019;173(3):743-7.
[17] Enger SM, Ross RK, Paganini-Hill A, Bernstein L. Breastfeeding experience and breast cancer risk among postmenopausal women. Cancer 1998;7(5):365-9.
[18] Yaghjyan L, Colditz GA. Estrogens in the breast tissue: a systematic review. Cancer Causes Control 2011;22(4):529-40.
[19] Smalley M, Ashworth A. Stem cells and breast cancer: a field in transit. Nat Rev Cancer 2003; 3(11):832-44.
[20] Beral V, Reeves G, Bull D, Green J. Million Women Study Collaborators. Breast cancer risk in relation to the interval between menopause and starting hormone therapy. J Natl Cancer Inst 2011; 103(4):296-305.
[21] Faupel-Badger JM, Arcaro KF, Balkam JJ, Eliassen AH, Hassiotou F, Lebrilla CB,… Watson CJ. Postpartum remodeling, lactation, and breast cancer risk: summary of a National Cancer Institute-sponsored workshop. J Natl Cancer Inst 2013;105(3):166-74.
[22] Islami F, Liu Y, Jemal A, Zhou J, Weiderpass E, Colditz G,… Weiss M. Breastfeeding and breast cancer risk by receptor status—a systematic review and meta-analysis. Ann Oncol 2015;26(12): 2398-407.

[23] Ma H, Ursin G, Xu X, Lee E, Togawa K, Duan L,… Simon MS. Reproductive factors and the risk of triple-negative breast cancer in white women and African-American women: a pooled analysis. Breast Cancer Res 2017;19(1):6.

[24] Chlebowski RT, Manson JE, Anderson GL, Cauley JA, Aragaki AK, Stefanick ML,… Qi L. Estrogen plus progestin and breast cancer incidence and mortality in the Women's Health Initiative Observational Study. J Natl Cancer Inst 2013;105(8):526-35.

[25] Gaudet MM, Gierach GL, Carter BD, Luo J, Milne RL, Weiderpass E,… Wolk A. Pooled analysis of nine cohorts reveals breast cancer risk factors by tumor molecular subtype. Cancer Res 2018; 78(20):6011-21.

[26] Li K, Anderson G, Viallon V, Arveux P, Kvaskoff M, Fournier A,… Chirlaque MD. Risk prediction for estrogen receptor-specific breast cancers in two large prospective cohorts. Breast Cancer Res 2018;20(1):147.

[27] Manson JE, Chlebowski RT, Stefanick ML, Aragaki AK, Rossouw JE, Prentice RL,… Wactawski-Wende J. Menopausal hormone therapy and health outcomes during the intervention and extended poststopping phases of the Women's Health Initiative randomized trials. JAMA 2013;310(13):1353-68.

[28] Chlebowski RT, Rohan TE, Manson JE, Aragaki AK, Kaunitz A, Stefanick ML,… Adams-Campbell LL. Breast cancer after use of estrogen plus progestin and estrogen alone: analyses of data from 2 women's health initiative randomized clinical trials. JAMA Oncol 2015;1(3):296-305.

[29] LaCroix AZ, Chlebowski RT, Manson JE, Aragaki AK, Johnson KC, Martin L,… Howard BV. Health outcomes after stopping conjugated equine estrogens among postmenopausal women with prior hysterectomy: a randomized controlled trial. JAMA 2011;305(13): 1305-14.

[30] Bakken K, Fournier A, Lund E, Waaseth M, Dumeaux V, Clavel-Chapelon F,… Slimani N. Menopausal hormone therapy and breast cancer risk: impact of different treatments. The European Prospective Investigation Into Cancer and Nutrition. Int J Cancer 2011;128(1):144-56.

[31] Calle EE, Feigelson HS, Hildebrand JS, Teras LR, Thun MJ, Rodriguez C. Postmenopausal hormone use and breast cancer associations differ by hormone regimen and histologic subtype. Cancer 2009; 115(5):936-45.

[32] Pelucchi C, Levi F, La Vecchia C. The rise and fall in menopausal hormone therapy and breast cancer incidence. Breast 2010;19(3):198-201.

[33] Bassuk SS, Manson JE. Oral contraceptives and menopausal hormone therapy: relative and attributable risks of cardiovascular disease, cancer, and other health outcomes. Ann Epidemiol 2015; 25(3):193-200.

[34] Mørch LS, Skovlund CW, Hannaford PC, Iversen L, Fielding S, Lidegaard Ø. Contemporary hormonal contraception and the risk of breast cancer. N Engl J Med 2017;377(23):

2228-39.

[35] Westhoff CL, Pike MC. Hormonal contraception and breast cancer. Contraception 2018; 98(3): 171-3.

[36] Cao Y, Hou L, Wang W. Dietary total fat and fatty acids intake, serum fatty acids and risk of breast cancer: a meta-analysis of prospective cohort studies. Int J Cancer 2016;138(8):1894-904.

[37] Chen M, Rao Y, Zheng Y, Wei S, Li Y, Guo T, Yin P. Association between soy isoflavone intake and breast cancer risk for pre-and post-menopausal women: a meta-analysis of epidemiological studies. PLoS One 2014;9(2):1-10.

[38] Bakker MF, Peeters PH, Klaasen VM, Bueno-de-Mesquita HB, Jansen EH, Ros MM,…Rinaldi S. Plasma carotenoids, vitamin C, tocopherols, and retinol and the risk of breast cancer in the European Prospective Investigation into Cancer and Nutrition cohort, 2. Am J Clin Nutr 2016;103(2):454-64.

[39] Farvid MS, Chen WY, Rosner BA, Tamimi RM, Willett WC, Eliassen AH. Fruit and vegetable consumption and breast cancer incidence: repeated measures over 30 years of follow-up. Int J Cancer 2019;144(7):1496-510.

[40] Ogimoto I, Shibata A, Fukuda K. World Cancer Research Fund/American Institute of Cancer Research 1997 recommendations: applicability to digestive tract cancer in Japan. Cancer Causes Control 2000;11(1):9-23.

[41] Jiralerspong S, Goodwin PJ. Obesity and breast cancer prognosis: evidence, challenges, and opportunities. J Clin Oncol 2016;34(35):4203-16.

[42] Iyengar NM, Arthur R, Manson JE, Chlebowski RT, Kroenke CH, Peterson L,…Nassir R. Association of body fat and risk of breast cancer in postmenopausal women with normal body mass index: a secondary analysis of a randomized clinical trial and observational study. JAMA Oncol 2019; 5(2):155-63.

[43] Picon-Ruiz M, Morata-Tarifa C, Valle-Goffin JJ, Friedman ER, Slingerland JM. Obesity and adverse breast cancer risk and outcome: mechanistic insights and strategies for intervention. CA Cancer J Clin 2017;67(5):378-97.

[44] Chlebowski RT, Luo J, Anderson GL, Barrington W, Reding K, Simon MS,…Strickler H. Weight loss and breast cancer incidence in postmenopausal women. Cancer 2019;125(2):205-12.

[45] Nelson HD, Zakher B, Cantor A, Fu R, Griffin J, O'Meara ES,…Mandelblatt JS. Risk factors for breast cancer for women aged 40 to 49 years: a systematic review and meta-analysis. Ann Intern Med 2012;156(9):635-48.

[46] Assi N, Rinaldi S, Viallon V, Dashti SG, Dossus L, Fournier A,…Boeing H. Mediation analysis of the alcohol-postmenopausal breast cancer relationship by sex hormones in the EPIC cohort. Int J Cancer 2020;146(3):759-68.

[47] Jung S, Wang M, Anderson K, Baglietto L, Bergkvist L, Bernstein L,…Falk R. Alcohol

consumption and breast cancer risk by estrogen receptor status: in a pooled analysis of 20 studies. Int J Epidemiol 2016;45(3):916-28.

[48] Kerr J, Anderson C, Lippman SM. Physical activity, sedentary behaviour, diet, and cancer: an update and emerging new evidence. Lancet Oncol 2017;18(8):e457-71.

[49] McTiernan ANNE, Friedenreich CM, Katzmarzyk PT, Powell KE, Macko R, Buchner D,... George SM. Physical activity in cancer prevention and survival: a systematic review. Med Sci Sports Exerc 2019;51(6):1252-61.

[50] Moore SC, Lee IM, Weiderpass E, Campbell PT, Sampson JN, Kitahara CM,... Adami HO. Association of leisure-time physical activity with risk of 26 types of cancer in 1.44 million adults. JAMA Intern Med 2016;176(6):816-25.

[51] Pizot C, Boniol M, Mullie P, Koechlin A, Boniol M, Boyle P, Autier P. Physical activity, hormone replacement therapy and breast cancer risk: a meta-analysis of prospective studies. Eur J Cancer 2016;52:138-54.

[52] Beebe-Dimmer JL, Yee C, Cote ML, Petrucelli N, Palmer N, Bock C,... Simon MS. Familial clustering of breast and prostate cancer and risk of postmenopausal breast cancer in the Women's Health Initiative study. Cancer 2015;121(8):1265-72.

[53] Tung N, Lin NU, Kidd J, Allen BA, Singh N, Wenstrup RJ,... Garber JE. Frequency of germline mutations in 25 cancer susceptibility genes in a sequential series of patients with breast cancer. J Clin Oncol 2016;34(13):1460.

[54] Ehrhardt MJ, Howell CR, Hale K, Baassiri MJ, Rodriguez C, Wilson CL,... Wang Z. Subsequent breast cancer in female childhood cancer survivors in the St Jude Lifetime Cohort Study (SJLIFE). J Clin Oncol 2019;37(19):1647.

[55] Schaapveld M, Aleman BM, van Eggermond AM, Janus CP, Krol AD, van der Maazen RW,... Van Imhoff GW. Second cancer risk up to 40 years after treatment for Hodgkin's lymphoma. N Engl J Med 2015;373(26):2499-511.

[56] Ahern TP, Broe A, Lash TL, Cronin-Fenton DP, Ulrichsen SP, Christiansen PM,... Damkier P. Phthalate exposure and breast cancer incidence: a Danish nationwide cohort study. J Clin Oncol 2019;37(21):1800-9.

[57] Gaudet MM, Deubler EL, Kelly RS, Ryan Diver W, Teras LR, Hodge JM,... Palli D. Blood levels of cadmium and lead in relation to breast cancer risk in three prospective cohorts. Int J Cancer 2019; 144(5):1010-6.

[58] Rodgers KM, Udesky JO, Rudel RA, Brody JG. Environmental chemicals and breast cancer: an updated review of epidemiological literature informed by biological mechanisms. Environ Res 2018;160:152-82.

[59] Cordina-Duverger E, Menegaux F, Popa A, Rabstein S, Harth V, Pesch B,... Erren TC. Night shift work and breast cancer: a pooled analysis of population-based case-control studies with complete work history. Eur J Epidemiol 2018;33:369-79.

[60] Hansen J. Night shift work and risk of breast cancer. Curr Environ Health Rep 2017;4

(3):325-39.

[61] Wegrzyn LR, Tamimi RM, Rosner BA, Brown SB, Stevens RG, Eliassen AH,... Schernhammer ES. Rotating night-shift work and the risk of breast cancer in the nurses' health studies. Am J Epidemiol 2017;186(5):532-40.

[62] Colquhoun A, Arnold M, Ferlay J, Goodman KJ, Forman D, Soerjomataram I. Global patterns of cardia and non-cardia gastric cancer incidence in 2012. Gut 2015;64(12): 1881-8.

[63] Memon A, Bannister P. Epidemiology of cervical cancer. In: Uterine cervical cancer. Cham: Springer; 2019. p. 1-16.

[64] Huang FY, Kwok YK, Lau ET, Tang MH, Ng TY, Ngan HY. Genetic abnormalities and HPV status in cervical and vulvar squamous cell carcinomas. Cancer Genet Cytogenet 2005;157(1):42-8.

[65] Khazaei Z, Dehkordi AH, Amiri M, Adineh HA, Sohrabivafa M, Darvishi I,... Goodarzi E. The incidence and mortality of endometrial cancer and its association with body mass index and human development index in Asian population. World Cancer Res J 2018; 5 (4):11.

[66] Kumar R, Rai AK, Das D, Das R, Kumar RS, Sarma A,... Ramteke A. Alcohol and tobacco increases risk of high risk HPV infection in head and neck cancer patients: study from North-East Region of India. PLoS One 2015;10(10)e0140700 https://doi.org/10.1371/journal.pone.0140700.

[67] Merrill RM, Fugal S, Novilla LB, Raphael MC. Cancer risk associated with early and late maternal age at first birth. Gynecol Oncol 2005;96(3):583-93.

[68] Bidus MA, Elkas JC. Berek & Novak's gynecology. Philadelphia, PA: Lippincott Williams & Wilkins; 2007.

[69] Bruni L, Diaz M, Castellsagué M, Ferrer E, Bosch FX, de Sanjosé S. Cervical human papillomavirus prevalence in 5 continents: meta-analysis of 1 million women with normal cytological findings. J Infect Dis 2010;202(12):1789-99.

[70] Wardak S. Human papillomavirus (HPV) and cervical cancer. Med Dosw Mikrobiol 2016; 68(1):73-84.

[71] Zur Hausen H. Papillomaviruses and cancer: from basic studies to clinical application. Nat Rev Cancer 2002;2(5):342-50.

[72] Crosbie EJ, Einstein MH, Franceschi S, Kitchener HC. Human papillomavirus and cervical cancer. Lancet 2013;382(9895):889-99.

[73] De Sanjosé S, Diaz M, Castellsagué X, Clifford G, Bruni L, Muñoz N, Bosch FX. Worldwide prevalence and genotype distribution of cervical human papillomavirus DNA in women with normal cytology: a meta-analysis. Lancet Infect Dis 2007;7(7):453-9.

[74] Galani E, Christodoulou C. Human papilloma viruses and cancer in the post-vaccine era. Clin Microbiol Infect 2009;15(11):977-81.

[75] Gunnell AS, Tran TN, Torrång A, Dickman PW, Sparén P, Palmgren J, Ylitalo N. Synergy between cigarette smoking and human papillomavirus type 16 in cervical cancer in situ development. Cancer 2006;15(11):2141-7.

[76] Ferenczy A, Coutlée F, Franco E, Hankins C. Human papillomavirus and HIV coinfection and the risk of neoplasias of the lower genital tract: a review of recent developments. CMAJ 2003; 169(5):431-4.

[77] Palefsky J. Human papillomavirus infection in HIV-infected persons. Top HIV Med 2007; 15(4):130-3.

[78] Mbulawa ZZ, Marais DJ, Johnson LF, Boulle A, Coetzee D, Williamson AL. Influence of human immunodeficiency virus and CD4 count on the prevalence of human papillomavirus in heterosexual couples. J Gen Virol 2010;91(12):3023-31.

[79] Pantanowitz L, Michelow P. Review of human immunodeficiency virus (HIV) and squamous lesions of the uterine cervix. Diagn Cytopathol 2011;39(1):65-72.

[80] Strickler HD, Palefsky JM, Shah KV, Anastos K, Klein RS, Minkoff H,... Fazzari M. Human papillomavirus type 16 and immune status in human immunodeficiency virus-seropositive women. J Natl Cancer Inst 2003;95(14):1062-71.

[81] Koskela P, Anttila T, Bjørge T, Brunsvig A, Dillner J, Hakama M,... Luostarinen T. Chlamydia trachomatis infection as a risk factor for invasive cervical cancer. Int J Cancer 2000;85(1):35-9.

[82] Smith JS, Bosetti C, Munoz N, Herrero R, Bosch FX, Eluf-Neto J,... Peeling RW. Chlamydia trachomatis and invasive cervical cancer: a pooled analysis of the IARC multicentric case-control study. Int J Cancer 2004;111(3):431-9.

[83] Silva J, Cerqueira F, Medeiros R. Chlamydia trachomatis infection: implications for HPV status and cervical cancer. Arch Gynecol Obstet 2014;289(4):715-23.

[84] Hildesheim A, Herrero R, Castle PE, Wacholder S, Bratti MC, Sherman ME,... Helgesen K. HPV co-factors related to the development of cervical cancer: results from a population-based study in Costa Rica. Br J Cancer 2001;84(9):1219-26.

[85] Kim J, Kim BK, Lee CH, Seo SS, Park SY, Roh JW. Human papillomavirus genotypes and cofactors causing cervical intraepithelial neoplasia and cervical cancer in Korean women. Int J Gynecol Cancer 2012;22(9):1570-6.

[86] International Collaboration of Epidemiological Studies of Cervical Cancer. Carcinoma of the cervix and tobacco smoking: collaborative reanalysis of individual data on 13,541 women with carcinoma of the cervix and 23,017 women without carcinoma of the cervix from 23 epidemiological studies. Int J Cancer 2006;118(6):1481-95.

[87] Jensen KE, Schmiedel S, Norrild B, Frederiksen K, Iftner T, Kjaer SK. Parity as a cofactor for high-grade cervical disease among women with persistent human papillomavirus infection: a 13-year follow-up. Br J Cancer 2013;108(1):234-9.

[88] Castellsagué X, Bosch FX, Muñoz N. The male role in cervical cancer. Salud Publica Mex

2003;45:345-53.

[89] Liu ZC, Liu WD, Liu YH, Ye XH, Chen SD. Multiple sexual partners as a potential independent risk factor for cervical cancer: a meta-analysis of epidemiological studies. Asian Pac J Cancer Prev 2015; 16(9):3893-900.

[90] Silins I, Ryd W, Strand A, Wadell G, Törnberg S, Hansson BG, ... Persson K. Chlamydia trachomatis infection and persistence of human papillomavirus. Int J Cancer 2005;116(1):110-5.

[91] Winer RL, Hughes JP, Feng Q, O'Reilly S, Kiviat NB, Holmes KK, Koutsky LA. Condom use and the risk of genital human papillomavirus infection in young women. N Engl J Med 2006;354(25): 2645-54.

[92] Vanakankovit N, Taneepanichskul S. Effect of oral contraceptives on risk of cervical cancer. Med J Med Assoc Thailand 2008;91(1):7.

[93] Moreno V, Bosch FX, Muñoz N, Meijer CJ, Shah KV, Walboomers JM,... International Agency for Research on Cancer (IARC) Multicentric Cervical Cancer Study Group. Effect of oral contraceptives on risk of cervical cancer in women with human papillomavirus infection: the IARC multicentric case-control study. Lancet 2002;359(9312):1085-92.

[94] Lacey Jr. JV, Swanson CA, Brinton LA, Altekruse SF, Barnes WA, Gravitt PE,... Schwartz PE. Obesity as a potential risk factor for adenocarcinomas and squamous cell carcinomas of the uterine cervix. Cancer 2003;98(4):814-21.

[95] Lee JK, So KA, Piyathilake CJ, Kim MK. Mild obesity, physical activity, calorie intake, and the risks of cervical intraepithelial neoplasia and cervical cancer. PLoS One 2013;8(6) https://doi.org/10.1371/journal.pone.0066555.

[96] Poorolajal J, Jenabi E. The association between BMI and cervical cancer risk: a meta-analysis. Eur J Cancer Prev 2016;25(3):232-8.

[97] González CA, Travier N, Luján-Barroso L, Castellsagué X, Bosch FX, Roura E, ... Sacerdote C. Dietary factors and in situ and invasive cervical cancer risk in the European prospective investigation into cancer and nutrition study. Int J Cancer 2011; 129 (2): 449-59.

[98] Tomita LY, Filho AL, Costa MC, Andreoli MAA, Villa LL, Franco EL, Cardoso MA. Diet and serum micronutrients in relation to cervical neoplasia and cancer among low-income Brazilian women. Int J Cancer 2010;126(3):703-14.

[99] Ghosh C, Baker JA, Moysich KB, Rivera R, Brasure JR, McCann SE. Dietary intakes of selected nutrients and food groups and risk of cervical cancer. Nutr Cancer 2008;60(3): 331-41.

[100] Fonseca-Moutinho JA. Smoking and cervical cancer. ISRN Obstet Gynecol 2011;2011: https://doi.org/10.1371/journal.pone.0066555.

[101] Roura E, Castellsagué X, Pawlita M, Travier N, Waterboer T, Margall N, ... Tjønneland A. Smoking as a major risk factor for cervical cancer and pre-cancer: results from the EP-

IC cohort. Int J Cancer 2014;135(2):453-66.

[102] Plummer M, Herrero R, Franceschi S, Meijer CJ, Snijders P, Bosch FX,… Muñoz N. Smoking and cervical cancer: pooled analysis of the IARC multi-centric case-control study. Cancer Causes Control 2003;14(9):805-14.

[103] Bray F, Ferlay J, Soerjomataram I, Siegel RL, Torre LA, Jemal A. Global cancer statistics 2018: GLOBOCAN estimates of incidence and mortality worldwide for 36 cancers in 185 countries. CA Cancer J Clin 2018;68(6):394-424.

[104] Coburn SB, Bray F, Sherman ME, Trabert B. International patterns and trends in ovarian cancer incidence, overall and by histologic subtype. Int J Cancer 2017;140(11): 2451-60.

[105] Yoneda A, Lendorf ME, Couchman JR, Multhaupt HA. Breast and ovarian cancers: a survey and possible roles for the cell surface heparan sulfate proteoglycans. J Histochem Cytochem 2012; 60(1):9-21.

[106] Chornokur G, Amankwah EK, Schildkraut JM, Phelan CM. Global ovarian cancer health disparities. Gynecol Oncol 2013;129(1):258-64.

[107] Mohammadian M, Ghafari M, Khosravi B, Salehiniya H, Aryaie M, Bakeshei FA, Mohammadian-Hafshejani A. Variations in the incidence and mortality of ovarian cancer and their relationship with the human development index in European Countries in 2012. Biomed Res Ther 2017;4(8): 1541-57.

[108] Chan JK, Urban R, Cheung MK, Osann K, Husain A, Teng NN,… Leiserowitz GS. Ovarian cancer in younger vs older women: a population-based analysis. Br J Cancer 2006; 95(10):1314-20.

[109] Poole EM, Merritt MA, Jordan SJ, Yang HP, Hankinson SE, Park Y,… Terry KL. Hormonal and reproductive risk factors for epithelial ovarian cancer by tumor aggressiveness. Cancer 2013; 22(3):429-37.

[110] Walsh T, Casadei S, Lee MK, Pennil CC, Nord AS, Thornton AM,… Norquist B. Mutations in 12 genes for inherited ovarian, fallopian tube, and peritoneal carcinoma identified by massively parallel sequencing. Proc Natl Acad Sci 2011;108(44):18032-7.

[111] Toss A, Tomasello C, Razzaboni E, Contu G, Grandi G, Cagnacci A,… Cortesi L. Hereditary ovarian cancer: not only BRCA 1 and 2 genes. BioMed Res Int 2015; https://doi.org/10.1155/2015/341723.

[112] Nakamura K, Banno K, Yanokura M, Iida M, Adachi M, Masuda K,… Tominaga E. Features of ovarian cancer in Lynch syndrome. Mol Clin Oncol 2014;2(6):909-16.

[113] Helder-Woolderink JM, Blok EA, Vasen HFA, Hollema H, Mourits MJ, De Bock GH. Ovarian cancer in Lynch syndrome; a systematic review. Eur J Cancer 2016;55:65-73.

[114] Holschneider CH, Berek JS. Ovarian cancer: epidemiology, biology, and prognostic factors. Semin Surg Oncol 2000;19(1):3-10.

[115] Soegaard M, Jensen A, Høgdall E, Christensen L, Høgdall C, Blaakær J, Kjaer SK.

Different risk factor profiles for mucinous and nonmucinous ovarian cancer: results from the Danish MALOVA study. Cancer Epidemiol Prev Biomarkers 2007;16(6):1160-6.

[116] Tsilidis KK, Allen NE, Key TJ, Dossus L, Lukanova A, Bakken K,... Tjønneland A. Oral contraceptive use and reproductive factors and risk of ovarian cancer in the European Prospective Investigation Into Cancer and Nutrition. Br J Cancer 2011;105(9):1436-42.

[117] Tung KH, Goodman MT, Wu AH, McDuffie K, Wilkens LR, Kolonel LN,... Sobin LH. Reproductive factors and epithelial ovarian cancer risk by histologic type: a multiethnic case-control study. Am J Epidemiol 2003;158(7):629-38.

[118] Riman T, Dickman PW, Nilsson S, Correia N, Nordlinder H, Magnusson CM, Persson IR. Risk factors for epithelial borderline ovarian tumors: results of a Swedish case-control study. Gynecol Oncol 2001;83(3):575-85.

[119] La Vecchia C, Franceschi S. Oral contraceptives and ovarian cancer. Eur J Cancer Prev 1999;8:297-304.

[120] Zhou J, Chng WJ. Roles of thioredoxin binding protein (TXNIP) in oxidative stress, apoptosis and cancer. Mitochondrion 2013;13(3):163-9.

[121] Lacey Jr. JV, Mink PJ, Lubin JH, Sherman ME, Troisi R, Hartge P,... Schairer C. Menopausal hormone replacement therapy and risk of ovarian cancer. JAMA 2002;288(3):334-41.

[122] Risch HA, Marrett LD, Jain M, Howe GR. Differences in risk factors for epithelial ovarian cancer by histologic type: results of a case-control study. Am J Epidemiol 1996;144(4):363-72.

[123] Mørch LS, Løkkegaard E, Andreasen AH, Krüger-Kjær S, Lidegaard Ø. Hormone therapy and ovarian cancer. JAMA 2009;302(3):298-305.

[124] Goodman MT, Wu AH, Tung KH, McDuffie K, Kolonel LN, Nomura AM,... Hankin JH. Association of dairy products, lactose, and calcium with the risk of ovarian cancer. Am J Epidemiol 2002;156(2):148-57.

[125] Mori M, Harabuchi I, Miyake H, Casagrande JT, Henderson BE, Ross RK. Reproductive, genetic, and dietary risk factors for ovarian cancer. Am J Epidemiol 1988;128(4):771-7.

[126] McCann SE, Freudenheim JL, Marshall JR, Graham S. Risk of human ovarian cancer is related to dietary intake of selected nutrients, phytochemicals and food groups. J Nutr 2003;133(6):1937-42.

[127] McCann SE, Moysich KB, Mettlin C. Intakes of selected nutrients and food groups and risk of ovarian cancer. Nutr Cancer 2001;39(1):19-28.

[128] Bandera EV, Lee VS, Qin B, Rodriguez-Rodriguez L, Powell CB, Kushi LH. Impact of body mass index on ovarian cancer survival varies by stage. Br J Cancer 2017;117(2):282-9.

[129] Delort L, Kwiatkowski F, Chalabi N, Satih S, Bignon YJ, Bernard-Gallon DJ. Central

adiposity as a major risk factor of ovarian cancer. Anticancer Res 2009;29(12):5229-34.

[130] Anderson JP, Ross JA, Folsom AR. Anthropometric variables, physical activity, and incidence of ovarian cancer: the Iowa Women's Health Study. Cancer 2004; 100 (7): 1515-21.

[131] Beehler GP, Sekhon M, Baker JA, Teter BE, McCann SE, Rodabaugh KJ, Moysich KB. Risk of ovarian cancer associated with BMI varies by menopausal status. J Nutr 2006;136 (11):2881-6.

[132] Parkin DM, Bray FI, Devesa SS. Cancer burden in the year 2000. The global picture. Eur J Cancer 2001;37:4-66.

[133] Ferlay J, Soerjomataram I. GLOBOCAN: cancer incidence and mortality worldwide: IARC cancer base no. 11. International Agency for Research on Cancer; 2013.

[134] Fitzmaurice C, Akinyemiju TF, Al Lami FH, Alam T, Alizadeh-Navaei R, Allen C,… Aremu O. Global, regional, and national cancer incidence, mortality, years of life lost, years lived with disability, and disability-adjusted life-years for 29 cancer groups, 1990 to 2016: a systematic analysis for the global burden of disease study. JAMA Oncol 2018;4 (11):1553-68.

[135] Bray F, dos Santos Silva I, Moller H, Weiderpass E. Endometrial cancer incidence trends in Europe: underlying determinants and prospects for prevention. Cancer 2005;14(5): 1132-42.

[136] Purdie DM, Green AC. Epidemiology of endometrial cancer. Best Pract Res Clin Obstet Gynaecol 2001;15(3):341-54.

[137] Dossus L, Rinaldi S, Becker S, Lukanova A, Tjonneland A, Olsen A,… Clavel-Chapelon F. Obesity, inflammatory markers, and endometrial cancer risk: a prospective case-control study. Endocr Relat Cancer 2010;17(4):1007.

[138] Killackey MA. Endometrial adenocarcinoma in breast cancer patients receiving antiestrogens. Cancer Treat Rep 1985;69:237-8.

[139] Fearnley EJ, Marquart L, Spurdle AB, Weinstein P, Webb PM. Australian Ovarian Cancer Study Group and Australian National Endometrial Cancer Study Group: Polycystic ovary syndrome increases the risk of endometrial cancer in women aged less than 50 years: an Australian case-control study. Cancer Causes Control 2010;21(12):2303-8.

[140] Navaratnarajah R, Pillay OC, Hardiman P. Polycystic ovary syndrome and endometrial cancer. Semin Reprod Med 2008;26(01):062-71.

[141] Schumer ST, Cannistra SA. Granulosa cell tumor of the ovary. J Clin Oncol 2003;21(6): 1180-9.

[142] Chang ET, Lee VS, Canchola AJ, Clarke CA, Purdie DM, Reynolds P,… Pinder R. Diet and risk of ovarian cancer in the California Teachers Study cohort. Am J Epidemiol 2007; 165(7):802-13.

[143] Simpson ER, Brown KA. Obesity, aromatase and breast cancer. Expert Rev Endocrinol

Metab 2011;6(3):383-95.

[144] Friberg E, Orsini N, Mantzoros CS, Wolk A. Diabetes mellitus and risk of endometrial cancer: a metaanalysis. 1365-74.

[145] Nagamani M, Stuart CA. Specific binding and growth-promoting activity of insulin in endometrial cancer cells in culture. Am J Obstet Gynecol 1998;179(1):6-12.

[146] Lucenteforte E, Bosetti C, Talamini R, Montella M, Zucchetto A, Pelucchi C,... La Vecchia C. Diabetes and endometrial cancer: effect modification by body weight, physical activity and hyperten sion. Br J Cancer 2007;97(7):995-8.

[147] Sjögren LL, Mørch LS, Løkkegaard E. Hormone replacement therapy and the risk of endometrial cancer: a systematic review. Maturitas 2016;91:25-35.

[148] Moore RG, MacLaughlan S, Bast Jr. RC. Current state of biomarker development for clinical application in epithelial ovarian cancer. Gynecol Oncol 2010;116(2):240-5.

[149] Lu KH, Dinh M, Kohlmann W, Watson P, Green J, Syngal S,... Terdiman J. Gynecologic cancer as a "sentinel cancer" for women with hereditary nonpolyposis colorectal cancer syndrome. Obstet Gynecol 2005;105(3):569-74.

[150] Zucchetto A, Serraino D, Polesel J, Negri E, De Paoli A, Dal Maso L,... Talamini R. Hormonerelated factors and gynecological conditions in relation to endometrial cancer risk. Eur J Cancer Prev 2009;18(4):316-21.

第 5 章
基于量子点纳米抗体的三阴性乳腺癌治疗技术

Rama Rao Malla

Cancer Biology Lab,Department of Biochemistry and Bioinformatics,Institute of Science,GITAM(Deemed to be University),Visakhapatnam,Andhra Pradesh,India

摘要

三阴性乳腺癌是全世界女性的一个重要的健康问题,因此,我们需要寻求一种创新且可靠的治疗方法。随着量子点(quantum dot,QD)等光学和化学方法的出现,基于量子点的纳米技术在癌症成像领域受到了特别的关注。本文重点介绍纳米技术在三阴性乳腺癌成像、靶向定位和治疗中的应用,以及在乳腺癌治疗中可使用的各种纳米抗体。

关键词

癌症成像,纳米抗体,量子点,三阴性乳腺癌

缩略词

BRET	生物发光共振能量转移
EGFR	表皮生长因子受体
FA	叶酸
HA	透明质酸
MRI	磁共振成像
NIR	近红外
NP	纳米颗粒
PDT	光动力疗法
PEI	聚乙烯亚胺
QD	量子点
SLN	前哨淋巴结
TNBC	三阴性乳腺癌

一、概述

三阴性乳腺癌(triple negative breast cancer, TNBC)侵袭性强、预后差,对全球女性的健康构成严重威胁[1]。由于缺乏特异性标志物和有效的治疗方法,TNBC难以被完全控制。从长期来看,早期诊断可以显著降低TNBC患者的死亡率,然而TNBC的分期(如侵袭和转移)非常复杂,需要深入探讨以便更好地进行诊断和评估预后。其复杂性主要在于了解肿瘤细胞与微环境之间的复杂相互作用。因此,需要开发典型癌症的检测和诊断方法,将复杂的分子数据转化为成像信号[2]。癌细胞的早期诊断是预后最关键的部分。

在全球范围内,研究人员已经研究了各种诊断TNBC的方法,包括钼靶X线检查、磁共振成像(magnetic resonance imaging,MRI)、超声、计算机体层成像、正电子发射体层成像和组织活检。这些非侵入性成像工具与组织活检相结合,可以有效观察实体肿瘤、确认肿瘤的存在,以及对TNBC的原发和继发部位进行定位。然而,这些技术存在一些局限性,包括在微观水平上检测异常的灵敏度和特异度较差、难以识别肿瘤的初期阶段及难以检测分子层面的癌前病变,同时不适用于年轻女性[3]。因此,寻找新的检测方法及进行实时监测对了解TNBC的发病机制至关重要。

二、具有生物医学应用价值的量子点

量子点(quantum dot,QD)等光学和化学方法在癌症成像领域备受关注,因为它们具有独特的尺寸和表面特征及潜在的生物医学应用价值,比如原位多重成像[4]。人们为了探索QD的独特性质,已经开发了基于QD的原位多重成像设备,用于对肿瘤组织标本进行定量分析。QD是一种工程荧光纳米颗粒(nanoparticle,NP),拥有独特的光学和化学特性,使其成为生物医学应用的理想平台。在靶向治疗中,早期诊断和标志物识别变得尤为重要。光学方法用于检查腋窝淋巴结以评估转移,是TNBC预后评估的第一步。本章总结了QD在TNBC临床研究中的生物医学应用(图5-1)。

三、量子点的构造

QD是尺寸在2～10 nm范围内的纳米晶体,表面涂覆颗粒以增强溶解性、降低毒性,并且高度选择性地靶向识别肿瘤标志物。QD的核心主要包含Ⅱ/Ⅳ族金

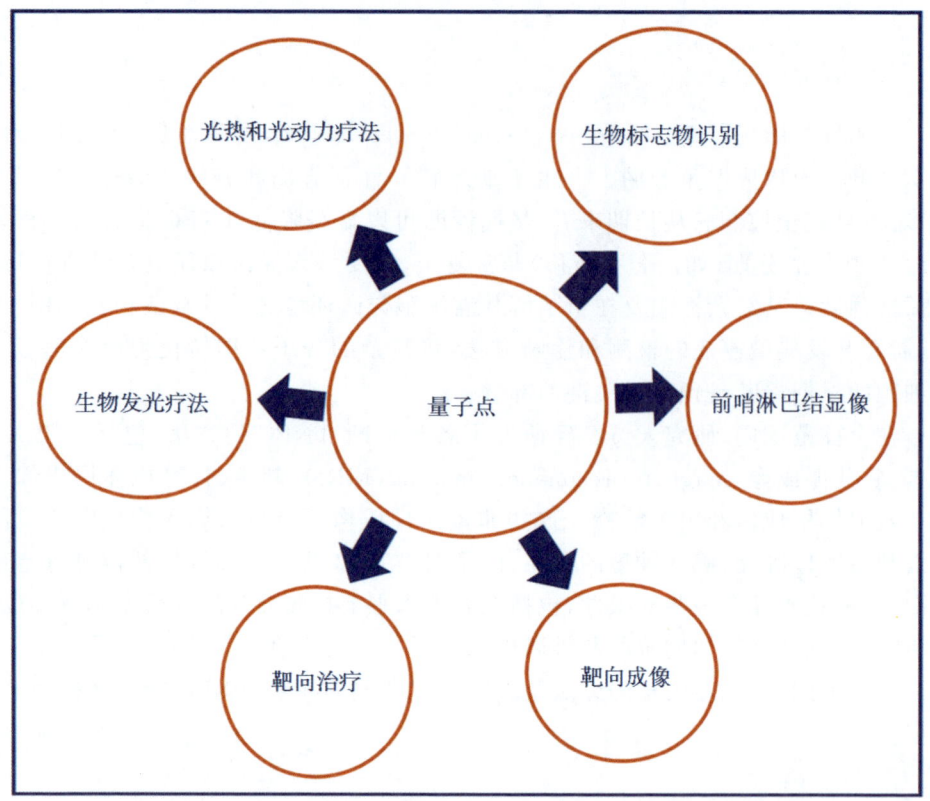

图 5-1　三阴性乳腺癌临床研究中量子点的生物医学应用

注：量子点可以用于靶向治疗、靶向成像、前哨淋巴结显像、生物标志物识别、光热和光动力疗法，以及生物发光疗法。

属，包括镉/硒或镉/碲，而外壳则主要由硫化锌（ZnS）或硫化镉（CdS）制成。当前使用的 QD 不含镉，而是由铟/钯制成，使其具有更高的生物相容性。

QD 的构建方法包括将纳米颗粒嵌入纳米球体中，在纳米球体形成过程中加入纳米颗粒，将纳米颗粒组装到纳米球体表面，或在纳米球体的孔内原位合成纳米颗粒（图 5-2）。

纳米球和纳米颗粒是通过嵌入或结合的方法分别制备的，然后再组合在一起。在另外两种方法中，组合是在纳米球或纳米颗粒的形成过程中发生的[5]。表 5-1 总结了多种比较方法。

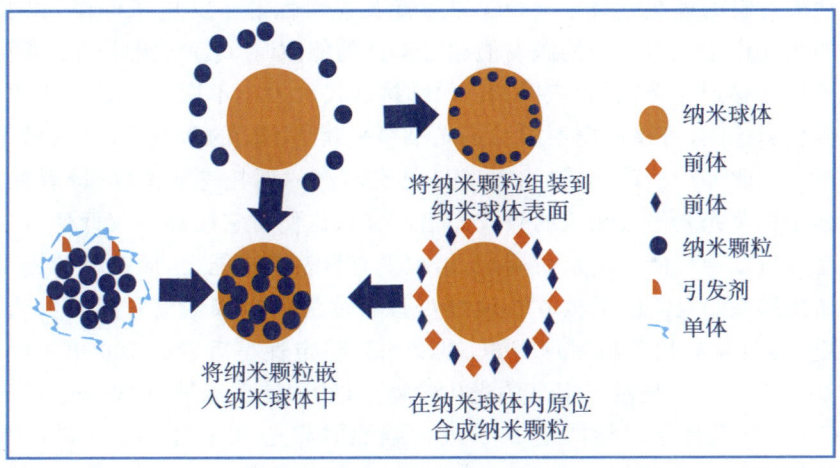

图 5-2 生物医学应用中量子点的构建方法

注:量子点可以通过将纳米颗粒嵌入纳米球体中,或在纳米球体形成过程中将纳米颗粒纳入其中,也可以将纳米颗粒组装到纳米球体表面,或在纳米球体的孔内原位合成纳米颗粒等方法构建。

表 5-1 量子点构建方法总结

项目	嵌入方法	合并方法	组装方法	原位合成
操作过程	非常方便	方便	非常枯燥	方便
操作条件	超声破碎	用力搅拌	温和摇晃	高温
操作时间	1 h	超过 1 h	超过 1 h	超过 1 h
纳米颗粒分布	不均匀	均匀	均匀	均匀
纳米颗粒聚合	部分	部分	少	很少
负载能力	相对低	中等	非常高	高
编码类型	丰富	中等	非常丰富	简单
可控性	相对随机	相对可控	非常可控	可控
稳定性	极性溶液中稳定	稳定	稳定	稳定
复合物大小	纳米级	纳米级	纳米级	微米级

四、量子点的独特特性

QD 由于量子效应和尺寸效应而具有特定的光学和电学特性。纳米颗粒的这些特性包括尺寸、介电、量子约束和表面效应,使得 QD 成为生物领域中作为荧光探针和功能材料的理想选择[5]。QD 的独特荧光特性源于其电子间隙,以及与周围构型的相互作用。当光子的激发能超过 QD 的能隙时,QD 将吸收光子并将电子从价电子层转移到导带,然后依据 QD 的结构和尺寸发出不同的荧光。相比之下,为了获得色彩区间,可以使用不同的荧光染料来获得不同的激发光,这是昂贵且复杂的分析[6]。此外,与有机染料相比,QD 具有较高的斯托克斯位移(译者注:斯托克斯位移是指荧光光谱较相应的吸收光谱红移),这使得它能够在较低信号强度下进行光谱分析成为可能[7]。众所周知,组织具有自发荧光能力,而有机荧光染料的斯托克斯位移较小,因此,需要在检测器处设置滤波器以降低信号强度的质量[8]。QD 的荧光强度是有机染料罗丹明 6G 的 20 倍,稳定性是后者的 100 倍。此外,修饰后的 CdS/ZnS QD 显示出很高的光化学稳定性,即使在能量为 500 mW、激发波长为 488 nm 的条件下也能持续 14 h 发出强烈的荧光,并在生物分子之间表现出长时间的细胞相互作用[9]。

五、用于生物标志物检测的量子点

当前尚无用于鉴定 TNBC 亚型特征(即高侵袭性与低侵袭性、转移性与非转移性)的检测方法。高通量基因组学和蛋白质组学研究已鉴定了一些用于区分 TNBC 亚型的生物标志物。生物标志物在诊断、预后、治疗和长期管理方面越来越受到重视。癌症生物标志物是癌症发展过程中生物状态变化的细胞指标。众所周知,致癌转化可导致生物分子或生物标志物分泌到体液中的水平升高或异常[10]。因此,生物标志物可以提供有关癌症发病率和进展的信息。已确认多种蛋白质作为不同癌症的独特生物标志物,例如,前列腺癌的前列腺特异性抗原、卵巢癌的 CA125[11]、肠癌的癌胚抗原和乳腺癌的 HER2[12]。识别 TNBC 的生物标志物对于早期诊断至关重要。高通量基因组学、蛋白质组学和代谢组学技术的进步已经发现了 mRNA 或蛋白质表达的改变,以及不同水平的代谢物[13],这些生物标志物可用于诊断、预后评估、风险评估、复发预测及治疗反应评估。

在寻求生物标志物的敏感检测方面,纳米技术大有前途。QD 可以同时检测血液和组织活检样本中的 10~100 种癌症生物标志物[14]。实际上,QD 扩展了细胞、组织和全身多重生物标志物在癌症成像的应用。QD 还有望建立个性化的治疗模式,提高癌症诊断和治疗的能力[15]。

六、前哨淋巴结显像技术

前哨淋巴结(sentinel lymph node,SLN)是肿瘤的主要引流区域,也是肿瘤转移的第一个部位。SLN 显像对于包括乳腺癌在内的各种癌症的手术治疗至关重要。现代 SLN 显像方法包括引入酸性硫放射胶体和蓝色染料,在手术中使用光子探针监控,偶尔结合 X 射线寻找 SLN。许多研究报告都建议将 SLN 显像视为"金标准"。目前,有机染料和放射性胶体是 SLN 显像的首选材料,但 SLN 显像具有一些局限性,如电离辐射暴露和局部组织损伤。

QD 可以应用于 SLN 显像而无须活检。手术切除原发灶是乳腺癌早期诊断的理想方法。然而,由于难以区分肿瘤边界和残留癌细胞,肿瘤可能频繁复发。带有功能基团的 QD 可用于图像引导手术切除肿瘤。光稳定的近红外(near-infrared,NIR)QD 具有良好的组织穿透性。尽管 QD 可能存在延迟清除而导致积累的问题,但无镉 QD 的临床试验结果令人鼓舞,并展现了它们在癌症检测和治疗方面的潜力[16]。铟基 QD 已被应用于小鼠乳腺癌模型,结果表明它不会通过淋巴系统扩散。

一种聚乙二醇化的 QD 从肿瘤原发灶迁移到 SLN,可以通过上皮细胞进行无创定位[17]。具有透明质酸(hyaluronic acid,HA)和阴离子糖胺聚糖共轭的 QD 可用于淋巴循环成像。研究表明,它们在淋巴循环中的毒性较小,疗效较高,并且 HA 的共轭物可提高肿瘤的渗透性。尺寸小于 10 nm 的分子能够扩散到淋巴结,故适用于基于 SLN 的显像,而尺寸在 50~100 nm 范围内的颗粒表现出混合作用,对淋巴管的穿透性较差。但尺寸为 10 nm 的聚乙二醇化 QD 不适用于 SLN 显像[18]。

七、量子点在三阴性乳腺癌靶向成像中的应用

基于荧光的肿瘤靶向成像是诊断体内局部实体癌的一种很有前景的方法。与传统成像技术相比,这是一种方便且成本低廉的方法。该方法利用具有明亮稳定的近红外荧光的成像剂对肿瘤进行高效成像。例如,将近红外 QD 连接到抗体上,可获得高荧光量子产率和光稳定性。封装有 QD 和 siRNA 的适配偶联脂质纳米载体具有治疗 TNBC 的潜力。

磷酸铟核/硫化锌壳 QD(InP/ZnS QD)具有近红外荧光,并已应用于生物分布研究。抗表皮生长因子受体(epidermal growth factor receptor,EGFR)纳米抗体的共轭增强了基于 QD 的胶束的细胞摄取和细胞毒性。与氨基黄酮(aminoflavone,AF)包被的非靶向胶束类似,AF 包被的纳米抗体(nanobody,Nb)共轭胶束在 TNBC 模型中沉积在肿瘤中的水平更高,且无全身毒性。因此,基于 QD 的 Nb 共轭胶束可用作 TNBC 的新型纳米治疗平台[19]。

八、用于三阴性乳腺癌生物发光成像的自发光量子点

基于近红外的荧光成像具有各种优势,包括出色的生物安全性、灵敏度、操作简便和实时成像。然而,与基于光学成像的近红外荧光成像相比,基于生物发光共振能量转移(bioluminescence resonance energy transfer,BRET)的QD-BRET系统具有一些优势,特别是在深层组织检测方面[20]。QD-BRET系统通过与底物co-elenterazine(译者注:腔肠素,一种天然的荧光素,可作为许多荧光素酶的底物)相互作用,结合 *Rotylenchulus reniformis* 荧光素酶(Luc8)突变体而发出蓝色荧光。这种基于生物发光的成像可用于检测深层组织而不受肿瘤组织自身荧光的干扰[21]。也可利用多模态荧光和生物发光成像技术检测TNBC肺转移灶[22]。

九、量子点在三阴性乳腺癌微转移检测中的应用

为预防术后癌症复发,需确保消灭所有癌细胞。近期研究表明,术中荧光成像可用于乳腺肿瘤的手术显像,术中实时荧光成像有望增强乳腺肿瘤的成像效果[20]。目前常见的癌症成像模式是磁共振成像,但无法检测到早期癌细胞和隐匿癌细胞。免疫组化结合反转录聚合酶链反应通常用于微转移的成像,但其局限性在于耗时且无法提供即时结果[21]。因此,针对转移性疾病推荐采用新型疗法。将与cRGD生物共轭的QD静脉注射到肿瘤部位,利用近红外荧光成像技术已在肿瘤手术中取得成功。标记有环-Arg-Gly-Asp-Tyr(c-RGDY)的QD可靶向整合素肿瘤细胞,有助于微转移的检测[23]。

十、用于三阴性乳腺癌免疫疗法的量子点

大多数TNBC患者EGFR高表达,它是乳腺癌的预后和预测标志物[24]。HER2阳性乳腺癌具有侵袭性且预后较差。EGFR靶向治疗是个性化精准医疗最成功的一步(图5-3)。针对EGFR的人源化单克隆抗体(monoclonal antibodies,mAb)已证明联合化疗药物可提高生存率。据报道,相较于传统方法,EGFR生物共轭QD与免疫组化的结合可提高单细胞的可视化灵敏度和疗效,同时成本更低。QD抗癌共轭物可用于标记细胞水平的定量分析。而与QD共轭抗体功能化的微珠可用于靶向癌症抗原。QD与特异性抗体的耦合可用于药物的主动和被动靶向,从而提高药物的渗透性和持久性[25]。

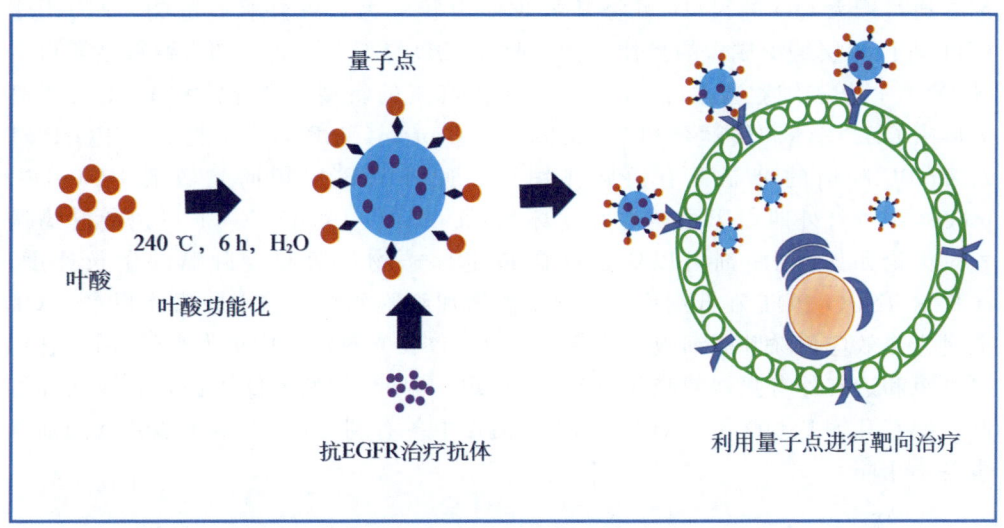

图 5-3　QD 在三阴性乳腺癌 EGFR 靶向治疗中的应用
注：量子点与特异性抗体偶联可用于药物的主动靶向和被动靶向。

十一、用于基因治疗的量子点

叶酸(folic acid, FA)-QD 复合物已被应用在乳腺癌治疗中，因为叶酸受体在乳腺癌中表达高，并且作为一种低分子量的靶向分子在乳腺癌中发挥作用。经过羧基衍生的 FA 复合物具有与叶酸受体持久结合的能力。小分子、毒素、化疗药物、放射治疗药物、聚合物包裹的治疗药物、基因递送剂、抑制性原药及免疫治疗药物基本上都能够通过共价结合与叶酸形成复合物[26]。

由于 d-dot/PAH 纳米复合物在较高浓度下具有很高的生物相容性，因此使用 d-dot/聚合物纳米复合物转染 siRNA 来靶向突变致癌 KRAS 基因在癌症治疗中备受关注。最近，QD-Forster 共振能量转移被应用于免疫测定及设计纳米药物释放的纳米传感器[27]。纳米抗体介导的乳腺癌免疫活化疗法的最佳解释是 TNBC 细胞表面的选择性抗二硝基苯(anti-DNP)抗体。此外，针对人类 STAT3 开发的 SBT-100(抗 STAT3 B VHH13)可抑制 p-STAT3 的功能[28]。

十二、用于三阴性乳腺癌光动力和光热疗法的量子点

光敏剂的光动力疗法(photodynamic therapy, PDT)是临床医疗实践中的一种辅助疗法。要提 PDT 的效率，必须使用高质量的具有近红外吸收能力的光敏

剂。通过增大 QD 的尺寸，可将其吸收能力转变为近红外吸收能力，成为用于 PDT 进行深层组织成像的最佳选择。此外，QD 释放单线态氧和有毒重金属可诱导 DNA 损伤和细胞凋亡（图 5-4）。基于大麻素的新型联合疗法和 PDT 可提高大麻素 CB2 受体和转运蛋白（translocator protein，TSPO）的活性。TSPO-PDT 对 TNBC 肿瘤的抑制具有协同作用[29]。此外，CB2R 靶向光敏剂 IR700DX-mbc94 在近红外照射下可诱导肿瘤坏死，而 TSPO-IR700DX-6T 可诱导肿瘤凋亡。无论如何，光敏剂可以通过靶向特定标志物显著减慢肿瘤的生长速度。cCB2R-TSPO-PDT 在低剂量的情况下能增加细胞死亡并缩小肿瘤体积[30]。QD 通过光热效应消除肿瘤细胞。棕色或黑色 QD 在光热疗法中更为有效，因为它们对红色和近红外有强烈的吸收，能深入组织。因此，这些 QD 能够有效地破坏细胞。镉基和铜基 QD 在 TNBC 的 PDT 治疗中各有利弊，在生物医学领域的前景也各不相同。

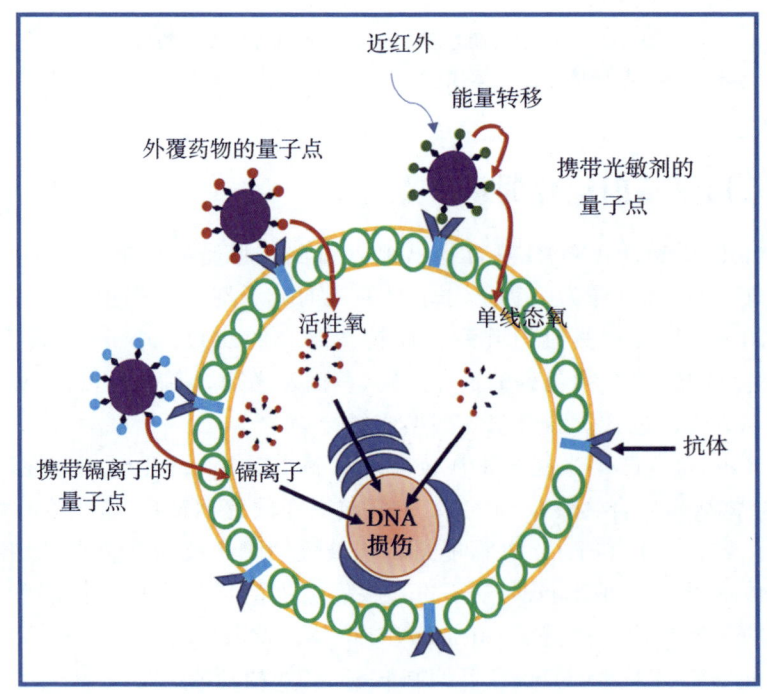

图 5-4 量子点在 TNBC 光动力疗法中的可能机制

注：量子点能有效地产生单线态氧并释放有毒离子，尤其是重金属阳离子。单线态氧和重金属离子都能损伤 DNA，诱导细胞凋亡。

十三、用于三阴性乳腺癌靶向治疗的纳米抗体

在乳腺癌治疗中,聚合 NP 可被用作细胞毒性药物的载体,将药物输送到靶点(图 5-5)。此系统中的最佳例子是将皂草素输送到细胞中,皂草素在细胞中具有特定的靶点,但不会被内化。对于 HER2 阳性乳腺癌细胞,可以使用聚乙二醇化的多聚(乳酸-羟基乙酸-羟基甲基羟基乙酸)NP 作为载体,其表面覆盖有针对 HER2 受体而不是 HER2-TNBC 细胞的 11A4 纳米抗体。使用纳米抗体可以防止被特异性摄取。研究表明,皂草素-11A4 NP 与光化学内化相结合,可通过诱导细胞凋亡显著降低细胞的增殖率和存活率[31]。

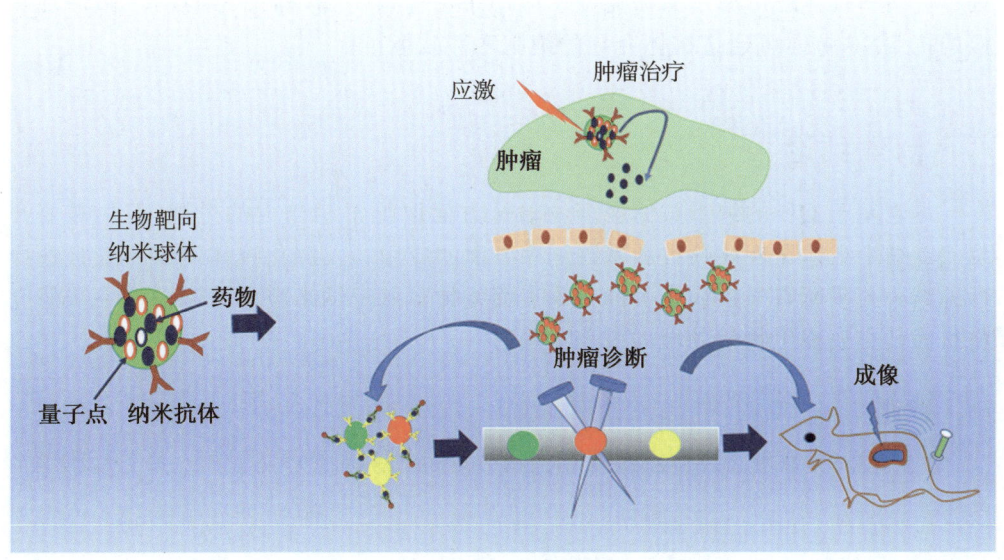

图 5-5 量子点纳米抗体介导的诊断和治疗
注:纳米抗体共轭的量子点装载药物后可内化和释放药物,也可用于癌症诊断。

此外,纳米抗体还可用于基因递送和靶向转录。通常情况下,抗 HER2 纳米抗体的可变结构域与聚乙烯亚胺(polyethylenimine polymer,PEI)和聚乙二醇[poly(ethylene glycol),PEG]共价连接,形成了 PEI-PEG NP 中的 NHS-PEG3500 的远端[32]。在癌症干细胞(cancer stem cell,CSC)治疗中,用抗 HER2 纳米抗体结合聚酰胺多聚物可以靶向 HER2 过表达的 TNBC 细胞系,对 CSC 表现出很高的效率[33]。对 PD-1/PD-L1 免疫检查点的抗 PD-L1 mAb 具有抗肿瘤活性,PD-L1 Nb(纳米抗体)具有竞争性结合抑制作用,并模拟了分子动力学[34]。

重组免疫毒素因其特异性而在肿瘤治疗中备受关注。融合了 Nb-Fc(纳米抗体的 Fc 段)的曲妥珠单抗(HER2 抗体)重链可用于治疗 HER2 阳性乳腺癌。Intein 是一种融合的外毒素 A,将其作为结合蛋白与麦芽糖表达融合[35]。融合了纳米抗体的磁性油小体可将油基亲脂类药物用于乳腺癌治疗[36]。此外,使用 At 标记的 sdAb 结合物,特别是 iso-[211At] SAGMB-5F7,对表达 HER2 的乳腺癌进行 α 粒子靶向放射治疗效果显著[37]。

为了治疗 TNBC,设计出一种与表皮生长因子受体 N 带 AF(氨基黄酮)共轭的 QD 胶束[38]。此外,中和肿瘤微环境中的 TNF-α 是使用纳米抗体的新方法,它能增强紫杉醇疗法并抑制乳腺癌的转移。一项研究证明,通过使用缺氧靶向荧光纳米抗体,tCAIX 特异性纳米抗体-IRDye800CW 可用作浸润性乳腺癌的快速成像剂[5]。纳米抗体还可通过激活免疫反应应用于治疗。例如,标记为 HER2 阳性乳腺癌的抗 DNP 抗体可通过抗体介导的细胞毒性破坏目标[40]。

十四、结论

尽管基于 QD 的纳米载体在药物输送方面取得了相当大的进展,但仍需要开发 QD 纳米载体在疾病筛查和基因测序方面的应用。人源化抗体能够有效且选择性地结合几乎所有与疾病相关的细胞表面受体。基于纳米技术检测的进一步研究将扩大其在癌症生物学领域的应用范围。

致谢

作者感谢印度新德里 DST-EMR(EMR/2016/002694,日期:2017 年 8 月 21 日)对该项目的支持。

利益冲突

作者声明不存在利益冲突。

参 考 文 献

[1] Fang M, Peng CW, Pang DW, Li Y. Quantum dots for cancer research: current status, remaining issues, and future perspectives. Cancer Biol Med 2012;9(3):151-63.

[2] Sanz-Moreno V, Marshall CJ. The plasticity of cytoskeletal dynamics underlying neoplastic cell migration. Curr Opin Cell Biol 2010;22(5):690-6.

[3] Zhao MX, Zeng EZ. Application of functional quantum dot nanoparticles as fluorescence probes in cell labeling and tumor diagnostic imaging. Nanoscale Res Lett 2015;10:171.

[4] He X, Ma N. An overview of recent advances in quantum dots for biomedical applications. Colloids Surf B Biointerfaces 2014;124:118-31.

[5] Wen CY, Xie HY, Zhang ZL, Wu LL, Hu J, Tang M, Wu M, Pang DW. Fluorescent/magnetic micro/nano-spheres based on quantum dots and/or magnetic nanoparticles: preparation, properties, and their applications in cancer studies. Nanoscale 2016;8(25): 12406-29.

[6] Bai M, Bornhop DJ. Recent advances in receptor-targeted fluorescent probes for in vivo cancer imaging. Curr Med Chem 2012;19(28):4742-58.

[7] Jaiswal JK, Mattoussi H, Mauro JM, Simon SM. Long-term multiple color imaging of live cells using quantum dot bioconjugates. Nat Biotechnol 2003;21(1):47-51.

[8] Viswanath AK. From clusters to semiconductor nanostructures. J Nanosci Nanotechnol 2014;14(2):1253-81.

[9] Smith AM, Nie S. Semiconductor nanocrystals: structure, properties, and band gap engineering. Acc Chem Res 2010;43(2):190-200.

[10] Mason JN, Farmer H, Tomlinson ID, Schwartz JW, Savchenko V, DeFelice LJ, Rosenthal SJ, Blakely RD. Novel fluorescence-based approaches for the study of biogenic amine transporter localization, activity, and regulation. J Neurosci Methods 2005;143(1):3-25.

[11] Rosenblum LT, Kosaka N, Mitsunaga M, Choyke PL, Kobayashi H. Optimizing quantitative in vivo fluorescence imaging with near-infrared quantum dots. Contrast Media Mol Imaging 2011;6(3):148-52.

[12] Doré-Savard L, Barriére DA, Midavaine É, B elanger D, Beaudet N, Tremblay L, Beaudoin JF, Turcotte EE, Lecomte R, Lepage M, Sarret P. Mammary cancer bone metastasis follow-up using multimodal small-animal MR and PET imaging. J Nucl Med 2013;54(6): 944-52.

[13] Fisher B, Bauer M, Wickerham DL, Redmond CK, Fisher ER, Cruz AB, Foster R, Gardner B, Lerner H, Margolese R, et al. Relation of number of positive axillary nodes to the prognosis of patients with primary breast cancer. An NSABP update. Cancer 1983;52(9): 1551-7.

[14] Hulvat M, Rajan P, Rajan E, Sarker S, Schermer C, Aranha G, Yao K. Histopathologic characteristics of the primary tumor in breast cancer patients with isolated tumor cells of the sentinel node. Surgery 2008;144(4):518-24 discussion 524.

[15] Wu X, Wu M, Zhao JX. Recent development of silica nanoparticles as delivery vectors for cancer imaging and therapy. Nanomedicine 2014;10(2):297-312.

[16] Bakalova R, Zhelev Z, Kokuryo D, Spasov L, Aoki I, Saga T. Chemical nature and structure of organic coating of quantum dots is crucial for their application in imaging diagnostics. Int J Nanomedicine 2011;6:1719-32.

[17] Chowbay B, Jada SR, Wan Teck DL. Correspondence re: Cecchin et al. , Carboxylesterase isoform 2 mRNA expression in peripheral blood mononuclear cells is a predictive marker of

the irinotecan to SN38 activation step in colorectal cancer patients. Clin Cancer Res 2005; 11:6901-7. Clin Cancer Res 2006;12(6):1942 author reply 1942-3.

[18] Meyer JS. Sentinel lymph node biopsy: strategies for pathologic examination of the specimen. J Surg Oncol 1998;69(4):212-8.

[19] Lin G, Ouyang Q, Hu R, Ding Z, Tian J, Yin F, Xu G, Chen Q, Wang X, Yong KT. In vivo toxicity assessment of non-cadmium quantum dots in BALB/c mice. Nanomedicine 2015;11(2):341-50.

[20] Tsoi KM, Dai Q, Alman BA, Chan WC. Are quantum dots toxic? Exploring the discrepancy between cell culture and animal studies. Acc Chem Res 2013;46(3):662-71.

[21] Shukur A, Rizvi SB, Whitehead D, Seifalian A, Azzawi M. Altered sensitivity to nitric oxide donors, induced by intravascular infusion of quantum dots, in murine mesenteric arteries. Nanomed Nanotechnol Biol Med 2013;9(4):532-9.

[22] Miao P, Han K, Tang Y, Wang B, Lin T, Cheng W. Recent advances in carbon nanodots: synthesis, properties and biomedical applications. Nanoscale 2015;7(5):1586-95.

[23] Huang X, Zhang F, Zhu L, Choi KY, Guo N, Guo J, Tackett K, Anilkumar P, Liu G, Quan Q, Choi HS, Niu G, Sun YP, Lee S, Chen X. Effect of injection routes on the biodistribution, clearance, and tumor uptake of carbon dots. ACS Nano 2013;7(7):5684-93.

[24] Abdullah Al N, Lee JE, In I, Lee H, Lee KD, Jeong JH, Park SY. Target delivery and cell imaging using hyaluronic acid-functionalized graphene quantum dots. Mol Pharm 2013; 10(10):3736-44.

[25] Zheng XT, Ananthanarayanan A, Luo KQ, Chen P. Glowing graphene quantum dots and carbon dots: properties, syntheses, and biological applications. Small 2015;11(14): 1620-36.

[26] Schneider R, Schmitt F, Frochot C, Fort Y, Lourette N, Guillemin F, Muller JF, Barberi-Heyob M. Design, synthesis, and biological evaluation of folic acid targeted tetraphenylporphyrin as novel photosensitizers for selective photodynamic therapy. Bioorg Med Chem 2005;13(8):2799-808.

[27] Zhang G, Gao J, Qian J, Zhang L, Zheng K, Zhong K, Cai D, Zhang X, Wu Z. Hydroxylated mesoporous nanosilica coated by polyethylenimine coupled with gadolinium and folic acid: a tumortargeted T(1) magnetic resonance contrast agent and drug delivery system. ACS Appl Mater Interfaces 2015;7(26):14192-200.

[28] Lee SJ, Shim YH, Oh JS, Jeong YI, Park IK, Lee HC. Folic-acid-conjugated pullulan/poly(DL-lactideco-glycolide) graft copolymer nanoparticles for folate-receptor-mediated drug delivery. Nanoscale Res Lett 2015;10:43.

[29] Shao D, Li J, Pan Y, Zhang X, Zheng X, Wang Z, Zhang M, Zhang H, Chen L. Noninvasive theranostic imaging of HSV-TK/GCV suicide gene therapy in liver cancer by folate-targeted quantum dotbased liposomes. Biomater Sci 2015;3(6):833-41.

[30] Yuan Y, Zhang J, An L, Cao Q, Deng Y, Liang G. Oligomeric nanoparticles functional-

ized with NIR-emitting CdTe/CdS QDs and folate for tumor-targeted imaging. Biomaterials 2014;35(27):7881-6.

[31] Yoo HS, Park TG. Folate-receptor-targeted delivery of doxorubicin nano-aggregates stabilized by doxorubicin-PEG-folate conjugate. J Control Release 2004;100(2):247-56.

[32] Martínez-Jothar L, Beztsinna N, van Nostrum CF. Selective cytotoxicity to HER2 positive breast cancer cells by saporin-loaded nanobody-targeted polymeric nanoparticles in combination with photochemical internalization. Mol Pharm 2019;16(4):1633-47.

[33] Saqafi B, Rahbarizadeh F. Polyethyleneimine-polyethylene glycol copolymer targeted by anti-HER2 nanobody for specific delivery of transcriptionally targeted tBid containing construct. Artif Cells Nanomed Biotechnol 2019;47(1):501-11.

[34] Reshadmanesh A, Rahbarizadeh F, Ahmadvand D, Jafari Iri Sofla F. Evaluation of cellular and transcriptional targeting of breast cancer stem cells via anti-HER2 nanobody conjugated PAMAM dendrimers. Artif Cells Nanomed Biotechnol 2018;46(Suppl 3):S105-15.

[35] Sun X, Yan X, Zhuo W, Gu J, Zuo K, Liu W, Liang L, Gan Y, He G, Wan H, Gou X, Shi H, Hu J. PD-L1 nanobody competitively inhibits the formation of the PD-1/PD-L1 complex: comparative molecular dynamics simulations. Int J Mol Sci 2018;19(7):1984-94.

[36] Pirzer T, Becher KS, Rieker M, Meckel T. Generation of potent anti-HER1/2 immunotoxins by protein ligation using split inteins. ACS Chem Biol 2018;13(8):2058-66.

[37] (a) Mazzega E, de Marco A. Engineered cross-reacting nanobodies simplify comparative oncology between humans and dogs. Vet Comp Oncol 2018;16(1):E202-6; (b) Choi J, Vaidyanathan G, Koumarianou E, Kang CM, Zalutsky MR. Astatine-211 labeled anti-HER2 5F7 single domain antibody fragment conjugates: radiolabeling and preliminary evaluation. Nucl Med Biol 2018;56:10-20.

[38] (a) Wang Y, Wang Y, Chen G, Li Y, Xu W, Gong S. Quantum-dot-based theranostic micelles conjugated with an anti-EGFR nanobody for triple-negative breast cancer therapy. ACS Appl Mater Interfaces 2017;9(36):30297-305; (b) Ji X, Peng Z, Li X, Yan Z, Yang Y, Qiao Z, Liu Y. Neutralization of TNFα in tumor with a novel nanobody potentiates paclitaxel-therapy and inhibits metastasis in breast cancer. Cancer Lett 2017;386:24-34.

[39] (a) van Brussel AS, Adams A, Oliveira S, Dorresteijn B, El Khattabi M, Vermeulen JF, van der Wall E, Mali WP, Derksen PW, van Diest PJ, Van Bergen En Henegouwen PM. Hypoxia-targeting fluorescent nanobodies for optical molecular imaging of pre-invasive breast cancer. Mol Imaging Biol 2016;18(4):535-44; (b) Gray MA, Tao RN, DePorter SM, Spiegel DA, McNaughton BR. A nanobody activation immunotherapeutic that selectively destroys HER2-positive breast cancer cells. Chembiochem 2016;17(2):155-8.

[40] Gray MA, Tao RN, DePorter SM, Spiegel DA, McNaughton BR. A nanobody activation immunotherapeutic that selectively destroys HER2-positive breast cancer cells. Chembiochem 2016;17(2):155-8.

第 6 章
纳米技术在卵巢癌领域的进展

Kiranmayi Patnala[a], Rama Rao Malla[b], Soumya Vishwas[a]

[a] Department of Biotechnology, Institute of Science, GITAM (Deemed to be University), Visakhapatnam, Andhra Pradesh, India
[b] Cancer Biology Lab, Department of Biochemistry and Bioinformatics, Institute of Science, GITAM (Deemed to be University), Visakhapatnam, Andhra Pradesh, India

摘要

卵巢癌是女性特有的一种弥漫性生长且早期无症状的癌症。早期卵巢癌没有任何症状，因此，卵巢癌发现时大多数处于晚期。这类患者的生存率主要取决于癌症的分期。虽然患者在接受各种药物治疗后可能会初步康复，但在大多数情况下，长期用药可能会导致耐药。卵巢癌可以通过传统的肿瘤细胞减灭手术进行治疗，即清除肿瘤细胞，抑或是通过纳米技术将化疗药物输送到特定的肿瘤部位进行治疗。尽管在Ⅰ期卵巢癌可以完全切除肿瘤，但所有分期的卵巢癌都必须使用化疗药物进行治疗。这就为开发高效纳米抗癌制剂提供了更大的空间。本章总结了基于纳米技术的新型治疗策略和制剂，以及这些策略和制剂在卵巢癌成像、检测和治疗方面的成果。

关键词

纳米颗粒，卵巢癌，诊断，成像，治疗，临床前开发，化疗药物，新型疗法

缩略词

ADCT	两亲性树突状共聚物
Apo	脂蛋白
Au-NP	金纳米颗粒
CA	癌抗原
CE	癌胚抗原
DNA	脱氧核糖核酸
DOPC	二油酰基磷脂酰胆碱
EGFR	表皮生长因子受体
EGP	乙二醇-谷氨酸-苯丙氨酸
ELISA	酶联免疫吸附试验

EOC	上皮性卵巢癌
EPR	增强渗透性和保持力
FDA	美国食品药品管理局
FILIP1L	丝胶 1A 互作蛋白 1
Gd-B-dendrimer	生物素共轭树枝状聚合物与钆螯合物
HA-E1A	人类腺病毒 5 型早期区域 1A
HE4	人类附睾蛋白
Heparin-PE	肝素-聚乙烯亚胺
HER	人表皮生长因子受体
HPMA	N-(2-羟基丙基)甲基丙烯酰胺
HSulf-1	硫酸肝素-6-O-内硫酸酯酶 1
ID4	DNA 结合抑制剂 4
IL-12	白介素 12
IO-NP	氧化铁纳米颗粒
IP	腹腔内
IV	静脉内
LHR	促黄体素受体
LHRHan	(译者注:应为:LHRHa)促黄体素释放素类似物
MEMS	微机电系统
MRI	磁共振成像
MUC	黏蛋白
NIR	近红外
NP	纳米颗粒
PA	光声
PAMAM	聚酰胺-胺
PDT	光动力疗法
PEG	聚乙二醇
PEI	聚乙烯亚胺
PLA	聚乳酸
PLGA	聚(D,L-乳酸-共聚乙醇酸)
QD	量子点
RES	网状内皮系统
ROMA	卵巢恶性肿瘤风险指数
RONDEL	RNAi/寡核苷酸纳米颗粒传输

ROS	活性氧
RRM2	核糖核苷酸还原酶的 M2 亚基
scFV	单链可变片段
SELDI-TOF-MS	表面增强激光解析/电离飞行时间质谱仪
shRNA	短发夹核糖核酸
siRNA	干扰小 RNA
SPECT	单光子发射计算机体层成像
SR-B1	清道夫受体 B1 型
STAT3	信号转导及转录活化因子 3
TP	肿瘤蛋白
VEGF	血管内皮生长因子

一、概述

卵巢癌是全球女性的常见死因。一项研究显示,2018 年登记的 295 414 例卵巢癌患者中,有 184 799 人死亡[1]。早期卵巢癌(在转移到腹膜或累及其他器官之前发现的卵巢癌)预后相对较好。晚期患者的 5 年生存率较早期下降了 20%。在过去的 30 年里,卵巢癌患者的生存率没有改善。这是因为超过 60% 的病例发现时已经是Ⅲ期以上[2]。超过 90% 的卵巢癌是上皮起源的,称为上皮性卵巢癌(epithelial ovarian cancer,EOC)。这些 EOC 分为黏液性、透明细胞、低级别浆液性、高级别浆液性和子宫内膜样,在腹腔内(intraperitoneal,IP)定位上具有相似性,并伴随各种症状[2]。根据组织起源和基因组分析结果,这些疾病存在明显区别。表 6-1 展示了基因突变与不同类型卵巢癌之间的关系[2-7]。

表 6-1 EOC 及其相关基因突变

癌症亚型	EOC 病例报道*	报告的基因突变	起源组织
Ⅰ型:黏液性	<5%	KRAS(75%)	—
Ⅰ型:透明细胞	10%	ARIK1A(50%)、PIK3CA(50%)、PTEN(20%)	子宫内膜
Ⅰ型:浆液性、低级别	<5%	BRAF/KRAS(50%)、ERBB2(9%)	输卵管伞部
Ⅱ型:浆液性、高级别	70%	TP53(96%)、BRCA1/BRCA2(22%)	输卵管伞部
Ⅰ型——低级别和Ⅱ型——高级别:子宫内膜样	10%	CTNNB1(40%) PIK3CA(20%)、PTEN(20%)	子宫内膜

* 译者注:占比。

目前,卵巢浆液性癌在女性中发病率较高,且患者群体庞大。因此,学术界正致力于开发新的卵巢浆液性癌的治疗方法。修复损伤的脱氧核糖核酸(deoxyribonucleic acid,DNA)通常需要 BRCA1/2 基因参与,这两个基因的胚系突变导致了 22%的高级别卵巢浆液性癌[8]。已知子宫内膜异位症最终会引起透明细胞癌,但黏液亚型的起源仍未明确[6]。妊娠、子宫切除手术及避孕药的使用降低了子宫内膜样癌的风险[9]。早期的研究误将排卵期女性卵巢的外上皮认为是卵巢癌的起源部位,但随后的研究表明输卵管上皮才是导致严重卵巢癌形成的原因之一,并且大多数情况下与 BRCA1/2 基因组变异有关[10]。排卵过程中,当卵巢上皮发生破损时,输卵管伞状突更接近破损位置,并促使了卵巢癌前体病变形成。卵巢癌一般在腹腔内种植扩散,如浆液性 II 型癌,经常在腹腔内广泛转移后才得到诊断[7,11]。III 期和 IV 期癌症患者表现为腹腔内液体过度积聚,进而出现腹痛或腹胀。上述情况预示患者预后不佳[12]。

二、诊断和临床治疗现况

卵巢癌被称为"沉默的杀手",因为在早期阶段没有任何症状。有 3/4 的卵巢癌病例在进展到 III 或 IV 期后才被诊断[9],也就是说,卵巢癌只有在发生远处转移时才能确诊。目前尚无有效的生物标志物来检测早期卵巢癌,急需开拓新的研究领域。蛋白质组学研究揭示了许多从患者血清中识别出的新型卵巢肿瘤标志物[13]。Bast 等从卵巢癌上皮细胞系中提取出来一种抗原性蛋白质黏蛋白 16(mucin16,MUC16)[14],也称为癌抗原(cancer antigen,CA)125。然而,CA125 用于筛查时,有大量的假阳性和假阴性结果,在肝病和妊娠期间也会表达,导致误诊。研究表明,卵巢癌患者血清中蛋白质(11N-聚糖)的糖基化增加,与 CA125 相比具有更好的灵敏度和特异度[15-18]。然而,这些肿瘤标志物对癌症的诊断仍不够有效。一项研究表明,约 50%的卵巢癌患者可以检测到分泌性糖蛋白人附睾蛋白 4(human epididymis4,HE4)的表达,而这部分患者体内 CA125 水平较低。因此,这种蛋白质可能最大限度地减少假阴性结果[19]。在绝经期女性中,相比单独使用 CA125 进行筛查,卵巢恶性肿瘤风险指数(risk of ovarian malignancy algorithm,ROMA)(结合 HE4 和 CA125)显示出多样化且更好的结果。美国食品药品管理局(Food and Drug Administration,FDA)批准 OVA1 用于卵巢癌患者的筛查,该检测使用转铁蛋白、脂蛋白(apolipoprotein,Apo)A1、转甲状腺素蛋白、CA125 和微球蛋白-2 等血清标志物组合来运算,表面增强激光解吸/电离飞行时间质谱仪(surface-enhanced laser desorption/ionization time of flight mass spectrometry,SELDI-TOF-M)可以识别上述标志物。然而,在卵巢癌筛查方面,使用该检测与单纯使用 CA125 相比并无显著差别[20,21]。理想的治疗模式是针对肿瘤对特定蛋白质表达水平的变化进行筛查，以助于肿瘤靶向治疗的发展。

目前，肿瘤细胞减灭术是卵巢癌治疗的标准方法。肿瘤切除术也被称为减瘤术，在过去50年一直是常规的治疗手段。在减瘤术后，患者通常接受基于铂类药物的静脉内（intravenous，IV）化疗6~8周。在此期间，患者对卡铂或顺铂等化疗药物表现出良好的反应。然而，大多数患者在健康状态改善一段时间后会复发，并对铂类药物产生耐药。各种经批准用于卵巢癌患者的联合化疗方案如博来霉素-依托泊苷-顺铂、吉西他滨和紫杉醇及多西他赛和卡铂都显示出良好的效果。已经获得批准用于卵巢癌治疗的联合化疗包括卡铂和多西他赛、吉西他滨和紫杉醇以及博来霉素-依托泊苷-顺铂。由于卵巢肿瘤多局限于腹腔内，多年来肿瘤学家已经通过IP途径给药[22]。该途径将导管放置在患者体内给药，某种程度上给患者带来了不便。此外，IP治疗还可能引起非预期并发症，如胃肠道问题或腹腔内感染[23]。值得注意的是，与其他治疗方式相比而言，IP途径能够减轻全身毒性并增强对肿瘤的靶向作用。因此，可以利用纳米技术对IP途径进行探索，用于癌症的成像和治疗。

三、纳米技术在诊断和成像中的应用

近年来，基于微机电系统（microelectromechanical system，MEMS）和各种基于纳米颗粒的技术在诊断领域取得了显著进展。这些进展主要集中在改善成像对比剂和生物标志物检测方法方面。最近有报道称CA125、间皮素和HE4在多项检测中展现出很好的应用前景。它们作为诊断方法表现出了更好的性能和可靠性[24,25]。众所周知，高质量生物标志物的可用性对于诊断至关重要，而纳米技术可以为诊断带来更多改善。基于纳米技术的检测和传感器快速、可靠、具有成本效益，可用于癌症的多重筛查[26-29]。

2009年，Jokerst等开发了一种基于抗原-抗体反应的检测方法，并将其整合到量子点上[30]。该系统利用量子点标记CA125抗体，在微流控纳米平台上进行操作。该平台包含一组孔洞，每个孔洞都能够捕获一个单独的琼脂糖颗粒，并且这些琼脂糖颗粒含有固定化抗体以捕获特定抗原分子。一旦捕获到目标抗原分子，另一个量子点标记抗体则允许荧光信号可视化。这种琼脂糖珠被成功地应用于人类表皮生长因子受体（human epidermal growth factor receptor，HER）2和CA125等多个标志物的同时检测，与酶联免疫吸附试验（enzyme-linked immunosorbent assay，ELISA）相比，该系统对癌胚抗原（carcinoembryonic，CE）的反应性更强。随着"可编程生物纳米芯片"的进一步开发完善，该方法将适用于卵巢癌筛查[31]。

现有诊断手段检测血清 CA125 的阈值应达到 35 U/ml。而通过采用丝网打印金纳米颗粒（gold nanoparticle，Au-NP）电极检测血清 CA125，能够检测到 6.7 U/ml 的无标记检测[32]。

一抗标记的氧化铁纳米颗粒与树突状分子或鲁米诺改变的二抗也作为发光传感平台。该平台检测到的 CA125 浓度可低至 0.03 μU/ml[33,34]。基于各种纳米颗粒、芯片、MEMS 和其他平台的系统有望用于卵巢癌的筛查，并在其诊断中发挥至关重要的作用。

在众多的成像模式中，光学成像、超声和磁共振成像（magnetic resonance imaging，MRI）是卵巢癌最常用的 3 种成像方法。然而，大多数临床诊断都倾向于采用经阴道超声检查。表 6-2 总结了用于卵巢癌成像的纳米颗粒（nanoparticles，NP）。

表 6-2　用于卵巢癌成像的纳米颗粒

成像方式	纳米颗粒	靶点	药物	样本*	细胞系
光学	量子点	CA125 抗体	N	异种移植	HO8910
	量子点	EPR	N	异种移植	HEYA8
	量子点	HER2 抗体	N	体外	SKOV-3
	量子点	MUC1-适体	Y	异种移植	A2780
	聚甲基丙烯酸酯酸（可见光）	HER2 抗体		体外	SKOV-3
	脂蛋白（NIR）	叶酸		异种移植	—
	PEG-PLA（NIR）	EPR		异种移植	A2780
	聚乙二醇脂质（NIR）	EPR		异种移植	SKOV-3
	NaYF$_4$:Yb^{3+}/Er^{3+}@二氧化硅	—		体外	SKOV-3
磁共振	树状聚物	生物素		异种移植	SHIN3
	脂质体	叶酸		异种移植	IGROV-1, OVCAR-3
	铁矿石	叶酸		体外	SKOV-3
	氧化铁/钆	EPR		异种移植	SKOV-3
影像声学	金纳米棒	EPR		异种移植	2008, HEY, SKOV-3
超声	脂质体 微气泡	—		体外	不适用的

*译者注：应为样本来源。

在超声成像中,人们将高频声波定向到探头朝向的组织。来自内部器官的反射声波用于图像构建。对于超声检查,内部组织的声学特性必须存在差异。超声中常用的对比剂是具有全氟碳填充或空气填充核心的颗粒。2种商用超声对比剂 OPTISON 和 Definity 都被用于检查和记录卵巢肿瘤的微血管变化。OPTISON 由白蛋白稳定化全氟丙烯颗粒制备而成,Definity 含有全氟丙烯脂质微球[35,36]。彩色多普勒、3D 超声检查及微管造影是有前景的超声技术,目前正用于卵巢癌的成像或诊断[37]。

未来,多种 NP 组件将在 MRI 癌症成像中发挥重要作用,可以提供更好的对比度。T_1 加权像可利用各种 NP(如树突状分子、胶束和脂质体),而 T_2 加权像常使用氧化铁纳米颗粒(iron oxide nanoparticles, IO-NP)。Gd-B-树突状分子最初应用于癌症异种移植物的体内 MRI[38]。含有叶酸修饰的 Gd^{3+} 脂质体也被用于体内成像[39]。SKOV-3 卵巢细胞的体外 T_2 加权像可通过叶酸移植的聚甘油修饰 IO-NP 表面来实现[40,41],而 T_1 加权像可通过两性离子表面的 IO-NP 来实现。这些 NP 的半衰期约为 1 h,在循环系统中通过增强渗透性和保持力(enhanced permeability and retention, EPR)积累[42]。近期观察到,在使用 MRI 和单光子发射计算机体层成像(single-photon emission computerized tomography, SPECT)双重系统时,右旋糖酐包被的 IO-NP 联合标记的间皮素抗体在 A431-K5(译者注:人表皮癌细胞)异种移植物中产生了有效的成像[43]。如果相同受体在卵巢癌细胞中高表达,则类似颗粒可用于影像诊断。

用于近红外光学成像的探针应具备光稳定性、高量子产率、高摩尔吸附系数和大斯托克斯位移。大量树状分子、脂质体和聚合物 NP 整合了这些近红外染料,以评估小鼠移植瘤 HT29(结肠)和 A2780(卵巢)细胞系中的肿瘤的分布与积累。该染料首先被装入聚乙二醇-聚乳酸(polyethylene glycol-polylactic acid, PEG-PLA)共聚物 NP 中,注射后实现长达 2 天的成像,随后被网状内皮系统(reticuloendothelial system, RES)清除。111 nm 颗粒比 166 nm 颗粒表现出更合适的 RES 清除率和更高的肿瘤积累效应[44]。在一项研究中,将 ICG(近红外染料)与坦螺旋霉素和紫杉醇一起封装在 PEG 化胶束中,在 SKOV-3 移植瘤小鼠体内引入这些封装胶束,比游离药物表现出更好的疗效。这些 NP 通过 EPR 效应在肿瘤组织中积累,实现长达 2 天的成像效果[45]。

量子点(QD)是一种无机纳米颗粒。与其他几种粒子相比,QD 具有更优异的光学特性,例如,较大的斯托克斯位移、有限的发射窗口、宽激发范围及低光漂白现象[46-48]。类似于聚合物纳米颗粒,QD 也被应用于 A2780 癌症移植物治疗。其发射波长约为 500 nm。当与黏蛋白 1(mucin1, MUC1)(靶向适配体)和药物多柔比星结合时,QD 不仅可用于成像,还可用于卵巢癌治疗[49]。

与超声成像一样,光声(photoacoustic,PA)成像是利用近红外辐射通过局部加热来生成基于声波的图像。在此过程中,可以通过应用纳米材料或微小分子实现局部加热效果。例如,在近红外辐射下,金纳米棒不仅产生局部加热效应,还能增强对比度。这些金纳米棒已应用于小鼠卵巢癌移植物 PA 成像。注入这些纳米棒后,180 min 后显示出最强信号,持续至 48 h。研究表明,长宽比为 3.5 的金纳米棒是体内成像的理想选择[50]。

四、化疗中的纳米技术

基于纳米技术的脂质体结合制剂具有增加药物积累、药物保留时间和药物相容性的巨大优势。例如,多柔比星脂质体是 FDA 批准的用于复发性癌症患者的 NP 配方。这种获批的配方基于含有多柔比星药物的聚乙二醇化脂质体,目前与吉西他滨联合用于治疗铂类耐药的癌症患者。与使用未修饰的多柔比星治疗的患者相比,使用 NP 脂质体配方治疗的患者显示出更长的血浆半衰期和更高的肿瘤内积累。这些脂质体在给药后能够持续保持数天[51]。多柔比星脂质体的 Ⅱ 期试验表明,与游离多柔比星相比,多柔比星脂质体毒性更低[52]。使用托泊替康和吉西他滨进行标准治疗的复发性或难治性卵巢癌患者在使用多柔比星脂质体治疗时能够获益[53-56]。这一研究还显示出铂类耐药患者存活率增加,疾病无进一步进展[55,56]。另一项针对铂类敏感癌症患者的研究表明,多柔比星脂质体与卡铂联合治疗同紫杉醇与卡铂的标准治疗产生了类似的结果。对铂类部分耐药的患者采用多柔比星脂质体-卡铂治疗后,未发现疾病进展[57]。此外,相较于单独使用多柔比星脂质体,多柔比星脂质体与曲妥珠单抗联合使用时,部分或完全铂类耐药的癌症患者的生存率有所提高[58,59]。多柔比星脂质体在治疗卵巢癌方面的成功为使用各种纳米制剂进行新的临床试验开辟了前景。然而,另一种药物托泊替康在治疗复发或再发性卵巢转移性癌方面显示出与多柔比星脂质体和紫杉醇类似的疗效[60]。含有托泊替康的脂质体正在进行 Ⅰ 期临床试验。使用 PEG 化脂质体托泊替康与托泊替康相比未显示出明显的改善[61]。此外,由于引起过度的血液清除而对大鼠造成了有害的影响[62]。勒托替康是基于脂质体的另一种制剂,与游离药物相比,暴露量增加。尽管有这种特性,但该药必须在极量下才能发挥最佳效果。这一特性导致了不良反应增多,尤其是已经接受其他药物治疗的人群。由于它无法在这类患者中表现出显著疗效,所以无法获得临床使用批准[63]。

abraxane 是一种经 FDA 批准用于治疗乳腺癌、肺癌和 Ⅰ 期胰腺癌的药物。它是白蛋白结合型紫杉醇或白蛋白结合型紫杉醇与 NP 结合物的商品名[64]。相较于其他紫杉醇制剂,白蛋白结合型紫杉醇具有更多优势。白蛋白可以稳定近 130 nm

大小的紫杉醇颗粒。普通紫杉醇制剂则需要合成溶剂来携带和递送药物至靶细胞,并可能引起过敏反应[65]。2006 年首次将 abraxane 应用于卵巢癌患者,以减少由紫杉醇引起的过敏反应,这些患者接受三轮治疗的过程中未出现不良反应[66]。自此以后,白蛋白结合型紫杉醇一直处于铂类敏感性和铂类耐药性卵巢癌患者Ⅱ期临床试验中。每周向铂类耐药患者注射 abraxane 一次,平均无进展生存期达 135 天[67]。该药对铂类敏感患者的反应率达到 64%。针对这两类患者的研究结果证明了 abraxane 的有效性,因此可以进行Ⅲ期临床试验[68]。xyotax 是一种紫杉醇药物制剂,它是一种纳米级无溶剂制剂,在进入细胞代谢之前会从紫杉醇偶联物降解为 L-谷氨酸。在单药Ⅰ期和Ⅱ期临床试验中显示出令人振奋的疗效[69]。xyotax 在Ⅱ期临床试验中对复发性卵巢癌患者展示了良好的疗效。该药物用于卵巢癌二线或三线治疗时,其活性属于中等水平,但仍有成为维持用药选择的前景[70]。与卡铂联合应用于一线治疗也是一种可行方案。其他药物配方包括 nanotax——处于Ⅰ期临床试验阶段的紫杉醇 NP 混悬液,以及 etirinotecan pegol——一种可能用于治疗铂类耐药型卵巢癌患者的聚合物偶联物(NKTR-102,nektar)。在 etirinotecan pegol 分子中,一种可分解的拓扑异构酶Ⅰ抑制剂将 PEG-NP 与伊立替康连接在一起,当两者分解时被激活。在Ⅰ期临床试验中,该药物对一组接受过治疗的患者展现出抗癌活性[71]。Ⅱ期临床试验显示出该药对铂类耐药卵巢癌患者表现出高度活性。每个月给药一次就能将生存期提高平均 5.4 个月。这一结果进一步推动了针对乳腺癌和卵巢癌的Ⅲ期临床试验[72]。另一项Ⅰ期临床试验表明,喜树碱(拓扑异构酶抑制剂)与环化 PEG-NP 的结合物制剂比游离喜树碱更为有效[73]。与 PEG 类似,N-(2-羟基丙基)甲基丙烯酰胺[N-(2-hydroxypropyl)methacrylamide,HPMA]也可用于药物递送。作为兼容聚合物,它可以通过与酸敏感连接分子结合来运载卡铂类似物或奥沙利铂类似物。ProLindac(与 HPMA 结合的奥沙利铂类似物)在临床预试验中的疗效优于顺铂,结果显示,它在癌细胞的累积量是顺铂的 16 倍。尽管其表现出较高耐受性,但Ⅰ期临床试验效果不及奥沙利铂[74]。单药Ⅱ期临床试验显示,在接受大剂量治疗后,2/3 的晚期卵巢癌患者达到了稳定状态,为进一步联合临床研究打开了道路。此外,在Ⅰ期和Ⅱ期临床试验中使用 HPMA 结合卡铂类似物也呈现令人振奋的毒理特征[75,76]。表 6-3 列示了正进行的针对卵巢癌的纳米配方的相关临床试验证据。

表 6-3 卵巢癌纳米制剂的临床试验

复合物名称	配方	活性剂	阶段	实验编号
多柔比星脂质体	聚乙二醇化脂质体多柔比星	多柔比星	FDA 认可的	NCT00945139 NCT00862355 NCT00248248
—	脂质体托泊替康	托泊替康	第一阶段	NCT00765973
OSI-211	勒托替康脂质体	勒托替康	第二阶段	NCT00010179
abraxane，ABI-007	纳米颗粒结合白蛋白结合型紫杉醇	紫杉醇	第二阶段	批准用于乳腺癌、小细胞癌和胰腺癌 NCT00466986 NCT00407563
xyotax	紫杉醇 poliglumex	紫杉醇	第二阶段	NCT00060359 NCT00017017
nanotax	纳米颗粒	紫杉醇	第一阶段	NCT00666991
NKTR-102	etirinotecan pegol	拓扑异构酶Ⅰ抑制剂	第二阶段	NCT00806156103
CRLX101	环糊精-PEG-喜树碱	喜树碱	第一阶段	NCT00333502 NCT01652079
proLindac（AP5346）	HPMA-奥沙利铂	奥沙利铂	第二阶段	文献[74,75]
AP5280	HPMA-卡铂酸盐	卡铂	第二阶段	文献[75,76]

五、临床前研究

NP 聚合物结构有助于药物靶向递送到肿瘤部位。一项研究表明,携带紫杉醇和顺铂的胶束具有细胞毒性。这种胶束由乙二醇-谷氨酸-苯丙氨酸(ethylene glycol-glutamic acid-phenylalanine, EGP)制成的核心包裹在 PEG 外壳中。该 NP 聚合物能够在组织蛋白酶 B 等蛋白水解酶作用下进行生物降解,在目标位点释放两种药物。卵巢癌在长期治疗后会逐渐产生多药耐药性。然而,与游离药物或仅携带单一药物的胶束相比,紫杉醇和顺铂联合纳米颗粒配方显示出良好疗效[77]。为了改善药代动力学特性,研究人员还开发了另一种共聚物胶束系统,这种新型 NP 系统由 PEG-聚 ε-己内酯-PEG 共聚物形成凝胶状态,在 IP 区域逐渐降解并释放多柔比星等药物,最后代谢出体外。尽管这是一个高治疗效率的可生物降解共聚物系统,但仍需要进一步临床试验验证[78]。与之相似,在小鼠移植瘤模型中测试时,使用棉花素和环丙胺抑制剂作为 IP 给药载体能够抑制肿瘤生长、减小肿瘤大小并提高存活率[79]。树突状分子如聚酰胺-胺(polyamidoamine,PAMAM)等不同半径的物质(1.3~2.9 nm)也被广泛应用于给药研究;携带顺铂的 PAMAM 表现出低毒性及更高耐受剂量的特点[80]。空间位阻、pH 敏感连接剂的使用或连接化学反应都会影响药物的靶向递送[81-83]。加州大学戴维斯分校癌症中心团队介绍了一种可用于卵巢癌治疗的两亲性树突状共聚物(amphiphilic dendritic copolymer telodendrimer,ADCT)。该系统核心和外壳均由 PEG、赖氨酸和胆汁酸组成,这一系统能够使结合后的紫杉醇具有水溶性;其体外活性与 abraxane 或紫杉醇相似;并且在小鼠模型实验中显示出了更强大的穿透力,以及比大多数 FDA 批准配方更显著的肿瘤抑制效果[84]。对其进行放射性标记显示,这种聚合物比紫杉醇代谢更慢,且在肿瘤部位表现出优先摄取,故可以作为药物载体进行进一步的临床试验[85,86]。还有一种用于在靶部位控制药物释放的聚合物 NP 系统,该系统包含 2 种药物成分:含有神经酰胺的缓释型聚(D,L-乳酸-共聚乙醇酸)[poly(D,L-lactic-co-glycolic acid),PLGA]和 pH 敏感型聚(β-氨基酯)包裹的紫杉醇。虽然它尚未应用于卵巢癌临床试验,但已显示出对异种移植瘤较好的减瘤效果[87]。

在卵巢癌细胞中,整合素、黏蛋白和紧密连接蛋白等表面蛋白高表达。受体蛋白[促黄体素受体(luteinizing hormone receptor,LHR)、EGFR 和 HER2]在卵巢癌细胞中的表达也会升高。目前最常用的肿瘤靶向和定位的技术是表面蛋白与抗体或多肽的结合技术。现在出现了另一种基于磁性 NP 的新型靶向技术。这种技术可以将顺铂药物装载至氧化铁颗粒中,并通过磁性定位使其靶向到卵巢癌细胞内部。该磁性定位系统可增加药物对肿瘤细胞近 110 倍的细胞毒性[88]。然而,该系统在临床试验中存在一个主要缺点:难以操控磁场,而磁场必须强大且精准靶向肿瘤细胞是这一系统发挥作用的必要条件。脂质体配方在卵巢癌的体内研究表明,脂质体制剂有望改善卵巢癌的治疗效果。当利用促黄体素释放素类似物(luteinizing hormone-releasing hormone analogue,LHRHa)将含多西他赛的胆固醇脂质体靶向至肿瘤部位时,肿瘤细胞内 1 h 药物累积量增加 9 倍,同时还减少了药物在脾脏和肝脏的积聚[89]。

在肿瘤细胞表面高表达的 A-3 整合素受体对"OA02"多肽具有显著亲和力。这些元素用于胶束载体,并有助于细胞摄取和 PEG 胶束的定位。携带紫杉醇的胶束复合物与紫杉醇制剂和非靶向 PEG 复合物相比能够降低全身毒性并提高肿瘤治疗效果。这些特征可能有助于减少化疗药物引起的不良反应[85,86]。

Nukolova 等设计了一种基于二嵌段共聚物的纳米凝胶,可实现叶酸在卵巢癌治疗中的靶向递送。利用该纳米凝胶在小鼠模型上对卵巢癌的影响进行研究发现,当携带多柔比星或顺铂时,该复合物特异性靶向肿瘤细胞并具有搅拌活性[90]。

在卵巢癌病例中,使用顺铂纳米凝胶靶向 LHRH 时,也观察到类似结果。该标志物也在前列腺癌和乳腺癌中高表达,因此这种凝胶还具备应用于其他癌症的前景[91]。

在含有多柔比星的聚胶束(L-组氨酸)中,叶酸再次被用作靶向配体。该系统在酸性 pH 下也展现出引人注目的药物控制释放效果。当在人类卵巢癌小鼠异种移植模型上进行测试时,胶束在肿瘤部位呈现更高程度的积累,并释放出高剂量药物。与游离多柔比星治疗相比,这些胶束使血浆半衰期延长了 5 倍,从而产生了更显著的治疗效果[92]。该团队还设计了一种叶酸修饰的胶束,通过受体介导内吞作用增强药物摄取。这些胶束能够抑制多药耐药肿瘤的生长,并且在动物实验中几乎没有观察到体重减轻[93]。当 pH 敏感性转变为 6.0 时,其对小鼠肿瘤表现出更强抑制效果,并持续近 2 个月[94]。

六、纳米技术在新疗法中的应用

尽管药物封装和药物靶向提高了肿瘤对药物的反应率,但可能导致癌症患者逐渐产生耐药性。许多 NP 介导的新型治疗方法正在取得进展。光动力疗法(photodynamic therapy,PDT)是一种用于卵巢癌治疗的新兴技术。在初步实验中,采用载有金丝桃素的聚乳酸 NP 对卵巢癌细胞进行体外 PDT[95],随后在大鼠体内进行研究。使用 NP 在大鼠上皮性卵巢癌细胞系进行的体内试验相比游离药物显示出更好的药物聚集性[96]。经过小鼠模型测试,含有氯光敏剂(Ce6)的 PEG 纳米配方对卵巢癌具有良好的疗效[33,34]。通过使用有效的光敏剂和近红外辐射,可以增加卵巢癌组织深度穿透能力。然而,在腹腔内应用 PDT 仍然面临挑战。一项在乳腺癌小鼠模型上进行的近红外与 NP 结合 Ce6 联合给药研究表明,PDT 表现出更好的组织穿透性和较低毒性[40,41]。

一种经过体外测试的卟啉光敏剂,在经过病毒衣壳包裹和靶向核仁素的适配体修饰后,能够具备特异性靶向乳腺癌细胞的能力[97]。这种核仁蛋白受体在卵巢癌细胞中也高度表达,扩大了类似系统靶向治疗的适应证。当接受可见光照射时,功能化富勒烯显示出产生活性氧(reactive oxygen species,ROS)的能力。根据这一特点,有研究对结肠腺癌小鼠模型进行了 IP PDT 测试,结果表明富勒烯作为有效光敏剂,无论是通过静脉注射还是暴露疗法,对细菌感染和纤维肉瘤都具备良好的疗效[98-100]。随着光敏剂技术不断改进,以及 NP 递送系统的进一步发展,未来 PDT 具有广阔的前景。

NP 系统由于具备更好的生物相容性,常被用于质粒和寡核苷酸递送。通常会对其电荷进行修饰使其与核苷酸有效结合,以实现药物递送[101-103]。目前已有多种基因递送方法利用功能化 NP 实现药物靶向递送至卵巢癌细胞[102]。

通过强有力地表达肿瘤抑制基因,可以将 DNA 质粒传递到癌细胞。由于大多数癌症病例中都能监测到肿瘤蛋白 53(tumor protein53,TP53)高频突变,目前正考虑采用 NP 靶向该抑制基因的方法进行临床试验。最近进行的"SGT-53"临床试验就是其中一项。SGT-53 是一种抗转铁蛋白受体单链可变片段(single-chain variable fragment,scFV)抗体,可与脂质体纳米载体结合,用于传递 TP53 基因。这项研究表明该技术能够稳定患者体内不同来源的肿瘤,同时并没有显著毒性,因此令人印象深刻[104]。几乎所有高级别卵巢浆液性癌患者都存在 TP53 突变,所以针对它的靶向治疗可能使这些患者获益。在 20 世纪 90 年代,曾尝试通过腺病毒靶向递送 TP53 基因(Ad-p53)进行临床试验。然而,该系统对患者的疗效并不显著,因为体内存在的抗体会将合并的病毒识别为外来颗粒而无法到达肿瘤部位[105]。NP 可用于将遗传物质传递到卵巢癌部位。在随后的Ⅰ期和Ⅱ期临床试验中,联合使用脂质体人类腺病毒 5 型早期区域 1A(human adenovirus type 5 early region 1A,HA-E1A)和紫杉醇治疗铂类耐药的卵巢癌患者时显示出较低毒性。但这种治疗方法的长期效果尚未报告[106]。2013 年进行了一项Ⅰ期临床试验,采用 PEG-聚乙烯亚胺[poly(ethylene imine),PEI]-胆固醇脂质体向腹腔内输送编码为白介素 12(interleukin 12,IL-12)(EGEN-001 试验)的质粒。这一试验的目的是唤起患者对癌细胞的局部免疫反应。患者通过增强 IL-12 刺激的细胞因子(γ干扰素和肿瘤坏死因子-α)产生积极反应,其毒性亦在可接受范围内[107]。目前正在进行Ⅱ期临床试验,探索 IP EGEN-001 或联合 IP Doxil 治疗复发性或难治性卵巢癌。

NP 已被应用于传递表达载体,以实现对卵巢癌细胞诱导抗肿瘤作用的成功摄取和表达。为了通过成功的摄取和表达引发抗肿瘤作用,NP 已被用于将表达载体传递到卵巢癌细胞。其中,纳米凝胶肝素-聚乙烯亚胺(heparin-polyethyleneimine,Heparin-PE)被用于传递携带硫酸肝素-6-O-内硫酸酯酶 1(heparin sulfate 6-O-endosulfatase 1,HSulf-1)[108]和丝胶 1A 互作蛋白 1(filamin A interacting protein 1-like,FILIP1L)[109]基因的 DNA 质粒,这些蛋白质在卵巢癌中通常受到负调控。将含有这些基因的 NP 表达载体通过腹腔注射到裸鼠异种移植物中后,观察到显著的细胞死亡、细胞增殖减少,以及血管生成停止等结果。此外,顺铂治疗能够进一步促使 $Hsulf-1$ 基因表达增强[108]。

NP 聚合物能够有效地递送干扰小 RNA(small interfering,siRNA)或短发夹核糖核酸(short hairpin RNA,shRNA)从而抑制致癌基因的表达。首个此类临床试验表明,肿瘤患者静脉注射 RNAi/寡核苷酸纳米颗粒传输(RNAi/oligonucleotide nanoparticle delivery,RONDEL)后核糖核苷酸还原酶的 M2 亚基(M2 subunit of ribonucleotide reductase，RRM2)水平显著降低[110]。这种基于聚乙二醇化环糊精的 NP 聚合物能够嵌入以其相应受体为靶点的转铁蛋白体。与其类似，另一项关于脂质体 siRNA 纳米载体向驱动蛋白纺锤体蛋白(ALN-VSP)和血管内皮生长因子(vascular endothelial growth factor，VEGF)肿瘤靶向递送的 II 期临床试验表明，NP 聚合物有较高的肿瘤靶向性和较低的毒性[111]。表 6-4 列出了一些有前景的基于 NP 的基因治疗的临床前研究。

表 6-4　基于 NP 的基因疗法的临床前研究

基因靶向肿瘤抑制因子	纳米颗粒组合		靶点	参考文献
人腺病毒 5 型 E1A 试验药物："tgDCC-E1"	质粒载体	脂质体	—	Phase I and II: NCT00102622[106,112]
	质粒载体	PEG-PEI-胆固醇脂质体	—	Phase I: NCT01489371 Phase I: NCT00473954 Phase II: NCT01118052[107]
硫酸肝素-6-O-内硫酸酯酶 1	质粒载体	肝素-聚乙烯亚胺纳米凝胶	—	Xenograft[108]
FILIP1L	质粒载体	肝素-聚乙烯亚胺纳米凝胶	—	Xenograft[109]
白喉毒素	质粒载体(卵巢特异性 HE 4 和 MSLN 启动子)	聚 β-氨基酯聚合物-DNA 复合物	—	Xenograft[113]
HIF1α	siRNA	脂质体	—	Xenograft[114]
PARP1	siRNA	脂质体	—	Xenograft[115]
Src	siRNA	壳聚糖	—	Xenograft[116]
Claudin-3	2 种 shRNA 质粒载体的共递送	PLGA 纳米颗粒	—	Xenograft[117]
CD44 and FAK	2 种 shRNA 质粒载体的共递送	PLGA 纳米颗粒	—	Xenograft[118]

续表

基因靶向肿瘤抑制因子	纳米颗粒组合		靶点	参考文献
EphA2 临床试验药物："siRNAEphA2-DOPC"	siRNA	负载 DOPC 脂质体的介孔硅	—	Xenograft[119,120] Phase Ⅰ：NCT01591356
EphA2 miR-520d-3p (targets EphB2)	与 miRNA 的共传递送的 siRNA	负载 DOPC 脂质体的介孔硅		Xenograft[121]
Jagged1	siRNA		—	Xenograft[122]
EGFR	siRNA		EphA2	Cell lines[123]
STAT3 and FAK	siRNA	HDL 纳米颗粒	SR-B1	Xenograft[124]
ID4	siRNA	Peptide 纳米颗粒	神经纤毛蛋白-1	Xenograft[108]
PLXDC1	siRNA	壳聚糖	整合蛋白	Xenograft[125]
—	非靶向 siRNA	聚乙烯亚胺纳米颗粒	聚乙烯亚胺纳米颗粒	Xenograft[126,127]

在卵巢癌中，酪氨酸激酶肝配蛋白（ephrin）受体 EphA2 的高表达与血管生成率和转移侵袭呈正相关[119,121,128-130]。

基于卵巢癌异种移植小鼠的试验表明，采用 NP 介导的 siRNA 递送抑制 EphA2 的表达后，可显著缩小肿瘤体积[119-121]。将 EphA2 siRNA 装载于硅颗粒上可以实现二油酰基磷脂酰胆碱（dioleoyl-phosphatidylcholine，DOPC）脂质体持续缓慢释放[131]，从而有效下调 EphA2 水平。这种下调进一步提高了 HeyA8 卵巢肿瘤对多西他赛的敏感性，同时，对于接受多西他赛和 siRNA 治疗的动物，还能起到抑制肿瘤生长的作用[119]。

一项癌症研究指出，在 DOPC 脂质体/硅纳米颗粒中，microRNA（miR-520d3p）和 EphA2 siRNA 的共传递能够提高针对异种移植物的抗肿瘤作用。miR 520d3p 通常通过靶向另一种 ephrin 受体 EphB2 来发挥作用，并与卵巢癌患者的预后相关[121]。

Dickerson 等开发了一种水凝胶 NP，可用于提高卵巢癌表皮生长因子受体（epidermal growth factor receptor，EGFR）siRNA 负荷。这些 NP 通过与 EphA2 肽受体结合而激活，在水凝胶中实现了对 EGFR 表达的下调，并增强了 EphA2 阳性细胞对多西他赛的敏感性[123]。尽管小分子靶向 EGFR 在临床试验中未发现获益,但利用 EphA2 特异性肽功能化的纳米颗粒可能有助于提高其在卵巢癌细胞中的定位。

清道夫受体 B1 型(scavenger receptor type B1,SR-B1)在肿瘤细胞中高度表达,并与脂蛋白结合以维持快速生长。当在结肠癌和卵巢癌小鼠模型中应用信号转导及转录活化因子 3(signal transducer and activator of transcription 3,STAT3)和黏附激酶的 siRNA 封装脂质体 NP 时,发现其能够增强肿瘤靶向性和蛋白沉默效果[124]。

DNA 结合抑制剂 4(inhibitor of DNA binding 4,ID4)是卵巢癌增殖所必需的转录调节因子[108]。siRNA 通过静电作用与串联肽序列结合可以降低 ID4 的表达水平。该肽由精氨酸结构域和肿瘤穿透结构域组成,形成环状纳米肽 LyP-1。已有研究证明,这种技术可以提高对肿瘤的靶向性和血管穿透能力[132]。将 ID4-siRNA 纳米复合物注射到异种移植物中,可抑制皮下肿瘤细胞生长。此外,在原位卵巢癌异种移植物中进行 IP 治疗也能够抑制肿瘤生长[108]。

同样,具有精氨酰甘氨酰天冬氨酸肽链的壳聚糖 NP 也已被开发出来,以实现靶向整合素受体,并特异性递送卵巢癌细胞增殖的基因的 siRNA。在小鼠移植瘤模型中进行测试时,结果显示,肿瘤生长得到抑制[125]。

此外,NP 基因治疗还被应用于调控肿瘤微环境。某些卵巢癌细胞和微环境中高表达 Notch 配体 Jagged1,可以采用壳聚糖作为载体来递送针对该配体的 siRNA。给予壳聚糖 NP 可以下调人类肿瘤细胞或小鼠基质细胞来源的 Jagged-1 表达,并有效减少了微环境诱导血管生成及移植物增殖[122]。

树突状细胞在肿瘤微环境中优先摄取聚乙烯亚胺基(PEI 基)NP。这些颗粒在装载非靶向 siRNA 时,可通过 Toll 样受体 5 诱导免疫反应[126,127]。大多数 NP 基因或 RNAi 递送策略仍处于Ⅰ或Ⅱ期临床试验中。然而,在不久的未来,它们作为新策略的应用备受期待。

七、结论

总而言之,当前 NP 在卵巢癌治疗中越来越受到青睐。由于它们的特性,NP 除在肿瘤检测和成像方面有巨大的应用外,还具有将治疗药物特异性递送到靶向部位的出色能力。无论如何,靶向和非靶向 NP 系统的进一步发展预计将很快进入临床试验阶段,同时基于 NP 的新策略将在不久的将来应用于卵巢癌的治疗。

致谢

作者感谢印度科学院生物技术系、印度科学院甘地技术与管理研究所,维萨卡帕特南,安得拉邦,印度。

利益冲突

作者声明不存在利益冲突。

参 考 文 献

[1] Bray F, Ferlay J, Soerjomataram I, Siegel RL, Torre LA, Jemal A. Global Cancer Statistics 2018: GLOBOCAN estimates of incidence and mortality worldwide for 36 cancers in 185 countries. CA Cancer J Clin 2018;68:394-424.

[2] Vaughan S, Coward JI, Bast Jr. RC, Berchuck A, Berek JS, Brenton JD, Coukos G, Crum CC, Drapkin R, Etemadmoghadam D, Friedlander M, Gabra H, Kaye SB, Lord CJ, Lengyel E, Levine DA, McNeish IA, Menon U, Mills GB, Nephew KP, Oza AM, Sood AK, Stonach EA, Walczak H, Bowtell DD, Balkwill FR. Rethinking ovarian cancer: recommendations for improving outcomes. Nat Rev Cancer 2011;11:719-25.

[3] Banerjee S, Kaye SB. New strategies in the treatment of ovarian cancer: current clinical perspectives and future potential. Clin Cancer Res 2013;19:961-8.

[4] Prat J. Ovarian carcinomas: five distinct diseases with different origins, genetic alterations, and clinicopathological features. Virchows Arch 2012;460:237-49.

[5] Berns EM, Bowtell DD. The changing view of high-grade serous ovarian cancer. Cancer Res 2012;72:2701-4.

[6] Kurman RJ, Shih IM. Molecular pathogenesis and extraovarian origin of epithelial ovarian cancer—shifting the paradigm. Hum Pathol 2011;42:918-31.

[7] Landen Jr. CN, Birrer MJ, Sood AK. Early events in the pathogenesis of epithelial ovarian cancer. J Clin Oncol 2008;26:995-1005.

[8] Cancer Genome Atlas Research Network. Integrated genomic analyses of ovarian carcinoma. Nature 2011;474:609-15.

[9] Jelovac D, Armstrong DK. Recent progress in the diagnosis and treatment of ovarian cancer. CA Cancer J Clin 2011;61:183-203.

[10] Piek JM, Verheijen RH, Kenemans P, Massuger LF, Bulten H, van Diest PJ. BRCA1/2-related ovarian cancers are of tubal origin: a hypothesis. Gynecol Oncol 2003;90:491.

[11] Tan DS, Agarwal R, Kaye SB. Mechanisms of transcoelomic metastasis in ovarian cancer. Lancet Oncol 2006;7:925-34.

[12] Davidson B. Ovarian carcinoma and serous effusions. Changing views regarding tumor progression and review of current literature. Anal Cell Pathol 2001;23:107-28.

[13] Husseinzadeh N. Status of tumor markers in epithelial ovarian cancer has there been any progress? A review. Gynecol Oncol 2011;120:152-7.

[14] Bast Jr. RC, Feeney M, Lazarus H, Nadler LM, Colvin RB, Knapp RC. Reactivity of a

monoclonal antibody with human ovarian carcinoma. J Clin Invest 1981;68:1331-7.

[15] Qian Y, Wang Y, Zhang X, Zhou L, Zhang Z, Xu J, Ruan Y, Ren S, Xu C, Gu J. Quantitative analysis of serum IgG galactosylation assists differential diagnosis of ovarian cancer. J Proteome Res 2013;12:4046-55.

[16] Biskup K, Braicu EI, Sehouli J, Fotopoulou C, Tauber R, Berger M, Blanchard V. Serum glycome profiling: a biomarker for diagnosis of ovarian cancer. J Proteome Res 2013;12: 4056-63.

[17] Li B, An HJ, Kirmiz C, Lebrilla CB, Lam KS, Miyamoto S. Glycoproteomic analyses of ovarian cancer cell lines and sera from ovarian cancer patients show distinct glycosylation changes in individual proteins. J Proteome Res 2008;7:3776-88.

[18] Saldova R, Royle L, Radcliffe CM, Abd Hamid UM, Evans R, Arnold JN, Banks RE, Hutson R, Harvey DJ, Antrobus R, Petrescu SM, Dwek RA, Rudd PM. Ovarian cancer is associated with changes in glycosylation in both acute-phase proteins and IgG. Glycobiology 2007;17:1344-56.

[19] Moore RG, McMeekin DS, Brown AK, DiSilvestro P, Miller MC, Allard WJ, Gajewski W, Kurman R, Bast Jr. RC, Skates SJ. A novel multiple marker bioassay utilizing HE4 and CA125 for the prediction of ovarian cancer in patients with a pelvic mass. Gynecol Oncol 2009;112:40-6.

[20] Moore LE, Pfeiffer RM, Zhang Z, Lu KH, Fung ET, Bast Jr. RC. Proteomic biomarkers in combination with CA 125 for detection of epithelial ovarian cancer using prediagnostic serum samples from the Prostate, Lung, Colorectal, and Ovarian (PLCO) Cancer Screening Trial. Cancer 2012;118:91-100.

[21] Zhang Z, Chan DW. The road from discovery to clinical diagnostics: lessons learned from the first FDA-cleared in vitro diagnostic multivariate index assay of proteomic biomarkers. Cancer Epidemiol Biomarkers Prev 2010;19:2995-9.

[22] Armstrong DK, Bundy B, Wenzel L, Huang HQ, Baergen R, Lele S, Copeland LJ, Walker JL, Burger RA, Gyencologic Oncology Group. Intraperitoneal cisplatin and paclitaxel in ovarian cancer. N Engl J Med 2006;354:34-43.

[23] Jaaback K, Johnson N, Lawrie TA. Intraperitoneal chemotherapy for the initial management of primary epithelial ovarian cancer. Cochrane Database Syst Rev 2011; CD005340.

[24] Nolen BM, Lokshin AE. Biomarker testing for ovarian cancer: clinical utility of multiplex assays. Mol Diagn Ther 2013;17:139-46.

[25] Sarojini S, Tamir A, Lim H, Li S, Zhang S, Goy A, Pecora A, Suh KS. Early detection biomarkers for ovarian cancer. J Oncol 2012;2012:709049.

[26] Swierczewska M, Liu G, Lee S, Chen X. Highsensitivity nanosensors for biomarker detection. Chem Soc Rev 2012;41:2641-55.

[27] Perfezou M, Turner A, Merkoci A. Cancer detection using nanoparticle-based sensors. Chem Soc Rev 2012;41:2606-22.

[28] Bellan LM, Wu D, Langer RS. Current trends in nanobiosensor technology. Rev Nanomed Nanobiotechnol 2011;3:229-46.

[29] Kimmel DW, LeBlanc G, Meschievitz ME, Cliffel DE. Electrochemical sensors and biosensors. Anal Chem 2011;84:685-707.

[30] Jokerst JV, Raamanathan A, Christodoulides N, Floriano PN, Pollard AA, Simmons GW, Wong J, Gage C, Furmaga WB, Redding SW, McDevitt JT. Nano-bio-chips for high performance multiplexed protein detection: determinations of cancer biomarkers in serum and saliva using quantum dot bioconjugate labels. Biosens Bioelectron 2009;24:3622-9.

[31] Raamanathan A, Simmons GW, Christodoulides N, Floriano PN, Furmaga WB, Redding SW, Lu KH, Bast Jr. RC, McDevitt JT. Programmable bio-nano-chip systems for serum CA125 quantification: toward ovarian cancer diagnostics at the point-of-care. Cancer Prev Res (Phila) 2012;5:706-16.

[32] Ravalli A, dos Santos GP, Ferroni M, Faglia G, Yamanaka H, Marrazza G. New label free CA125 detection based on gold nanostructured screen-printed electrode. Sens Actuators B 2013;179: 194-200.

[33] Li J, Xu Q, Fu C, Zhang Y. A dramatically enhanced electrochemiluminescence assay for CA125 based on dendrimer multiply labeled luminol on Fe_3O_4 nanoparticles. Sens Actuators B 2013;185: 146-53.

[34] Li Z, Wang C, Cheng L, Gong H, Yin S, Gong Q, Li Y, Liu Z. PEG-functionalized iron oxide nanoclusters loaded with chlorin e6 for targeted, NIR light induced, photodynamic therapy. Biomaterials 2013;34:9160-70.

[35] Fleischer AC, Lyshchik A, Andreotti RF, Hwang M, Jones HW, Fishman DA. Advances in sonographic detection of ovarian cancer: depiction of tumor neovascularity with microbubbles. Am J Roentgenol 2010;194:343-8.

[36] Fleischer AC, Lyshchik A, Jones Jr. HW, Crispens M, Loveless M, Andreotti RF, Williams PK, Fishman DA. Contrast-enhanced transvaginal sonography of benign versus malignant ovarian masses: preliminary findings. J Ultrasound Med 2008;27:1011-8.

[37] Fleischer AC, Lyshchik A, Hirari M, Moore RD, Abramson RG, Fishman DA. Early detection of ovarian cancer with conventional and contrast-enhanced transvaginal sonography: recent advances and potential improvements. J Oncol 2012;2012:11.

[38] Xu H, Regino CAS, Koyama Y, Hama Y, Gunn AJ, Bernardo M, Kobayashi H, Choyke PL, Brechbiel MW. Preparation and preliminary evaluation of a biotin-targeted, lectin-targeted dendrimer-based probe for dual-modality magnetic resonance and fluorescence imaging. Bioconjug Chem 2007;18:1474-82.

[39] Kamaly N, Kalber T, Thanou M, Bell JD, Miller AD. Folate receptor targeted bimodal liposomes for tumor magnetic resonance imaging. Bioconjug Chem 2009;20:648-55.

[40] Wang L, Neoh KG, Kang E-T, Shuter B. Multifunctional polyglycerol-grafted $Fe_3O_4@SiO_2$ nanoparticles for targeting ovarian cancer cells. Biomaterials 2011;32:2166-73.

[41] Wang C, Tao H, Cheng L, Liu Z. Near-infrared light induced in vivo photodynamic therapy of cancer based on upconversion nanoparticles. Biomaterials 2011;32:6145-54.

[42] Zhou Z, Wang L, Chi X, Bao J, Yang L, Zhao W, Chen Z, Wang X, Chen X, Gao J. Engineered iron-oxide-based nanoparticles as enhanced T1 contrast agents for efficient tumor imaging. ACS Nano 2013;7:3287-96.

[43] Misri R, Meier D, Yung AC, Kozlowski P, Häfeli UO. Development and evaluation of a dualmodality (MRI/SPECT) molecular imaging bioprobe. Nanomedicine 2012;8:1007-16.

[44] Schädlich A, Caysa H, Mueller T, Tenambergen F, Rose C, Goöpferich A, Kuntsche J, Mäder K. Tumor accumulation of NIR fluorescent PEG-PLA nanoparticles: impact of particle size and human xenograft tumor model. ACS Nano 2011;5:8710-20.

[45] Katragadda U, Fan W, Wang Y, Teng Q, Tan C. Combined delivery of paclitaxel and tanespimycin via micellar nanocarriers: pharmacokinetics, efficacy and metabolomic analysis. PLoS One 2013;8: e58619.

[46] Zdobnova TA, Dorofeev SG, Tananaev PN, Zlomanov VP, Stremovskiy OA, Lebedenko EN, Balalaeva IV, Deyev SM, Petrov RV. Imaging of human ovarian cancer SKOV-3 cells by quantum dot bioconjugates. Dokl Biochem Biophys 2010;430:41-4.

[47] Nathwani BB, Jaffari M, Juriani AR, Mathur AB, Meissner KE. Fabrication and characterization of silk-fibroin-coated quantum dots. IEEE Trans Nanobioscience 2009;8:72-7.

[48] Wang H-Z, Wang H-Y, Liang R-Q, Ruan K-C. Detection of tumor marker CA125 in ovarian carcinoma using quantum dots. Acta Biochim Biophys Sin 2004;36:681-6.

[49] Savla R, Taratula O, Garbuzenko O, Minko T. Tumor targeted quantum dot-mucin 1 aptamerdoxorubicin conjugate for imaging and treatment of cancer. J Control Release 2011;153:16-22.

[50] Jokerst JV, Cole AJ, Van de Sompel D, Gambhir SS. Gold nanorods for ovarian cancer detection with photoacoustic imaging and resection guidance via raman imaging in living mice. ACS Nano 2012;6:10366-77.

[51] Gabizon A, Catane R, Uziely B, Kaufman B, Safra T, Cohen R, Martin F, Huang A, Barenholz Y. Prolonged circulation time and enhanced accumulation in malignant exudates of doxorubicin encapsulated in polyethylene-glycol coated liposomes. Cancer Res 1994;54:987-92.

[52] Muggia FM, Hainsworth JD, Jeffers S, Miller P, Groshen S, Tan M, Roman L, Uziely B, Muderspach L, Garcia A, Burnett A, Greco FA, Morrow CP, Paradiso LJ, Liang LJ. Phase II study of liposomal doxorubicin in refractory ovarian cancer: antitumor activity and toxicity modification by liposomal encapsulation. J Clin Oncol 1997;15:987-93.

[53] Ferrandina G, Ludovisi M, Lorusso D, Pignata S, Breda E, Savarese A, Del Medico P, Scaltriti L, Katsaros D, Priolo D, Scambia G. Phase III trial of gemcitabine compared with pegylated liposomal doxorubicin in progressive or recurrent ovarian cancer. J Clin Oncol 2008;26:890-6.

[54] Mutch DG, Orlando M, Goss T, Teneriello MG, Gordon AN, McMeekin SD, Wang Y, Scribner Jr. DR, Marciniack M, Naumann RW, Secord AA. Randomized phase Ⅲ trial of gemcitabine compared with pegylated liposomal doxorubicin in patients with platinum-resistant ovarian cancer. J Clin Oncol 2007;25:2811-8.

[55] Gordon AN, Tonda M, Sun S, Rackoff W. Long-term survival advantage for women treated with pegylated liposomal doxorubicin compared with topotecan in a phase 3 randomized study of recurrent and refractory epithelial ovarian cancer. Gynecol Oncol 2004;95:1-8.

[56] Gordon AN, Fleagle JT, Guthrie D, Parkin DE, Gore ME, Lacave AJ. Recurrent epithelial ovarian carcinoma: a randomized phase Ⅲ study of pegylated liposomal doxorubicin versus topotecan. J Clin Oncol 2001;19:3312-22.

[57] Wagner U, Marth C, Largillier R, Kaern J, Brown C, Heywood M, Bonaventura T, Vergote I, Piccirillo MC, Fossati R, Gebski V, Lauraine EP. Final overall survival results of phase Ⅲ GCIG CALYPSO trial of pegylated liposomal doxorubicin and carboplatin vs paclitaxel and carboplatin in platinum-sensitive ovarian cancer patients. Br J Cancer 2012;107:588-91.

[58] Poveda A, Vergote I, Tjulandin S, Kong B, Roy M, Chan S, Filipczyk-Cisarz E, Hagberg H, Kaye SB, Colombo N, Lebedinsky C, Parekh T, Gómez J, Park YC, Alfaro V, Monk BJ. Trabectedin plus pegylated liposomal doxorubicin in relapsed ovarian cancer: outcomes in the partially platinumsensitive (platinum-free interval 6-12 months) subpopulation of OVA-301 phase Ⅲ randomized trial. Ann Oncol 2011;22:39-48.

[59] Monk BJ, Herzog TJ, Kaye SB, Krasner CN, Vermorken JB, Muggia FM, PujadeLauranine E, Lisyanskaya AS, Makhson AN, Rolski J, Gorbounova VA, Ghatage P, Bidzinski M, Shen K, Ngan HY, Vergote IB, Nam JH, Park YC, Lebedinsky CA, Poveda AM. Trabectedin plus pegylated liposomal doxorubicin in recurrent ovarian cancer. J Clin Oncol 2010;28:3107-14.

[60] Herzog TJ. Update on the role of topotecan in the treatment of recurrent ovarian cancer. Oncologist 2002;7(Suppl 5):3-10.

[61] Dadashzadeh S, Vali AM, Rezaie M. The effect of PEG coating on in vitro cytotoxicity and in vivo disposition of topotecan loaded liposomes in rats. Int J Pharm 2008;353:251-9.

[62] Ma Y, Yang Q, Wang L, Zhou X, Zhao Y, Deng Y. Repeated injections of PEGylated liposomal topotecan induces accelerated blood clearance phenomenon in rats. Eur J Pharm Sci 2012; 45:539-45.

[63] Dark GG, Calvert AH, Grimshaw R, Poole C, Swenerton K, Kaye S, Coleman R, Jayson G, Le T, Ellard S, Trudeau M, Vasey P, Hamilton M, Cameron T, Barrett E, Walsh W, Mcintosh L, Eisenhauer EA. Randomized trial of two intravenous schedules of the topoisomerase I inhibitor liposomal lurtotecan in women with relapsed epithelial ovarian cancer: a trial of the National Cancer Institute of Canada Clinical Trials Group. J Clin Oncol 2005;23:1859-66.

[64] Ma P, Russell J. Mumper, paclitaxel nano-delivery systems: a comprehensive review. J Nanomed Nanotechnol 2013;18:1000164-99.

[65] Mirtsching B, Cosgriff T, Harker G, Keaton M, Chidiac T, Min M. A phase II study of weekly nanoparticle albumin-bound paclitaxel with or without trastuzumab in metastatic breast cancer. Clin Breast Cancer 2011;11:121-8.

[66] Micha JP, Goldstein BH, Birk CL, Rettenmaier MA, Brown 3rd. JV. Abraxane in the treatment of ovarian cancer: the absence of hypersensitivity reactions. Gynecol Oncol 2006;100:437-8.

[67] Coleman RL, Brady WE, McMeekin DS, Rose PG, Soper JT, Lentz SS, Hoffman JS, Shahin MS. A phase II evaluation of nanoparticle, albumin-bound (nab) paclitaxel in the treatment of recurrent or persistent platinum-resistant ovarian, fallopian tube, or primary peritoneal cancer: a Gynecologic Oncology Group study. Gynecol Oncol 2011;122:111-5.

[68] Teneriello MG, Tseng PC, Crozier M, Encarnacion C, Hancock K, Messing MJ, Boehm KA, Williams A, Asmar L. Phase II evaluation of nanoparticle albumin-bound paclitaxel in platinum-sensitive patients with recurrent ovarian, peritoneal, or fallopian tube cancer. J Clin Oncol 2009;27:1426-31.

[69] Singer JW. Paclitaxel poliglumex (XYOTAX, CT-2103): a macromolecular taxane. J Control Release 2005;109:120-6.

[70] Sabbatini P, Sill MW, O'Malley D, Adler L, Secord AA, Gynecologic Oncology Group S. A phase II trial of paclitaxel poliglumex in recurrent or persistent ovarian or primary peritoneal cancer (EOC): a Gynecologic Oncology Group study. Gynecol Oncol 2008;111:455-60.

[71] Awada A, Garcia AA, Chan S, Jerusalem GH, Coleman RE, Huizing MT, Mehdi A, O'Reilly SM, Hamm JT, Barrett-Lee PJ, Cocquyt V, Sideras K, Young DE, Zhao C, Chia YL, Hoch U, Hannah AL, Perez EA; NKTR-102 Study Group. Two schedules of etirinotecan pegol (NKTR-102) in patients with previously treated metastatic breast cancer: a randomised phase 2 study. Lancet Oncol 2013;14:1216-25.

[72] Iqbal S, Tsao-Wei DD, Quinn DI, Gitlitz BJ, Groshen S, Aparicio A, Lenz HJ, El-Khoueiry A, Pinski J, Garcia AA. Phase I clinical trial of pegylated liposomal doxorubicin and docetaxel in patients with advanced solid tumors. Am J Clin Oncol 2011;34:27-31.

[73] Svenson S, Wolfgang M, Hwang J, Ryan J, Eliasof S. Preclinical to clinical development of the novel camptothecin nanopharmaceutical CRLX101. J Control Release 2011;153:49-55.

[74] Nowotnik DP, Cvitkovic E. ProLindac (AP5346): a review of the development of an HPMA DACH platinum polymer therapeutic. Adv Drug Deliv Rev 2009;61:1214-9.

[75] Duncan R. Development of HPMA copolymer-anticancer conjugates: clinical experience and lessons learnt. Adv Drug Deliv Rev 2009;61:1131-48.

[76] Lin X, Zhang Q, Rice JR, Stewart DR, Nowotnik DP, Howell SB. Improved targeting of

platinum chemotherapeutics. The antitumour activity of the HPMA copolymer platinum agent AP5280 in murine tumour models. Eur J Cancer 2004;40:291-7.

[77] Desale SS, Cohen SM, Zhao Y, Kabanov AV, Bronich TK. Biodegradable hybrid polymer micelles for combination drug therapy in ovarian cancer. J Control Release 2013;171: 339-48.

[78] Gong C, Yang B, Qian Z, Zhao X, Wu Q, Qi X, Wang Y, Guo G, Kan B, Luo F, Wei Y. Improving intraperitoneal chemotherapeutic effect and preventing postsurgical adhesions simultaneously with biodegradable micelles. Nanomedicine 2012;8:963-73.

[79] Cho H, Lai TC, Kwon GS. Poly(ethylene glycol)-block-poly(epsilon-caprolactone) micelles for combination drug delivery: evaluation of paclitaxel, cyclopamine and gossypol in intraperitoneal xenograft models of ovarian cancer. J Control Release 2013;166:1-9.

[80] Kirkpatrick GJ, Plumb JA, Sutcliffe OB, Flint DJ, Wheate NJ. Evaluation of anionic half generation 3.5-6.5 poly(amidoamine) dendrimers as delivery vehicles for the active component of the anticancer drug cisplatin. J Inorg Biochem 2011;105:1115-22.

[81] Zhu S, Hong M, Tang G, Qian L, Lin J, Jiang Y, Pei Y. Partly PEGylated polyamidoamine dendrimer for tumor-selective targeting of doxorubicin: the effects of PEGylation degree and drug conjugation style. Biomaterials 2010;31:1360-71.

[82] Zhu S, Hong M, Zhang L, Tang G, Jiang Y, Pei Y. PEGylated PAMAM dendrimerdoxorubicin conjugates: in vitro evaluation and in vivo tumor accumulation. Pharm Res 2010; 27:161-74.

[83] Kurtoglu YE, Mishra MK, Kannan S, Kannan RM. Drug release characteristics of PAMAM dendrimer-drug conjugates with different linkers. Int J Pharm 2010;384:189-94.

[84] Xiao K, Luo J, Fowler WL, Li Y, Lee JS, Xing L, Cheng RH, Wang L, Lam KS. A self-assembling nanoparticle for paclitaxel delivery in ovarian cancer. Biomaterials 2009; 30:6006-16.

[85] Xiao W, Luo J, Jain T, Riggs JW, Tseng HP, Henderson PT, Cherry SR, Rowland D, Lam KS. Biodistribution and pharmacokinetics of a telodendrimer micellar paclitaxel nanoformulation in a mouse xenograft model of ovarian cancer. Int J Nanomedicine 2012;7: 1587-97.

[86] Xiao K, Li Y, Lee JS, Gonik AM, Dong T, Fung G, Sanchez E, Xing L, Cheng HR, Luo J, Lam KS. "OA02" peptide facilitates the precise targeting of paclitaxel-loaded micellar nanoparticles to ovarian cancer in vivo. Cancer Res 2012;72:2100-10.

[87] Van Vlerken LE, Duan Z, Little SR, Seiden MV, Amiji MM. Augmentation of therapeutic efficacy in drug-resistant tumor models using ceramide coadministration in temporalcontrolled polymer-blend nanoparticle delivery systems. AAPS J 2010;12:171-80.

[88] Wagstaff AJ, Brown SD, Holden MR, Craig GE, Plumb JA, Brown RE, Schreiter N, Chrzanowski W, Wheate NJ. Cisplatin drug delivery using gold-coated iron oxide nanoparticles for enhanced tumour targeting with external magnetic fields. Inorg Chim Acta 2012;

393:328-33.

[89] Qin Y, Song Q-G, Zhang Z-R, Liu J, Fu Y, He Q, Liu J. Ovarian tumor targeting of docetaxelloaded liposomes mediated by luteinizing hormone-releasing hormone analogues. Arzneimittelforschung 2008;58:529-34.

[90] Nukolova NV, Oberoi HS, Cohen SM, Kabanov AV, Bronich TK. Folate-decorated nanogels for targeted therapy of ovarian cancer. Biomaterials 2011;32:5417-26.

[91] Nukolova NV, Oberoi HS, Zhao Y, Chekhonin VP, Kabanov AV, Bronich TK. LHRH-targeted nanogels as a delivery system for cisplatin to ovarian cancer. Mol Pharm 2013;10: 3913-21.

[92] Gao ZG, Lee DH, Kim DI, Bae YH. Doxorubicin loaded pH-sensitive micelle targeting acidic extracellular pH of human ovarian A2780 tumor in mice. J Drug Target 2005;13:391-7.

[93] Kim D, Lee ES, Park K, Kwon IC, Bae YH. Doxorubicin loaded pH-sensitive micelle: antitumoral efficacy against ovarian A2780/DOXR tumor. Pharm Res 2008;25:2074-82.

[94] Kim D, Gao ZG, Lee ES, Bae YH. In vivo evaluation of doxorubicin-loaded polymeric micelles targeting folate receptors and early endosomal pH in drug-resistant ovarian cancer. Mol Pharm 2009;6:1353-62.

[95] Zeisser-Labouebe M, Lange N, Gurny R, Delie F. Hypericin-loaded nanoparticles for the photodynamic treatment of ovarian cancer. Int J Pharm 2006;326:174-81.

[96] Zeisser-Labouébe M, Delie F, Gurny R, Lange N. Benefits of nanoencapsulation for the hypercinmediated photodetection of ovarian micrometastases. Eur J Pharm Biopharma 2009;71:207-13.

[97] Cohen BA, Bergkvist M. Targeted in vitro photodynamic therapy via aptamer-labeled, porphyrinloaded virus capsids. J Photochem Photobiol B 2013;121:67-74.

[98] Mroz P, Xia Y, Asanuma D, Konopko A, Zhiyentayev T, Huang YY, Sharma SK, Dai T, Khan UJ, Wharton T, Hamblin MR. Intraperitoneal photodynamic therapy mediated by a fullerene in a mouse model of abdominal dissemination of colon adenocarcinoma. Nanomedicine 2011;7:965-74.

[99] Liu J, Ohta S, Sonoda A, Yamada M, Yamamoto M, Nitta N, Murata K, Tabata Y. Preparation of PEG-conjugated fullerene containing Gd3+ ions for photodynamic therapy. J Control Release 2007;117:104-10.

[100] Tabata Y, Murakami Y, Ikada Y. Photodynamic effect of polyethylene glycol-modified fullerene on tumor. Jpn J Cancer Res 1997;88:1108-16.

[101] Heidel JD, Schluep T. Cyclodextrin-containing polymers: versatile platforms of drug delivery materials. J Drug Deliv 2012;2012:262731.

[102] Kim DH, Rossi JJ. Strategies for silencing human disease using RNA interference. Nat Rev Genet 2007;8:173-84.

[103] Mansouri S, Cuie Y, Winnik F, Shi Q, Lavigne P, Benderdour M, Beaumont E, Fernandes JC. Characterization of folate-chitosan-DNA nanoparticles for gene therapy. Bio-

materials 2006;27:2060-5.

[104] Senzer N, Nemunaitis J, Nemunaitis D, Bedell C, Edelman G, Barve M, Nunan R, Pirollo KF, Rait A, Chang EH. Phase I study of a systemically delivered p53 nanoparticle in advanced solid tumors. Mol Ther 2013;21:1096-103.

[105] Zeimet AG, Marth C. Why did p53 gene therapy fail in ovarian cancer? Lancet Oncol 2003;4:415-22.

[106] Madhusudan S, Tamir A, Bates N, Flanagan E, Gore ME, Barton DP, Harper P, Secki M, Thomas H, Lemoine NR, Charnock M, Habib NA, Lechler R, Nicholls J, Pignatelli M, Ganesan TS. A multicenter phase I gene therapy clinical trial involving intraperitoneal administration of E1A-lipid complex in patients with recurrent epithelial ovarian cancer overexpressing HER-2/neu oncogene. Clin Cancer Res 2004;10:2986-96.

[107] Anwer K, Kelly FJ, Chu C, Fewell JG, Lewis D, Alvarez RD. Phase I trial of a formulated IL-12 plasmid in combination with carboplatin and docetaxel chemotherapy in the treatment of platinum-sensitive recurrent ovarian cancer. Gynecol Oncol 2013;131: 169-73.

[108] Ren Y, Cheung HW, von Maltzhan G, Agrawal A, Cowley GS, Weir BA, Boehm JS, Tamayo P, Karst AM, Liu JF, Hirsch MS, Mesirov JP, Drapkin R, Root DE, Lo J, Fogal V, Ruoslahti E, Hahn WC, Bhatia SN. Targeted tumor-penetrating siRNA nanocomplexes for credentialing the ovarian cancer oncogene ID4. Sci Transl Med 2012; 4: 147ra12.

[109] Xie C, Gou ML, Yi T, Deng H, Li ZY, Liu P, Qi XR, He X, Wei Y, Zhao X. Efficient inhibition of ovarian cancer by truncation mutant of FILIP1L gene delivered by novel biodegradable cationic heparin-polyethyleneimine nanogels. Human Gene Ther 2011;22: 1413-22.

[110] Davis ME, Zuckerman JE, Choi CH, Seligson D, Tolcher A, Alabi CA, Yen Y, Heidel JD, Ribas A. Evidence of RNAi in humans from systemically administered siRNA via targeted nanoparticles. Nature 2010;464:1067-70.

[111] Tabernero J, Shapiro GI, LoRusso PM, Cervantes A, Schwartz GK, Weiss GJ, PazAres L, Cho DC, Infante JR, Alsina M, Gounder MM, Falzone R, Harrop J, White AC, Toudjarska I, Bumcrot D, Meyers RE, Hinkle G, Svrzikapa N, Hutabarat RM, Clausen VA, Cehelsky J, Nochur SV, Gamba-Vitalo C, Vaishnaw AK, Sah DW, Gollob JA, Burris 3rd HA. First-in-humans trial of an RNA interference therapeutic targeting VEGF and KSP in cancer patients with liver involvement. Cancer Discov 2013;3:406-17.

[112] Xing X, Zhang S, Chang J, Tucker SD, Chen H, Huang L, Hung MC. Safety study and characterization of E1A-liposome complex gene-delivery protocol in an ovarian cancer model. Gene Ther 1998;5:1538-44.

[113] Huang YH, Zugates GT, Peng W, Holtz D, Dunton C, Green JJ, Hossain N, Chernick MR, Padera Jr RF, Langer R, Anderson DG, Sawicki JA. Nanoparticle-delivered suicide

gene therapy effectively reduces ovarian tumor burden in mice. Cancer Res 2009;69:6184-91.

[114] Wang Y, Liu Y, Malek SN, Zheng P, Liu Y. Targeting HIF1α eliminates cancer stem cells in hematological malignancies. Cell Stem Cell 2011;8:399-411.

[115] Goldberg MS, Xing D, Ren Y, Orsulic S, Bhatia SN, Sharp PA. Nanoparticle-mediated delivery of siRNA targeting Parp1 extends survival of mice bearing tumors derived from Brca1-deficient ovarian cancer cells. Proc Natl Acad Sci U S A 2011;108:745-50.

[116] Kim HS, Han HD, Armaiz-Pena GN, Stone RL, Nam EJ, Lee JW, Shahzad MM, Nick AM, Lee SJ, Roh JW, Nishimura M, Mangala LS, Bottsford-Miller J, Gallick GE, LopezBerestein G, Sood AK. Functional roles of Src and Fgr in ovarian carcinoma. Clin Cancer Res 2011;17:1713-21.

[117] Sun C, Yi T, Song X, Li S, Qi X, Chen X, Lin H, He X, Li Z, Wei Y, Zhao X. Efficient inhibition of ovarian cancer by short hairpin RNA targeting claudin-3. Oncol Rep 2011;26:193-200.

[118] Zou L, Song X, Yi T, Li S, Deng H, Chen X, Li Z, Bai Y, Zhong Q, Wei Y, Zhao X. Administration of PLGA nanoparticles carrying shRNA against focal adhesion kinase and CD44 results in enhanced antitumor effects against ovarian cancer. Cancer Gene Ther 2013;20:242-50.

[119] Shen H, Rodriguez-Aguayo C, Xu R, Gonzalez Villasana V, Mai J, Huang Y, Zhang G, Guo X, Bai L, Qin G, Deng X, Li Q, Erm DR, Aslan B, Liu X, Sakamoto J, Chavez-Reyes A, Han HD, Sood AK, Ferrari M, Lopez-Berestein G. Enhancing chemotherapy response with sustained EphA2 silencing using multistage vector delivery. Clin Cancer Res 2013;19:1806-15.

[120] Hasan N, Mann A, Ferrari M, Tanaka T. Mesoporous silicon particles for sustained gene silencing. Methods Mol Biol 2013;1049:481-93.

[121] Nishimura M, Jung EJ, Shah MY, Lu C, Spizzo R, Shimizu M, Han HD, Ivan C, Rossi S, Zhang X, Nicoloso MS, Wu SY, Almeida MI, Bottsford-Miller J, Pecot CV, Zand B, Matsuo K, Shahzad MM, Jennings NB, Rodriguez Aguayo C, Lopez-Berestein G, Sood AK, Calin GA. Therapeutic synergy between microRNA and siRNA in ovarian cancer treatment. Cancer Discov 2013;3:1302-15.

[122] Steg AD, Katre AA, Goodman B, Han HD, Nick AM, Stone RL, Coleman RL, Alvarez RD, Lopez Berestein G, Sood AK, Landen CN. Targeting the notch ligand JAGGED1 in both tumor cells and stroma in ovarian cancer. Clin Cancer Res 2011;17:5674-85.

[123] Dickerson EB, Blackburn WH, Smith MH, Kapa LB, Lyon LA, McDonald JF. Chemosensitization of cancer cells by siRNA using targeted nanogel delivery. BMC Cancer 2010;10:10.

[124] Shahzad MM, Mangala LS, Han HD, Lu C, Bottsford-Miller J, Nishimura M, Mora EM, Lee JW, Stone RL, Pecot CV, Thanapprapasr D, Roh JW, Gaur P, Nair MP, Park

YY, Sabnis N, Deavers MT, Lee JS, Ellis LM, LopezBerestein G, McConathy WJ, Prokai L, Lacko AG, Sood AK. Targeted delivery of small interfering RNA using reconstituted highdensity lipoprotein nanoparticles. Neoplasia 2011;13:309-19.

[125] Han HD, Mangala LS, Lee JW, Shahzad MM, Kim HS, Shen D, Nam EJ, Mora EM, Stone RL, Lu C, Lee SJ, Roh JW, Nick AM, LopezBerestein G, Sood AK. Targeted gene silencing using RGD-labeled chitosan nanoparticles. Clin Cancer Res 2010; 16: 3910-22.

[126] Cubillos-Ruiz JR, Engle X, Scarlett UK, Martinez D, Barber A, Elgueta R, Wang L, Nesbeth Y, Durant Y, Gewirtz AT, Sentman CL, Kedl R, Conejo-Garcia JR. Polyethylenimine-based siRNA nanocomplexes reprogram tumor-associated dendritic cells via TLR5 to elicit therapeutic antitumor immunity. J Clin Invest 2009;119:2231-44.

[127] Cubillos-Ruiz JR, Baird JR, Tesone AJ, Rutkowski MR, Scarlett UK, Camposeco Jacobs AL, Anadon-Arnillas J, Harwood NM, Korc M, Fiering SN, Sempere LF, Conejo Garcia JR. Reprogramming tumor-associated dendritic cells in vivo using miRNA mimetics triggers protective immunity against ovarian cancer. Cancer Res 2012;72:1683-93.

[128] Pasquale EB. Eph receptor signalling casts a wide net on cell behaviour. Nat Rev Mol Cell Biol 2005;6:462-75.

[129] Thaker PH, Deavers M, Celestino J, Thornton A, Fletcher MS, Landen CN, Kinch MS, Kiener PA, Sood AK. EphA2 expression is associated with aggressive features in ovarian carcinoma. Clin Cancer Res 2004;10:5145-50.

[130] Lin YG, Han LY, Kamat AA, Merritt WM, Landen CN, Deavers MT, Fletcher MS, Urbauer DL, Kinch MS, Sood AK. EphA2 overexpression is associated with angiogenesis in ovarian cancer. Cancer 2007;109:332-40.

[131] Tanaka T, Mangala LS, Vivas-Mejia PE, Nieves-Alicea R, Mann AP, Mora E, Han HD, Shahzad MM, Liu X, Bhavane R, Gu J, Fakhoury JR, Chiappini C, Lu C, Matsuo K, Godin B, Stone RL, Nick AM, Lopez-Berestein G, Sood AK, Ferrari M. Sustained small interfering RNA delivery by mesoporous silicon particles. Cancer Res 2010; 70: 3687-96.

[132] Sugahara KN, Teesalu T, Karmali PP, Kotamraju VR, Agemy L, Greenwald DR, Ruoslahti E. Coadministration of a tumor-penetrating peptide enhances the efficacy of cancer drugs. Science 2010;328:1031-5.

第 7 章
乳腺癌的植物药疗法

Phaniendra Alugoju[a], Nyshadham S. N. Chaitanya[b], V. K. D. Krishna Swamy[a], Pavan Kumar Kancharla[c]

[a] Department of Biochemistry and Molecular Biology, School of Life Sciences, Pondicherry University, Puducherry, India
[b] Department of Animal Biology, School of Life Sciences, University of Hyderabad, Gachibowli, Hyderabad, India
[c] Department of Biotechnology, School of Life Sciences, Pondicherry University, Puducherry, India

摘要

乳腺癌是全世界导致人类死亡的主要原因之一,也是女性最常见的癌症类型。女性乳腺癌的发生有几种原因,已经报道的病因包括各种分子通路的干扰和伴随的分子标志物表达的改变。尽管手术、化疗和放疗等治疗方案对于乳腺癌有很好的治疗效果,但与这些方案相关的不良反应已促使科学界寻找替代方案。植物药疗法就是这样一种潜在的治疗策略。其中也包括使用传统药用植物针对不同的分子靶点治疗癌症,并且避免诱发不良反应。在这一章中,笔者将解读一些传统的印度药用植物对乳腺癌可能产生的有益作用。

关键词

乳腺癌,植物药疗法,危险因素,分子机制,药用植物

缩略词

ROS	活性氧
MAPK	丝裂原活化蛋白激酶
mTOR	哺乳动物雷帕霉素靶蛋白
PI3K	磷脂酰肌醇 3-激酶
ER	雌激素受体
PR	孕激素受体
DMBA	二甲基苯并蒽
MPTP	线粒体通透性转换孔
TNBC	三阴性乳腺癌

一、概述

癌症的特征是细胞不受控制的分裂和异常生长,肿瘤细胞可以通过侵入其他组织转移到身体的其他部位。癌症可能是由内部和外部因素引起并逐渐发生的。癌症的类型是以其来源的细胞类型命名的。例如,癌(上皮细胞)、肉瘤(骨和软组织)、白血病(血液组织)、淋巴瘤(由 B 或 T 淋巴细胞形成)、多发性骨髓瘤(浆细胞、骨髓瘤细胞)和黑色素瘤(黑色素细胞)。癌症类型也可以是基于其来源的器官或组织。例如,乳腺癌、血液癌、脑癌、肝癌、肺癌和皮肤癌。一份关于全球癌症负担的报告显示,2018 年估计全球有 1810 万癌症新发病例和 960 万死亡病例。

在全人群中肺癌是最常见的,第二常见的癌症是乳腺癌,这是女性常见的死亡原因[1]。与欠发达地区(中美洲、非洲、南美洲、密克罗尼西亚和波利尼西亚)(译者注:密克罗尼西亚和波利尼西亚均为太平洋岛国)相比,乳腺癌发病率在较发达地区(北美、澳大利亚、欧洲和日本)更高[2]。由于种族、卫生资源和生活方式的不同,乳腺癌的发病率差异很大[2-6]。在本章中,笔者将讨论乳腺癌的患病率、导致乳腺癌的因素、乳腺癌相关的分子机制,以及用于治疗乳腺癌的植物药疗法。

二、乳腺癌在印度的患病率

在印度女性中,乳腺癌是第二常见的癌症,确诊患者的病死率为 40%[7,8]。印度是全球癌症死亡率最高的国家[8,9],三阴性乳腺癌(triple negative breast cancer,TNBC)致死率最高,占死亡人数的 20%~43%[7,10-12]。在印度,患 TNBC 的高峰年龄是 40~55 岁,而在其他国家是 50~70 岁。报道显示,在班加罗尔[13]、海得拉巴[14]、斯利那加[15]和浦那[16]TNBC 在≤50 岁的女性中发病更为普遍。然而,德里是个例外,TNBC 在绝经后女性的发病率高于绝经前女性[17]。TNBC 在孟买的乳腺癌中占比最高,为 32.1%[18],其次是德里为 24.2%[17],海德拉巴为 22.8%[14]。最近的研究发现,TNBC 在年轻女性乳腺癌中发病占比为 31.57%,这一比例高于老年女性患者,且在印度女性、西班牙裔、华裔和非西班牙裔女性中都是最高的[19]。在印度年轻女性中雄激素受体亚型是最少的,而由原癌基因 neu 编码的人表皮生长因子受体 2 亚型(human epidermal growth factor receptor 2,HER2/neu)更为常见[20]。

三、乳腺癌发生的危险因素

乳腺癌发病的流行病学可以用细胞事件来解释,但具体发病原因并不清楚。

内源性类固醇性激素作为诱发因素的说法存在一定缺陷,唯一已知的诱发因素是辐射(ionizing radiation,IR)。女性性别、年龄、绝经年龄、初产年龄、从未生育过、是否哺乳和外源性雌激素等提示激素是诱发肿瘤的因素。但是,辐射、乳腺癌家族史、地域、营养因素、体重、身高、体型和良性乳腺疾病也可能是机制未知的乳腺癌的诱发因素[21]。癌症的病因是由多种因素导致的。包括:①无法修正的内源性危险因素,如 DNA 复制错误;②可修正的内/外源性危险因素,外源性因素包括辐射、化学致癌物、致癌病毒、吸烟、缺乏运动、营养失衡等,可部分修正的内源性因素包括生物性老化、DNA 修复机制、激素和炎症等[22]。

四、乳腺癌相关的分子机制

在乳腺癌中,早期乳腺细胞的生长失控可以通过乳腺钼靶 X 线检查诊断。而在晚期,癌细胞可能侵入腋窝淋巴结或身体的远处部位。乳腺癌可通过乳房皮肤或乳头的变化发现,并根据情况分为 Ⅰ~Ⅳ 期[23]。Ⅳ 期是转移性的,这意味着癌症已经从乳房扩散到腋窝淋巴结[24]。乳腺癌细胞可根据其蛋白表达的不同分为三类:雌激素受体(estrogen receptor,ER)、孕激素受体(progesterone receptor,PR),以及人表皮生长因子受体 2(HER2)。大多数癌细胞都表达 ER 或 PR 蛋白。高达 15%～20%的乳腺癌是 ERBB2 阳性(以前称为 HER2 阳性)。这 3 种蛋白都不表达的三阴性乳腺癌占乳腺癌的 15%[25]。癌症的分期和类型决定患者的预后和治疗。Ⅰ~Ⅲ 期治疗的目标是治愈,而 Ⅳ 期治疗的目标是控制肿瘤[26]。治疗不同类型的乳腺癌有不同的药物,治疗反应也有所不同。对于 ER/PgR 阳性的乳腺癌,抗雌激素类药物是有效的。对于 ERBB2 阳性的乳腺癌,需要静脉注射靶向药物。TNBC 需要采用静脉化疗。

癌症的复杂性是多因素和多维度的。癌症进展和转移的主要原因之一是氧化还原平衡被破坏[27]。活性氧(reactive oxygen species,ROS)的产生是由于细胞内 ROS 和环境因素引发氧化应激,氧化应激进一步导致了 DNA/蛋白质/脂质的降解[28],从而导致自噬、凋亡和炎症。细胞内大量的 ROS 激活磷脂酰肌醇-3-激酶(phosphoinositide 3-kinase,PI3K)/Akt、哺乳动物雷帕霉素靶蛋白(mammalian target of rapamycin,mTOR)、丝裂原活化蛋白激酶(mitogen-activated protein kinase,MAPK)信号转导通路,从而激活下游蛋白质,蜗牛转录因子和基质金属蛋白酶(matrix metalloproteinase,MMP)-2 和 MMP-9,导致上皮间充质转化(epithelial-mesenchymal transition,EMT),从而导致转移[29]。另一方面,缺氧诱导了血管内皮生长因子(vascular endothelial growth factor,VEGF)通过 PI3K/Akt/mTOR、磷酸酶-张力蛋白基因(phosphatase and tensin homolog,PTEN)、MAPK

信号通路表达,通过 HIF-1α 和 p70S6K1 的级联反应释放各种细胞因子、生长因子,且上调 MMP 导致血管生成[30]。氧化脂质配体不依赖缺氧,通过 TLR 激活 NF-κB。外源性或内源性产生的 ROS 激活细胞凋亡通路[31],并通过 MAPK、Bcl-2 和 Bax 的激活来介导[32](图 7-1)。

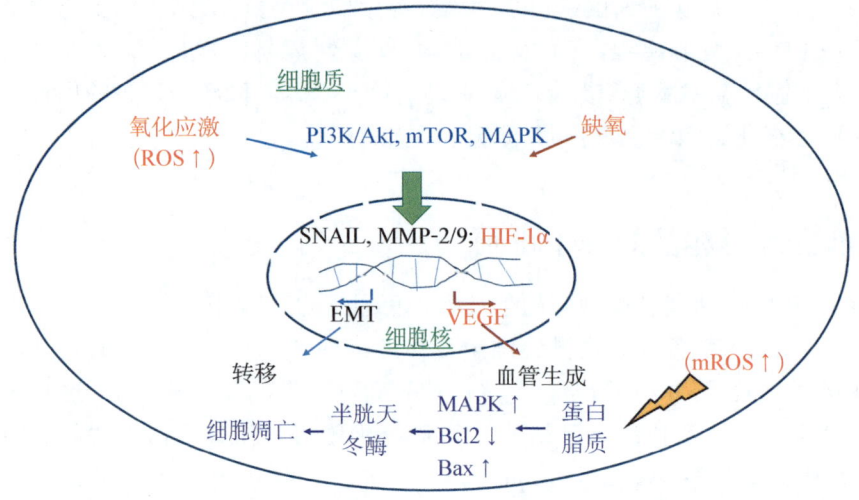

图 7-1 乳腺癌分子机制的概述

注:ROS. 活性氧;PI3K. 磷脂酰肌醇 3-激酶;mTOR. 哺乳动物雷帕霉素靶蛋白;MAPK. 丝裂原活化蛋白激酶;MMP. 基质金属蛋白酶;EMT. 上皮-间充质转化;VEGF. 血管内皮生长因子。

(一)氧化应激

有氧呼吸产生了多种对某些亚细胞事件至关重要的化合物,包括基因表达、信号转导、二硫键的形成和含半胱氨酸的天冬氨酸蛋白水解酶(caspase)活性的控制。黄嘌呤氧化酶和 NADPH 氧化酶复合物等酶作为氧化应激的内部来源,而紫外线辐射和化合物作为外部来源。根据包含原子的不同,反应物的种类可分为 ROS、活性氮(reactive nitrogen species,RNS)等[33]。这些机制和通路在哺乳动物细胞中是保守性的[33]。

(二)细胞凋亡

细胞凋亡可用于研究疾病的发病机制,同时也为治疗疾病提供了线索。在癌症中,细胞分裂和细胞死亡之间失去了原有的平衡。caspase 的激活包括内在和外在通路,以及鲜为人知的内在内质网通路[34]。[译者注:caspase(简称半胱天冬酶)

是一类在细胞质内引起细胞凋亡的关键酶。它们负责切割细胞内的特定蛋白质，从而启动和执行凋亡过程，一旦信号转导途径被激活，caspase 被活化，随后发生凋亡蛋白酶的级联反应]由于促凋亡和抗凋亡蛋白的平衡被打破，引起凋亡的减少或抗凋亡的增加，这在癌症的发生机制中起到了重要的作用[35]。因此，由于细胞分裂和细胞凋亡之间的失衡，乳腺癌细胞的凋亡明显减少[36]。

(三)MAPK 信号通路

MAPK 信号通路的作用是将细胞外信号与控制生长、增殖、迁移和凋亡的细胞内过程连接起来。在哺乳动物中发现的 MAPK 信号通路包括 MAPK/ERK 和 MAPK/JNK[37]。癌细胞形成肿瘤的过程主要是通过独立的增殖信号、高复制潜能、逃避凋亡、侵袭其他组织的能力和生成血管以供能来实现的[38]。MAPK 信号通路异常在癌症的发生和发展中发挥着作用[39]。同样，MAPK 信号通路在乳腺癌中被激活[40]。

(四)PI3K/AKT 信号通路

蛋白信号通路主要是调节细胞生长、分化和发育的，如 PI3K/Akt 信号通路。当信号通路受到频繁干扰，会在肿瘤组织中发生致癌变化[41]。在乳腺癌中 PI3K/Akt 信号通路的激活主要表现在内分泌治疗抵抗，并导致细胞生长和肿瘤增殖[42]。

(五)mTOR 信号通路

mTOR 信号通路在缺乏营养物质和生长因子的条件下，是细胞生长、存活和增殖所必需的[43]。体外和体内研究表明，mTOR 信号通路参与肿瘤生长、血管生成和转移[44]，上游蛋白如 HER2 和 IGFR，通过 PI3K 突变或 AKT 扩增抑制 PI3K/AKT 信号通路[45]。PTEN 是 PI3K 信号通路的负性调控因子，其在许多癌症中由于调控 miRNA 的表达、突变、甲基化和蛋白不稳定性而被下调[46]。PI3K/mTOR 信号通路在乳腺癌中被激活[47]。

此外，在乳腺癌中也有其他一些分子标志物的改变，包括周期蛋白依赖性激酶(cyclin-dependent kinase，CDK)/周期蛋白和多腺苷二磷酸核糖聚合酶(poly ADP-ribose polymerase，PARP)。

(六)CDK

CDK/周期蛋白家族在多种癌症的细胞周期、生长和增殖的失调中发挥作用[38,48]。CDK2 在喉癌、黑色素瘤和乳腺癌中过表达[49,50]。在一项敲除 CDK8 的研究中发现,乳腺癌细胞的增殖水平下降,这表明其在乳腺癌中发挥作用[51]。研究发现在乳腺癌、肺癌和甲状腺癌中存在伴侣周期蛋白,如周期蛋白 A 和 E 的过表达[52,53]。通过基因扩增或过表达,在乳腺癌中发现了高水平的周期蛋白 D1[54],而在细胞核中发现周期蛋白 E 水平较高[55]。

(七)PARP

PARP 家族包括 18 个成员,都具有催化 ADP 核糖转移到目标蛋白的作用,而且家族成员为了保守的催化域而具有共享的同源序列。PARP 在 DNA 修复过程、细胞凋亡和增殖中发挥作用[56]。端锚聚合酶 1(PARP 5a)在胃癌和乳腺癌中高表达[57]。

五、乳腺肿瘤发生的诱因

研究乳腺癌最有效的方法之一是建立实验动物模型。诱导乳腺组织发生肿瘤的方法之一是应用多环芳烃(polycyclic aromatic hydrocarbon,PAH)家族的化合物[58]。用于诱发乳腺肿瘤的化合物包括 7,12-二甲基苯并蒽[dimethylbenz(a)anthracene,DMBA][59]、N-甲基-N-亚硝基脲(N-nitroso-N-methylurea,NMU)[59]、2-氨基-1-甲基-6-苯基-咪唑[4,5-b]吡啶[2-amino-1-methyl-6-phenylimidazo(4,5-b)pyridine,PhIP][60]和 3-甲基胆蒽(3-methylcholanthrene,MC)[61]。DMBA 的代谢在肝脏的细胞色素 P450 系统中发生,产生自由基,从而导致 DNA 突变和 NF-κB 的激活。通过脱嘌呤破坏 DNA 的修复,最终导致细胞遗传物质的改变,从而诱导细胞凋亡通路和组织中肿瘤的发展[62]。NMU 通过甲基化 DNA 影响细胞蛋白的产生,并最终导致肿瘤。PhIP 是一种诱导突变和致癌的化合物,特别存在于肉类、鱼和卷烟烟雾中,直接影响乳腺、结肠和前列腺组织的 DNA[63]。MC 作为 AhR 的激动剂,诱导芳基烃受体(hydrocarbon receptor,AhR)-雌激素受体 α(estrogen receptor alpha,ERα)相互作用,从而诱导雌激素活性,增加原癌基因 c-fos 和 c-myc 的表达[64]。

六、用于乳腺癌研究的细胞系

第一个用于乳腺癌研究的细胞系建立于 1958 年,它被称为 BT-20[65]。细胞系由其来源命名,即实验室或患者或相同初始种群连续传代培养分离的亚种[66]。例如,HCC 细胞系来自哈蒙癌症中心(Hamon Cancer Center)[67],MDA 细胞系来自 MD 安德森医院和肿瘤研究所(MD Anderson Hospital and Tumor Institute)[68]。乳腺癌研究的细胞系包括 LY2、MCF7、MDAMB134、MDAMB134VI、T47D、ZR751、EFM192A、IBEP1、MDAMB330、MDAMB361、UACC812、ZR7527、

ZR7530、21MT1、OCUB-F、SKBR3、HMT3522、KPL-3C、MA11、MDAMB435、MDAMB436、MDAMB468、MFM223、SUM185PE、MDAMB231、SKBR7、SUM149PT 和 SUM159PT[66]。

七、乳腺癌的治疗策略

乳腺癌是女性最常见的癌症，约占所有癌症的 25.5%。这意味着如果要治疗乳腺癌，需要不断开发新药、联合用药和发掘有效的治疗策略。不同的治疗策略包括外科手术（外科医师切除癌症组织），放射治疗（通过高剂量的放射线破坏和缩小肿瘤的治疗方法），化学治疗（通过药物破坏癌细胞的治疗方法），激素治疗（通过使用激素抑制癌细胞生长的治疗方法）和精准治疗（基于对疾病遗传学分析的药物治疗方法）。然而，这些治疗策略会导致各种不良反应，并且往往对治疗癌症无效。因此，有必要寻找一些治疗癌症的替代方法，比如草药。

常见的癌症治疗因其导致许多有害的不良反应而不容易被接受，近年来抗肿瘤药物的耐药情况越来越严重。因此，现在人们关注的焦点已经转向了天然产品，如香料和植物。

八、植物药疗法

自古以来，植物就被用于治疗各种疾病。药用植物对于医疗健康有许多贡献，目前已有 100 多种植物衍生的化学物质被用作现代医学中的药物。需要注意的是，许多其他的药物都是对天然化学物质的简单合成修饰。植物药疗法是指利用植物提取物作为药物或保健品的研究[69]。在过去的数十年里，开展了越来越多的关于草药制剂和具有相关活性成分的化学物质对各类疾病的有效性的测试研究[70]。虽然植物制剂用于治疗癌症已有很多年的历史，然而目前还缺乏能在不伤害正常细胞的情况下选择性靶向作用于癌细胞的有效化合物。抗肿瘤药物的耐药性和某些肿瘤的异质性影响了肿瘤的治疗。尽管近期乳腺癌的化学治疗取得了一些进展，但仍然具有局限性。一方面，为了杀灭不敏感的肿瘤细胞而需要使用大剂量药物，这往往容易导致严重的不良反应。另一方面，小剂量药物使耐药的肿瘤细胞存活，导致对细胞抑制治疗无应答即形成难治性肿瘤，这对患者也是致命的。因此，需要找到不良反应最少的有效天然制剂，如草药和其他植物性配方。在下面的章节中，笔者将讨论具有抗乳腺癌活性的传统印度药用植物。此外，在表 7-1 中，列举了一些具有强大抗肿瘤活性的药用植物对乳腺癌不同的细胞系的作用。

表 7-1 具有抗乳腺癌活性的药用植物列表

植物名称	植物部位	活性成分	细胞系	作用机制	参考文献
Acacia nilotica 阿拉伯金合欢（豆科）	叶	γ-谷甾醇	MCF-7	· 细胞周期停滞在 G2/M 期 · ↓原癌基因 c-myc 的表达	[71]
Amoora rohituka（译者注：一种印度野生崖摩属植物）（楝科）	茎皮	Amooranin（译者注：一种三萜酸）	MCF-7, MCF-7/TH, MCF-10A	· 诱导细胞凋亡 · 诱导 DNA 阶梯形成 · ↑总 caspase 和 caspase-8 的活性	[72]
Andrographis paniculata 穿心莲（爵床科）	全株植物	穿心莲内酯	MDA-MB-231	· 诱导内部和外部的细胞凋亡通路 · 细胞周期停滞在 S 期和 G2/M 期 · ↑活性氧的产生 · ↑磷脂酰丝氨酸和 $\Delta\Psi_m$ 产生 · ↑caspase-3 和 caspase-9 · ↑Bax 和 Apaf-1 · ↓Bcl-2 和 Bcl-xL · ↓PI3 激酶/Akt 的激活 · 抑制血管生成因子，如 OPN 和 VEGF 的表达	[73-76]
Annona reticulata Linn. 牛心番荔枝（番荔枝科）	叶	T-47D		· ↓Bcl-2 · ↑Bax 和 Bak，以及 caspase 的激活 · 细胞周期停滞在 G2/M 期	[77]

续表

植物名称	植物部位	活性成分	细胞系	作用机制	参考文献
Artemisia absinthium 苦艾（菊科）	甲醇提取物		MDA-MB-231 和 MCF-7	• 核冷凝 • 细胞周期停滞在 sub-G1 期 • 激活 caspase-7 • ↑ Bax 和 Bcl-2 • ↑ MEK1/2 和 ERK1/2	[78]
Adiantum capillus veneris 盾叶铁线蕨（凤尾蕨科）			MCF7 和 BT47	粗提取物对 MCF7 和 BT47 细胞系具有抗增殖和诱导凋亡的作用	[79]
Aerva javanica（苋科）	叶		MCF-7	抗增殖活性	[80]
Anogeissus latifolia 宽叶榆绿木（使君子科）	全株植物		T47D 和 MCF-7	全株植物提取物抑制细胞增殖	[81]
Acacia catechu 儿茶（豆科）	全株植物		T47D 和 MCF-7	全株植物提取物抑制细胞增殖	[81]
Annona muricata L. 菠萝蜜（番荔枝科）	叶		MDA-MB-435S	细胞毒性	[82]
Annona muricata 刺果番荔枝（番荔枝科）	叶		MCF-7	抑制细胞增殖	[83]

续表

植物名称	植物部位	活性成分	细胞系	作用机制	参考文献
Anisochilus carnosus (L. f.) wall 耙草（唇形科）	叶		BT-549	对 BT-549 有强效细胞毒性	[84]
Artemisia nilagirica 南亚蒿（菊科）				提取物含有乙酸乙酯（AR-03）和己烷（AR-04）对乳腺癌细胞系具有最大的细胞毒性	[85]
Arisaema tortuosum (Wall.) Schott 曲序南星（天南星科）	根茎和叶			树叶提取的氯仿显著降低了 MCF-7 细胞系的活性	[86]
Allium atroviolaceum 石蒜科葱属植物（石蒜科）	花		MCF-7 和 MDA-MB-231	• 细胞周期停滞在 S 期、G2/M 期和 sub-G1 期 • ↓ Cdk1（作用于独立的 p53 通路） • ↓ Bcl-2 • caspase 介导的细胞凋亡	[87]
Butea monosperma 紫铆（蝶形花科）	树皮		MCF-7	• 提取物丁醇使细胞周期停滞在亚-G1 期 • ↑ 活性氧 • ↓ MMP 参与线粒体介导的细胞凋亡通路	[88]

续表

植物名称	植物部位	活性成分	细胞系	作用机制	参考文献
Phaseolus vulgaris L. 菜豆（豆科）	种子		MCF-7 和 MDA-MB-231	• 激活 caspase3/7 • ↑ Bax • ↓ Bcl-2 和 Bcl-xL • 细胞周期停滞在 S 期和 G2/M 期 • ↓ΔΨm 参与线粒体介导的细胞凋亡通路	[89]
Barleria buxifolia 假杜鹃（爵床科）	种子	barleriaquinone-Ⅰ (BQ-Ⅰ) 和 barleriaquinone-Ⅱ (BQ-Ⅱ)	MCF-7	• 细胞毒性 • 使 BQ-Ⅱ比 BQ-Ⅰ更活跃	[90]
Brassica juncea 芥菜（十字花科）	种子	芥子油苷	MCF-7 和 MDA-MB-231	• ↑ ROS • ↓ΔΨm 参与线粒体介导的细胞凋亡通路	[91]
Boerhaavia diffusa L. 黄细心（紫茉莉科）	全株植物		MCF-7	• ↓ pS2 中 mRNA 的表达 • 细胞周期停滞在 G0/1 期	[92]
Boswellia ovalifoliolata 橄榄科乳香树属植物（橄榄科）	叶		MDA-MB-231 和 MDA-MB-453	• 磷酸化-NF-κB (ser536)，PC-NA，Bcl-2 • ↑ Bax	[93]
Betula utilis 糙皮桦（桦木科）	树皮	桦木醇，白桦脂酸，羽扇豆醇，熊果酸，齐墩果酸和β-香树脂醇		• DR4, DR5 和 PARP 的裂解导致外部细胞凋亡通路 • ↑ ROS • ↓ΔΨm	[94]

续表

植物名称	植物部位	活性成分	细胞系	作用机制	参考文献
Cyperus rotundus 香附子（莎草科）	根茎		MCF-7、MDA-MB-231 和 MDA-MB-468	通过诱导细胞凋亡产生细胞毒作用，凋亡的产生与以下机制相关： • ↑死亡受体 4（DR4）、DR5 和促凋亡 Bax • ↓抗凋亡细胞生存素和 Bcl-2 • ↓Bid • 激活 caspase-8 和 caspase-9，其分别为外部和内部凋亡通路启动 caspase • ↑线粒体膜去极化与 caspase-3 的激活和 PARP 的裂解相关，PARP 是激活的 caspase-3 的重要底物	[95-97]
Chenopodium album 藜实（藜科）	叶		MCF-7 和 MDA-MB-468	树叶的甲醇提取物 C. album 表现出较大的抗癌活性	[98]
Costus pictus D. Don 闭鞘姜科（闭鞘姜科）	叶和根茎	木香烃内酯	MDA-MB-231 和 MCF10A	中度细胞毒性 • ↓NF-κB 亚基-p65,52 和 100	[99,100]
Cassia auriculate 耳叶番泻（云实科）	叶		MCF-7	核裂解和聚集 • ↓Bcl-2 蛋白 • ↑Bax 蛋白	[101]

续表

植物名称	植物部位	活性成分	细胞系	作用机制	参考文献
Centratherum anthelminticum (译者注：未查到中文名称，是一种类似于蓝冠菊的植物，又称苦孜然)（菊科）	种子	斑鸠菊大苦素和吲哚基乙基异腈	MCF-7, MDA-MB-231 和 LA7	• ↑ROS • ↓Bcl-2, Bcl-xL • ↓ΔΨm 和细胞色素 c 的释放 • 细胞色素 c 从线粒体中释放到细胞质触发 caspase 级联激活, PARP 裂解, DNA 损伤, 并最终通过凋亡导致细胞死亡 • 激活 FOXO 转录因子及其下游靶点（Bim, p27Kip1, p21Waf1/cip1, cyclinD1, cyclinE） • 下调 Akt 激酶活性, 导致 FOXO3a 累积 • 上调 p27Kip1 和 FOXO3a 水平, 下调 p-FOXO3a 水平 • 抑制 TNF-α 释放	[102-105]
Cephalotaxus griffithii 贡山三尖杉（紫杉科）			ZR751	↓hTERT, hTR 和 c-myc 的表达	[106]

续表

植物名称	植物部位	活性成分	细胞系	作用机制	参考文献
Citrullus colocynth L. 药西瓜（葫芦科）	果浆		MCF-7 和 MDA-MB-231	• ↓Bcl-2 和 Bcl-xL • ↑Bax 和 caspase 3 • ↑上皮基因角蛋白 19 • ↓间充质基因，波形蛋白，钙黏蛋白 N，Zeb1 和 Zeb2 • 提取物对上皮间充质转化（EMT）的抑制作用 • 干性相关基因 BMI-1 和 CD44	[107]
Caesalpinia sappan L. 苏木（豆科）	木芯和叶	巴西木素 A	MCF-7	诱导 MCF-7 细胞系细胞死亡	[108]
Dioscorea deltoidei 藏山药（薯蓣科）	植物材料	薯蓣皂苷配基		对 HBL100 细胞系具有显著的抗增殖作用	[109]
Drosera burmannii Vahl 锦地罗（茅膏菜科）	植株		MCF-7	• 细胞周期停滞在 G2/M 期 • ↓细胞周期蛋白 A1(cyclinA1)，cyclin B1 和 Cdk-1 • ↑p53，Bax/Bcl-2 导致 caspase 激活和 PARP 降解 • ↓iNOS，COX-2 和 TNF-α，以及抑制细胞内活 ROS 的产生，证实了提取物具有潜在的抗炎效果	[110]

续表

植物名称	植物部位	活性成分	细胞系	作用机制	参考文献
Dysoxylum binectariferum Hook. f 红果樫木（楝科）	树干树皮	罗希吐碱（rohitukine）		夫拉平度（flavopiridol）是强效的周期蛋白依赖性激酶（CDK）抑制剂	[111]
Eulophia nuda L. 紫花美冠兰（兰科）	甲醇提取物	9,10-二氢-2,5-二甲氧基菲-1,7-二醇（9,10-Dihydro-2,5-dimethoxyphenanthrene-1,7-diol）	MCF-7 和 MDA-MB-231	具有显著的抗增殖活性	[112]
Fraxinus micrantha（译者注：一种木樨科梣属植物，通常称小花白蜡马拉雅白蜡树）（木樨科）	树皮		MCF-7	↑NO 和 DNA 片段	[113]
Ficus religiosa 菩提树（桑科）	丙酮提取物			• 细胞周期阻滞在 G1 期 • 导致核染色质凝聚 • ↓ΔΨm 和诱导 caspase 的激活 • ↑ROS • ↑Bax 和 caspase9 的激活	[114]

续表

植物名称	植物部位	活性成分	细胞系	作用机制	参考文献
Glycyrrhiza glabra 光果甘草（豆科）	根	槲皮苷和光甘草醇（glabrol）		抑制 CYP1B1	[115]
Glycine max 大豆（豆科）	种子		MCF-7	大豆提取物是 MCF-7 细胞生长的启动子，胡芦巴提取物诱导细胞凋亡	[116]
Garcinia hombroniana 山凤果（金丝桃科）	树皮提取物			对 MCF-7 具有显著细胞毒性	[117]
Glycosmis pentaphylla (Retz.) DC 山小橘（芸香科）	干叶	羽扇豆醇、白杨素、槲皮素、β-谷甾醇和山柰酚	MCF-7 和 MDA-MB-231	激活 caspase-3/7，启动线粒体诱导的细胞凋亡	[118]
Juglans regia 胡桃（胡桃科）	根皮		MDA-MB-231	↑ Bax、caspase、tp53 和 TNF-α	[119]
Leptadenia reticulata ［译者注：未查到明确的中文名称，这是一种重要的阿育吠陀（一种古老的印度医学）草药，通常称为为吉万提］（萝藦科）			MCF-7	乙酸乙酯提取物有强细胞毒性	[120]

续表

植物名称	植物部位	活性成分	细胞系	作用机制	参考文献
Launaea procumbens 假小喙菊 (Asteraceae)（菊科；菊科植物）	叶		MCF-7	对乳腺癌 (MCF-7) 具有强大的细胞毒性	[121]
Trigonella foenumgraecum 香豆子（译者注：也称胡卢巴）(Fabaceae)（豆科）	种子		MCF-7	诱导细胞凋亡	[116]
Murraya koenigii Spreng 调料九里香 (Rutaceae)（芸香科）	叶		MCF-7 和 MDA-MB-231 & 4T1	• 细胞周期滞在 S 期 • 降低 26S 蛋白酶体的活性 • 抑制蛋白酶体的胰蛋白酶样蛋白水解活性，但不抑制糜蛋白酶样蛋白水解活性 • MK 可缩小肿瘤体积并减少肺转移 • 抑制 4T1 细胞的活性 • 降低 NO 和 iNOS、iCAM、NF-κB 和 c-myc 的水平	[122-124]
Morinda citrifolia L. 海滨木巴戟 (Rubiaceae)（茜草科）	果实与整株植物		MCF-7、MDA-MB-231 和 T47D	• 细胞周期停在 G1/S 期和 G0/1 期 • 抗增殖活性	[81,125]

续表

植物名称	植物部位	活性成分	细胞系	作用机制	参考文献
Mucuna pruriens (L.) DC 刺毛黧豆 (Fabaceae) (豆科)	种子	左旋多巴	T47D, MCF-7, MDA-MB-468, 和 MDA-MB-231	• 诱导 DNA 损伤 • 细胞周期停滞在 G1 期 • ↓ PRL 表达，进一步抑制 JAK2/STAT5A/cyclin D1 信号通路	[126]
Morus alba L. 桑白皮 (Moraceae) (桑科)	叶	凝集素	MCF-7	凝集素对 MCF-7 具有明显的抗增殖活性 • DNA 断裂 • caspase-3 激活 • ↓ NO • ↑ iNOS	[127,128]
Macrosolen parasiticus (L.) 鞘花属 (Loranthaceaea) (萝摩科)	茎		MCF-7	对 MCF-7 具有显著的细胞毒性活性	[129]
Maesa macrophylla 大叶鸢尾,大叶萱草 (Primulaceae) (报春花科)	叶		MCF-7 c	强大的细胞毒性	[130]
Madhuca indica 马杜鹃 (Sapotaceae) (山榄科)	花		MCF-7 和 MDA-MB-468	• ↑ caspase3/7 • ↓ COX-2 mRNA 和 COX-2 蛋白质	[131]

续表

植物名称	植物部位	活性成分	细胞系	作用机制	参考文献
Nardostachys jatamansi DC 甘松（Caprifoliaceae）（忍冬科）	根和根茎	Lupeol 和 β-谷甾醇（β-sitosterol）	MCF-7 和 MDA-MB-231	细胞周期停滞在 G2/M 期和 G0/1 期	[132]
Nyctanthes arbortristis Linn 夜花（译者注：是一种印度药用植物，也称帕瑞亚特）（Oleaceae）（木犀科）	种子	Arbortristoside-A(1) 和 7-O-trans-cinnamoyl 6β-hydroxyloganin(2)	MCF-7	具有中等体外抗癌活性	[133]
Oenothera biennis L. 月见草（Onagraceae）（柳叶菜科）	叶	oenotheralanosterol A 和 oenotheralanosterol B		显著的抗增殖活性	[134]
Orthosiphon pallidus 苍耳（Lamiaceae）（唇形科）			MCF-7 和 MDA-MB-231	显著的细胞毒性	[135]
Oroxylum indicum (L.) 木蝴蝶（Bignoniaceae）（紫葳科）			MDA-MB-231	诱导细胞凋亡和显著的抗转移活性	[136]

续表

植物名称	植物部位	活性成分	细胞系	作用机制	参考文献
Parmotrema reticulatum 粉网大叶梅(译者注:是一种阔叶绿藻型地衣)(Parmeliaceae)(梅衣科)	干地衣		MCF-7	• 细胞周期停滞在 S 期和 G2/M 期 • ↓周期蛋白 B1、Cdk-2 和 Cdc25C 以及 Cdk-1 和周期蛋白 A1 • ↑p53 和 p21 上调 • ↑Bax 和↓Bcl-2 的表达,导致 Bax/Bcl-2 比率升高和 caspase 级联激活,最终导致 PARP 降解,从而导致细胞凋亡	[137]
Psoralea corylifolia 补骨脂 (Fabaceae)(豆科)	种子		MCF7	• 通过诱导 caspase-9 和 caspase-7 的裂解诱导细胞凋亡 • ↑Bax 的上调,细胞色素 c 的释放 • ↑ROS • ↓ΔΨm • PARP 的裂解增加,导致细胞凋亡	[138]
Pithecellobium dulce 牛蹄豆 (Fabaceae)(豆科)	叶		MCF-7	• ↑Bax、p21、p53、TNF 和 fas 的 mRNA 表达。 • ↓Bcl-2、NF-κB 和 Cdk 的 mRNA 表达	[139]

续表

植物名称	植物部位	活性成分	细胞系	作用机制	参考文献
Pteris quadriureta 高山凤尾蕨 (Pteridaceae)(凤尾蕨科)			MCF7 和 BT47	对 MCF7 和 BT47 细胞系具有显著的抗增殖和诱导凋亡特性	[79]
Pomegranate 石榴 Punicaceae 石榴科	蒴果皮		MCF-7, MDA-MB-231	↓雌激素反应元件(ERE)介导的转录。PME 可与 27HC(27-hydroxycholesterol,27 羟胆固醇)竞争 ERα,并减少 27HC 诱导的 MCF-7 细胞增殖	[140]
Punica granatum 石榴 (Punicaceae)(石榴科)	果皮	多糖	MCF-7	细胞毒性	[141]
Picrorhiza kurroa Royle ex Benth 鼠牙草 (Scrophulariaceae)(玄参科)	根茎		MDA-MB-435S	细胞毒性和诱导细胞凋亡	[142]
Podophyllum hexandrum 桃儿七,鬼白 (Berberidaceae)(小檗科)	根茎		MCF-7	根茎的甲醇提取物和 70% 的乙醇提取物对 MCF-7 展现出最高的细胞毒性作用	[143]
Pteris vittata L. 蜈蚣凤尾蕨 (Pteridaceae)(凤尾蕨科)	甲醇		MCF-7	MCF-7 细胞活力的降低具有剂量依赖性	[144]

续表

植物名称	植物部位	活性成分	细胞系	作用机制	参考文献
Pongamia pinnata (L.) Pierre. 水黄皮 (Fabaceae)(豆科)	种子			细胞周期停滞在 G0/1 期 ↓周期蛋白 D1 水平	[145]
Polygonatum verticillatum (L.) 轮叶黄精 (Ruscaceae)(假叶树科)	根茎			氯仿提取物对人类乳腺癌细胞系 MCF-7 展示出最强的细胞毒性	[146]
Pyrenacantha volubilis 刺核藤 (Icacinaceae)(茶茱萸科)	种子	喜树碱		展示出最强的细胞毒性	[147]
Rheum emodi Wall. ex Meissn. 白牛尾七 (Polygonaceae)(蓼科)	根茎		MDA-MB-435S	诱导细胞凋亡	[148]
soybean (Fabaceae) and flaxseed (Linaceae) 大豆 (豆科)与亚麻籽 (亚麻科)	大豆籽和亚麻籽		MCF-7 和 MDA-MB-231	• ↓SOD 和 GPx • ↑细胞内 ROS 水平 • ↓MMP • 细胞周期停滞在 S 期、G2/M 期和亚 G1 期	[149]

续表

植物名称	植物部位	活性成分	细胞系	作用机制	参考文献
Semecarpus anacardium 肉托果（也称打印果）(Anacardiaceae)（漆树科）	坚果		T47D	• 细胞毒性源于诱导细胞凋亡 • 诱导细胞内储存的 Ca^{2+} 快速流动，这与线粒体跨膜电位的改变有关 • ↓Bcl-2 • ↑Bax，细胞色素 c，caspase 和 PARP 分裂	[150]
Semecarpus anacardium 肉托果 (Anacardiaceae)（漆树科）	根	全部生物碱和酚	MCF-7	生物碱部分具有最大的细胞毒性和凋亡诱导作用	[151]
Semecarpus lehyam 肉托果膏			MCF-7 和 MDA231	n-hexane 和氯仿馏分具有明显的细胞毒性	[152]
Syzygium aromaticum L. 丁香蒲桃 (Myrtaceae)（桃金娘科）			MCF-7 和 MDA-MB-231	最大的细胞毒性	[153]
Saraca indica 无忧树 (Caesalpiniaceae)（云实科）	树皮			抗乳腺癌活性	[154]

续表

植物名称	植物部位	活性成分	细胞系	作用机制	参考文献
Salacia oblonga（译者注：一种五层龙属植物）（Celastraceae）（卫矛科）	根部和气生部分		MCF7	显著的抗增殖活性	[155]
Tinospora cordifolia 波叶青牛胆（Menispermaceae）防己科			MDA-MB-231 和 MCF-7	↑ROS ↑Bax 和 ↓Bcl-2	[156]
Tiliacora racemosa 总状香料藤（Menispermaceae）防己科	根	全部生物碱和酚	MCF-7	最大的细胞毒性	[151]
Thespesia populnea 桐棉（Malvaceae）（锦葵科）		醌	MCF-7	细胞毒性	[157]
Terminalia bellerica 毗黎勒（Combretaceae）（使君子科）	整株植物		T47D 和 MCF-7	抗增殖活性	[81]
Taxus wallichiana 红豆杉（Taxaceae）（紫杉科）		紫杉脂素（taxiresinol）	MCF-7	细胞毒性	[158]

续表

植物名称	植物部位	活性成分	细胞系	作用机制	参考文献
Vernonia cinerea Less. 小花夜香牛（Asteraceae）（菊科）			MCF-7	· 诱导细胞凋亡 · 抑制 MDR 转运体（ABC-B1 和 ABC-G2）的功能活性，增强癌细胞对 DNR 的吸收	[159]
Wrightia tomentosa 脆木（Apocynaceae）（夹竹桃科）		齐墩果酸和熊果酸	MCF-7 和 MDA-MB-231	· 细胞周期阻滞在 G1 期 · ↑ROS · ↓MMP 和随后的细胞凋亡 · Bax/Bcl-2 比率 · Annexin V 阳性，caspase 8 激活和 DNA 断裂增强	[160]
Withania somnifera 睡茄（Solanaceae）（茄科）	根		MDA-MB-231	通过 ↑ROS，↑Bax/Bcl-2，↓MMP 和 caspase-3 激活诱导线粒体介导的细胞凋亡 · 细胞周期阻滞在 G2/M 期，核纤层蛋白 A/C 裂解	[161]
Zanthoxylum zanthoxyloides 肖花椒（Rutaceae）（芸香科）		花椒酸（Zantholic acid）		细胞毒性活性	[162]
体内研究					
Bacopa monnieri 假马齿苋（Plantaginaceae）（车前科）		Bacoside A, B 和葫芦素	艾氏腹水癌（EAC）肿瘤小鼠	显著减少肿瘤重量，血细胞比容，肿瘤体积和有活力的肿瘤细胞量	[163]

续表

植物名称	植物部位	活性成分	细胞系	作用机制	参考文献
Butea monosperma 紫矿（Fabaceae）（豆科）	花		甲基亚硝脲（Methylnitrosourea，MNU）诱导无雌激素的Sprague-Dawley大鼠患乳腺癌	• 雌激素和孕激素表达减少，核酸含量降低，潜伏期延长 • 诱导细胞凋亡，抑制血管生成和转移	[164]
Cedrus deodara 雪松（Pinaceae）（松科）	茎木	(−)-wikstromal，(−)-matairesinol（罗汉松脂素）和Benzylbutyrolactol（苯基丁内酯）		• 诱导体内肿瘤消退 • Annexin V 阳性细胞提示其诱导细胞凋亡的作用，诱导细胞内caspase，DNA 断裂和 DNA 细胞周期分析	[165]
Garcinia morella 莫雷拉藤黄（Clusiaceae）（藤黄科）		山竹子素（Garcinol）	MCF7，MDA-MB-231 和 SKBR3	• 诱导 P53 依赖性凋亡 • ↑ Bax • ↓ Bcl-xL	[166]
Murraya koenigii 调料九里香（Rutaceae）（芸香科）	叶		异种移植肿瘤小鼠模型	• 释放亚硝酸盐和 TNF-α 水平显著抑制爪部炎症 • 抑制内源性 26S 蛋白酶体活性。肿瘤生长的减少与蛋白酶体活性的降低有关 • ↑ caspase-3 活性和抗凋亡基因标记性细胞 • ↓ 血管生成和血管生成受到抑制，促进细胞凋亡 • 表明 TUNEL 阳	[167]

续表

植物名称	植物部位	活性成分	细胞系	作用机制	参考文献
Pyracantha fortuneana 火棘（Rosaceae）蔷薇科	干果实	含硒多糖	小鼠异种移植模型	・细胞周期停滞在 G2 期 ・抑制 CDC25C-cyclinB1/CDC2 通路 ・↑p53，Bax，Puma 和 Noxa ・↓Bcl-2 ・↑Bax/Bcl-2 增加 ・↑caspase 3/9 的活性 ・抑制肿瘤生长	[168]
Ricinus communis L. 蓖麻（Euphorbiaceae）大戟科	干果实		MCF-7 和侵袭性极强的三阴性 MDA-MB-231 乳腺癌细胞	・抑制迁移、黏附、侵袭、以及 MMP-2 和 MMP-9 的表达 ・↓Bcl-2 ・↑Bax 和 caspase-7 的表达，以及 PARP 的裂解 ・缩小肿瘤体积	[169]
Withania somnifera 睡茄（Solanaceae）茄科	叶提取物	Withaferin-A，一种睡茄交酯	异种移植小鼠肿瘤模型中的 HCT116 细胞	肿瘤体积缩小和重量显著减轻	[170]
Zizyphus Nummularia（译者注：一种鼠李科枣属小灌木）（Rhamnaceae）鼠李科	根皮		雌性瑞士白化小鼠的艾氏腹水癌（EAC）	缩少肿瘤体积和存活肿瘤细胞数量，增加体重和寿命	[171]

↓表示减少；↑表示增加。

(一)穿心莲

穿心莲(Andrographis paniculata)是一种一年生分枝草本植物,俗称"苦味之王"(king of bitter/mahatikta),属于爵床科(Acanthaceae)[172]。原生于印度和斯里兰卡,在孟加拉国、中国和印度尼西亚被广泛用作传统药物[173]。传统上用于治疗蛇咬伤、糖尿病、痢疾和疟疾。穿心莲的叶提取物也是治疗传染病、发热性疾病、绞痛、粪便不成形和腹泻的传统药物。据报道,它具有广泛的药理作用,如抗癌、抗肝炎、降血糖、抗炎、抗疟、抗氧化、治疗心血管疾病和性功能障碍。这种植物的生物活性成分包括二萜类(diterpenes)、黄酮类(flavonoids)、氧杂蒽酮(xanthones)和诺卡酮(nocardioides)[174]。穿心莲内酯(andrographolide)是从穿心莲中分离出来的一种二萜内酯,是穿心莲最重要的活性成分,据报道它具有多种生物活性,包括抗氧化、抗炎、细胞毒性、免疫调节、心脏保护、肝脏保护和神经调节作用。研究发现穿心莲内酯对多种细胞株具有抗癌活性。这种化合物的基本抗癌机制包括氧化应激、细胞周期停滞、抗炎、凋亡、坏死、自噬、抑制细胞黏附、增殖、迁移、侵袭和抗血管生成活性[175]。

穿心莲内酯可抑制乳腺癌细胞的增殖和迁移,使细胞周期停滞在 G2/M 期,并通过独立于 caspase 的途径诱导细胞凋亡。穿心莲内酯的抗肿瘤活性与抑制 PI3K/Akt 信号通路和血管生成分子,如骨桥蛋白(osteopontin, OPN)和血管内皮生长因子(vascular endothelial growth factor, VEGF)有关。它还能减弱肿瘤与内皮细胞的相互作用。因此,原位 NOD/SCID 小鼠的乳腺肿瘤生长受到抑制[73]。穿心莲内酯有利于乳腺上皮细胞的正常生长,其表现为处于 S 期和 G2/M 期的细胞数量增加。然而,对 p53 和 ER 失效的 MDA-MB-231(转移性乳腺癌细胞)却有抑制作用。抑制 MDA-MB-231 的肿瘤进展机制包括 ROS 生成增加、线粒体膜电位($\Delta\Psi$m)降低、磷脂酰丝氨酸外化、促凋亡(Bax/Apaf-1)信号通路激活和抗凋亡(Bcl-2/Bcl-xL)信号通路抑制,以及最终导致细胞凋亡的 caspase 3 和 caspase 9 的激活[74]。由于癌症特异性,穿心莲内酯及其类似物需要在与癌症化学预防相关的临床和生物医学研究中进一步研究。总之,可以认为穿心莲内酯在不久的将来可能会成为一种潜在的抗癌剂。

(二)睡茄

睡茄(Withania somnifera),也称南非醉茄(Ashwagandha),又名印度人参(Indian ginseng),是茄科(Solanaceae)多年生矮灌木。这种植物在印度医药中使用已久,其根部被用于 200 多种配方中[176]。植物化学物,如睡茄内酯(withanolide)、醉茄素(withaferin)、醉茄酮(withanone)和醉茄苷(withanoside),对肿瘤细胞系是有效的[177,178]。据报道,从这种植物中提取的糖蛋白和类凝集素蛋白可作为抗菌剂和抗蛇毒药物[179,180]。此外,一些临床前研究,如涉及神经保护、心脏保护、抗炎和抗糖尿病等研究也证实睡茄中多种植物成分的有效性。一种从睡茄(W. somnifera,WSPF)中提取的新型蛋白质组分对 MDA-MB-231 人类乳腺癌细胞具有显著的凋亡活性。MDA-MB-231 细胞凋亡的进展也是由这种成分介导的,可以将细胞周期停滞在 G2/M 期。后续发生一系列凋亡事件,包括 ROS 生成增加,以及随后的 $\Delta\Psi$m 丢失、Bax/Bcl-2 失调、caspase-3 激活和细胞死亡。此外,还观察到核纤层蛋白 A/C 蛋白的裂解和核形态变化。这凸显了 WSPF 对 TNBC 的治疗潜能[161]。同样,植物的根提取物可以抑制 MDA-MB-231 细胞的增殖,并使细胞周期停滞在亚 G1 期。并且通过减少细胞因子 CCL2(C-C motif Ligand 2)的表达来抑制异种移植的 MDA-MB-231 细胞增殖,从而缩小异种移植肿瘤的大小[181]。

醉茄素 A(withaferin A,WA)可以阻碍蛋白酶体降解系统并干扰自噬。当细胞内降解系统受到抑制时,泛素化蛋白质就会积累,进而在人类乳腺癌细胞系 MCF-7 和 MDA-MB-231 中展开蛋白质反应和 ER 应激介导的蛋白毒性。因此,WA 在抑制蛋白酶体系统和诱导自噬功能受损的同时,通过细胞蛋白毒性靶向抑制乳腺癌细胞[182]。

(三)波叶青牛胆

波叶青牛胆(Tinospora cordifolia),又名阿姆里塔(Amrita)和青牛胆茜草(Guduchi),属于防己科(Menispermaceae),常见于印度次大陆和中国。在阿育吠陀医学和民间医疗中,这种植物可单独使用也可与其他植物混合使用[183]。该植物的化学成分,包括生物碱(alkaloid)、萜类化合物(terpenoid)、木酚素(lignan)、类固醇(steroid)等。这些成分使其具有广泛的药理特性,如抗氧化、抗菌、抗糖尿病、抗应激活性、抗癌、抗艾滋病毒和免疫调节活性[184]。

波叶青牛胆(T. cordifolia,TcCF)的氯仿馏分中显示其含有芦丁(rutin)和槲皮素(quercetin)等药用活性成分,这使得该植物对乳腺癌细胞(MDA-MB-231 和 MCF7)具有抗癌特性。在经 TcCF 处理的乳腺癌细胞中观察到 ROS 增加、集落形成减少、促凋亡/抗凋亡基因表达比增加,最终导致细胞凋亡。然而,在抑制 ROS 后,凋亡机制被逆转,这显示了 ROS 生成在 TcCF 诱导乳腺癌细胞凋亡中的作用[156]。

从 TcCF 叶子的丁醇馏分中分离出的天然化合物 Bis(2-ethyl hexyl)1H-pyrrole-3,4-dicarboxylate(TCCP),具有促凋亡作用,可使 MDA-MB-231 细胞周期停滞在亚 G1 期。该机制涉及一系列事件,首先是线粒体膜电位降低、细胞内钙离子浓度升高、p53 磷酸化、内源性 ROS 生成、心磷脂过氧化、线粒体通透性转换孔

(mitochondrial permesbility transition pore,MPTP)形成、Bax/Bcl-2 比率增加、细胞色素在细胞质中释放、caspase 激活和凋亡的 DNA 断裂。此外,对小鼠艾氏腹水瘤(Ehrlich ascites tumor,EAT)的体内研究显示,小鼠存活率提高了 2 倍,而肝肾毒性却很小。因此,体外和体内研究显示 TCCP 能有效抑制 MDA-MB-231 细胞和小鼠 EAT 的肿瘤增殖[185]。

(四)调料九里香

调料九里香(*Murraya koenigii*,MK)又名咖喱叶(curry leave),属于芸香科(Rutaceae),广泛分布于亚洲东部。其药用特性在阿育吠陀医学中已有详细记载,药理学报告称其具有抗病毒、抗炎、抗糖尿病、抗利什曼原虫病和抗肿瘤活性[186-188]。对 26S 蛋白酶体的蛋白水解抑制是一种很有前景的癌症治疗方法,因为这种机制可选择性地杀死癌细胞,并提高它们对化疗药物的敏感性。MK 叶的总生物碱提取物和 mahanine(一种咔唑类生物碱)能抑制蛋白酶体的胰蛋白酶样蛋白水解活性,但不能抑制糜蛋白酶样蛋白水解活性[122]。富含水甲醇样多酚的 MK 叶提取物能诱导癌细胞的细胞周期停滞在 S 期,但不能诱导正常肺成纤维细胞的细胞周期停滞在 S 期。其机制涉及抑制癌细胞中的 26S 蛋白酶体,Annexin Ⅴ 结合的数据表明了由此导致的细胞凋亡[123]。对异种移植肿瘤小鼠模型进行进一步的体内研究,结果显示 MK 提取物对小鼠没有任何毒性作用。对提取物的分析表明,其中的黄酮类化合物,包括槲皮素(quercetin)、芹菜素(apigenin)、山奈酚(kaempferol)和芦丁(rutin),能有效抑制 MDA-MB-231 细胞中的内源性 26S 蛋白酶体。因此,肿瘤生长的抑制与蛋白酶体酶活性的降低有关。此外,caspase-3 活性增加、抗凋亡和血管生成基因表达下降也表明肿瘤进展受到抑制[167]。MK 通过降低硝酸盐和促炎性细胞因子(如 iNOS、iCAM、NF-κB 和 c-MYC)水平,减少了 4T1 乳腺癌小鼠的肿瘤大小和肺转移[124]。

(五)香附子

香附子[*Cyperus rotundus*,(CR)L.]又名梭梭草,是一种属于莎草科(Cyperaceae)的野生杂草。在阿育吠陀医学中,它被广泛用于治疗腹泻、糖尿病、炎症、疟疾和肠道疾病。同样,据报道,CR 在药理学上具有神经保护、心脏保护、肝脏保护、抗糖尿病、抗神经病变和抗惊厥等特性[189]。CR 根茎的甲醇提取物(methanolic extract of CR rhizome,MECR)可诱导 MCF7 细胞凋亡,而与 MECR 相比,乙醇提取物(ethanolic extract of CR rhizome,EECR)对 TNBC MDA-MB-231 的凋亡活性更高。TNBC 的细胞周期在 EECR 的作用下停滞在 G0/1 期。细胞凋亡的进展机制是死亡受体 4(death receptors4,DR4)、DR5 和促凋亡的 Bax 上调,而同时下调抗凋亡的 survivin 和 Bcl-2。caspase-8 和 caspase-9 的激活代表着外源性和内源性凋亡途径的启动。同样,效应分子 caspase-3 的激活与线粒体膜去极化和 PARP(活化的 caspase-3 的底物)的裂解有关[95,96,190]。此外,3-甲基腺嘌呤(3-methyladenine)可抑制 TNBC 细胞促存活自噬,并增加对 EECR 的敏感性[97]。

HC9 是一种多草药配方,阿育吠陀医师用它给哺乳期女性做母乳的清洁和解毒。CR 作为九种等比例药用植物之一被纳入 HC9。HC9 可使 MCF7 细胞系的细胞周期停滞在 S 期,MDA-MB-231 的细胞周期停滞在 G1 期。p53 和 p21 的上调可导致细胞周期停滞,而 MCF7 细胞周期停滞在 S 期的表现为 p16 的上调和 TNBC 肿瘤的停滞,MDA-MB-231 停滞在 G1 期的代表是 pRb 的上调。通过减少 MMP-2/9、HIF1α 和 VEGF 的表达,抑制 MCF7 和 MDA-MB-231 细胞系中的炎症标志物(NF-κB 和 COX-2),并改变染色质调节剂(SMAR1 和 CDP/Cux)的表达,HC9 明显降低了这两种细胞系的迁移。这种针对乳腺癌细胞的强效抗癌活性值得在未来进行临床前和临床研究[191]。

(六) *Centratherum anthelminticum*

Centratherum anthelminticum(L.)Kuntze,又称苦孜然(cumin),印地语中称为卡里吉利[译者注:音译,kalizeeri],属于菊科(Asteraceae),常见于印度、斯里兰卡和阿富汗。传统上,其种子用于治疗糖尿病,苦孜然还是一种用于全身恢复活力的制剂卡亚卡尔普[译者注:音译,Kayakalp]的主要成分。同样,据报道,其种子具有抗癌、抗糖尿病、抗炎、抗病毒、抗丝虫和抗菌等药理作用[192]。2004 年,Lambertini 等报道,80% 的 *C. anthelminticum* 种子乙醇提取物对 MCF7 和 MDA-MB-231 细胞系具有抗增殖作用。此外,用种子提取物处理这两种乳腺癌细胞系会诱导 ERα mRNA 的积累,这是乳腺肿瘤对内分泌治疗的一种确立的反应[102]。*C. anthelminticum* 的氯仿馏分(Chloroform fraction of *C. anthelminticum*,CACF)介导的对 MCF7 的抑制作用,可以观察到 MCF7 的形态学变化、细胞骨架结构破坏和 DNA 断裂。通过生物检测指导下的分馏,发现了 CACF 中的一种细胞毒性物质——vernodalin[103]。体外和体内报告显示,vernodalin 通过 PI3K-Akt/FOXO3a 途径介导乳腺癌细胞凋亡[104]。

(七) 胡桃

胡桃(*Juglans regia* L.),又称核桃,属于胡桃科(Juglandaceae)。原产于欧洲东南部、小亚细亚、印度和中国[193]。传统上,叶子可用于治疗静脉功能不全和痔疮的症状[194]。胡桃花具有一些生物活性复合物,如氮杂环吲哚(azacyclo-indole)、酚类(phenols)、生物碱(alkaloid)、黄酮(flavone)、四氢萘(tetralone)和萘醌(naphthoquinone)[195,196]。从胡桃壳中提取的胡桃苷(Juglanin)能抑制人类乳腺癌细胞的G2/M期生长,并通过ROS/JNK信号通路诱导细胞凋亡和自噬[197]。使用生物测定法从叶片氯仿提取物中分离出的5,7-二羟基-3,4′-二甲氧基黄酮(5,7-dihydroxy-3,4′-dimethoxyflavone)和核桃酮(regiolone)能诱导MCF7细胞中独立于caspase-3的凋亡途径,并使细胞周期停滞在G0/G1期[198,199]。胡桃的根皮(J. regia root bark,RBJR)氯仿提取物改善了MDA-MB-231细胞中Bax、caspase、p53和TNF-α介导的细胞毒性[119]。核桃油富含α-亚麻酸(alpha linolenic acid,ALA)和β-谷甾醇(β-sitosterol)。因此,从核桃油中提取的提取物与ALA和β-谷甾醇一样能减少MCF7的增殖。经ALA处理的小鼠乳腺癌细胞系TM2H显示出多个细胞靶标,包括PPAR、LXR和FXR靶基因。核桃油比其他测试过的核受体更广泛地提高了FXR的活性[200]。

(八)亚麻

亚麻(Flax)是一种食品膳食补充剂,常用于治疗更年期症状。亚麻籽富含植物雌激素-木酚素(phytoestrogen lignan)和ALA,其可能降低乳腺癌风险[201]。亚麻籽(flaxseed,FS)提取物诱导MCF7细胞凋亡介导的细胞毒性。细胞毒性机制始于ROS升高和线粒体膜电位丧失,最终以caspase级联反应介导的细胞凋亡结束[202]。在啮齿动物模型中,2.5%~10.0%的FS饮食或等量的木酚素或木酚油可抑制肿瘤的生长。同样,在临床试验中,补充FS(25 g/d,含50 mg木酚素,持续32天)可抑制乳腺癌患者的肿瘤生长,而以50 mg/d的剂量持续补充1年木酚素可降低绝经前女性患乳腺癌的风险[203]。此外,亚麻籽木酚素还能明显敏化SK-BR3和MDA-MB-231乳腺癌细胞系,增强多西他赛、多柔比星和卡铂等化疗药物的细胞毒性[204]。开环异落叶松树脂酚二葡萄糖苷(secoisolariciresinol diglucoside,SDG)是FS中一种含量较丰富的木酚素,在高雌激素环境中具有抗雌激素活性。采用SDG治疗可恢复乳腺组织中的多种生物标志物。此外,它不会促进卵巢上皮细胞癌前病变的进展[205]。亚麻秸秆中的黄酮C-葡萄糖苷(flavonoid C-glucosides)(如牡荆素、荭草苷和异荭草苷)及单独的提纯化合物对MCF7细胞具有细胞毒性。细胞凋亡与Bax/Bcl-2和caspases-7、caspases-8和caspases-9表达的增加有关[206]。FS新芽通过上调p53 mRNA,明显抑制了MCF7和MDA-MB-231细胞,而对MCF-10A中正常乳腺上皮细胞未观察到影响[译者注:原文为MCF-10A normal mammalian epithelial cell,mammalian可能为mammary的笔误(MCF-10A是一种上皮细胞系,于1984年从一名36岁患有纤维囊性乳腺病的白人女性的乳腺中分离出来)]。因此,这些研究表明,亚麻籽和亚麻秸秆中的植物成分具有抗癌潜力[207]。

(九)丁香蒲桃

丁香蒲桃(*Syzgium aromaticum*)又名丁香(cloves),是桃金娘科(Myrataceae)植物的芳香花蕾。丁香提取物对 MCF7 细胞有抗增殖和促凋亡作用。具体体现在细胞周期停滞在 S 期,随后线粒体膜电位降低,Bcl-2 表达受抑制和 caspase-7 升高。在一种由 N-亚硝基-N-甲基脲(*N*-nitroso-*N*-methylurea)诱导的乳腺癌模型中,将丁香的干花蕾与饮食一起给药,可降低大鼠癌细胞的肿瘤发生频率和脂质过氧化反应。它还抑制了抗凋亡基因 *Bcl-2* 和各种与转移和干性相关的基因,包括 Ki67、VEGFA、CD24 和 CD44。此外,它还能增加动物癌细胞中促凋亡基因 Bax、效应分子 caspase-3 和 ALDH1 的表达。补充丁香能增加癌细胞中组蛋白的赖氨酸三甲基化和乙酰化(H4K20me3、H4K16ac)。同样,在丁香处理的癌细胞中,肿瘤抑制基因 *TIMP3* 和 *RASSF1A* 的启动子岛的甲基化水平也发生了改变[208]。

丁香酚(eugenol)是丁香油的主要挥发性成分。在转染 *HRAS* 癌基因(MCF10A-ras)的细胞中,丁香酚通过抑制 c-Myc/PGC-1β/ERRα 信号通路,抑制氧化磷酸化复合物和脂肪酸氧化(fatty acid oxidizing,FAO)蛋白(如 PPARα、MCAD 和 CPT1C)的表达,从而显著降低细胞内 ATP 水平。这降低了 MCF10A-ras 细胞的氧化应激[209,210]。因此,丁香酚可通过调节能量代谢来预防乳腺癌。然而,在用丁香酚处理的正常 MCF10A 细胞中并没有发现这种机制。此外,丁香油对 MCF7 细胞也有最大的细胞毒性作用[211]。丁香提取物与纳米颗粒的结合也是一种很有前景的潜在癌症治疗方法[212]。

(十)肉托果

肉托果(*Semecarpus anacardium*,SA)的坚果提取物可通过一系列反应诱导 T47D 细胞凋亡,其中包括细胞内储存的 Ca^{2+} 增加、线粒体膜电位降低、Bcl-2/Bax 比率降低、细胞色素 c(cytosolic cytochrome c)增加、caspase 诱导的 PARP 分裂,最终导致 DNA 断裂[150]。多环芳烃(polycyclic aromatic hydrocarbon,PAH)是具有潜在遗传毒性作用的环境危险因素,乳腺组织中的外源物质代谢酶对此类化学致癌物的易感性和化疗反应都有影响。然而在 PAH 家族中的 7,12-二甲基苯并蒽[7,12-dimethylbenz(a)anthracene]诱导的啮齿动物乳腺癌模型中,用 SA 坚果提取物处理后,可恢复已改变的Ⅰ期生物转化酶(NADPH-细胞色素 P450 还原酶、NADPH-细胞色素 b5 还原酶和环氧化物水解酶)和Ⅱ期生物转化酶(谷胱甘肽-S-转移酶、谷胱甘肽过氧化物酶、葡糖醛酸还原酶、UDP 葡糖醛酸转移酶),并实现了对致癌物的完全解毒。同样,由于葡萄糖转运蛋白 1 和碳酸酐酶Ⅸ的表达减少,糖酵解酶的活性得到恢复,它还能延缓肿瘤的生长。此外,它还通过抑制 iNOS、

VEGF 和 HIF-1 来抑制血管生成活性,并通过抑制存活的细胞因子来防止内皮细胞增殖[213,214]。

kalpaamruthaa(KA)是一种悉达制剂[译者注:悉达(Siddha)是一种印度医学],成分包括肉托果(*Semecarpus anacardium*,SA)、余甘子(*Emblica officinalis*)(译者注:余甘子是一种印度硬毛猕猴桃)和蜂蜜。在 7,12-二甲基苯并蒽诱导的啮齿动物乳腺癌模型中,经 KA 和 SA 治疗后,血浆、肝脏和肾脏中胆固醇、磷脂、甘油三酯和游离脂肪酸水平的变化恢复正常。同样,SA 和 KA 治疗后,肿瘤大鼠体内的血管生成因子、脂质过氧化物和抗氧化剂水平也有所下降。此外,与 SA 相比,KA 的效果更好[215-217]。生物测定指导下分馏的肉托果膏己烷提取物(*Semecarpus lehyam* hexane extract,hSL)可有效敏化 ER 阳性的 MCF7 和 ER 阴性的 MDA-MB-231 癌细胞。(7;Z,10;Z)-3-十五碳-7,10-二烯基苯-1,2-二醇,(8;Z)3-戊二烯基-10-烯基苯-1,2-二醇,以及 3-十五烷基-苯-1,2-二醇[(7;Z,10;Z)-3-pentadeca-7,10-dienyl-benzene-1,2-diol;(8;Z)-3-pentadec-10-enyl-benzene-1,2-diol;3-pentadecyl-benzene-1,2-diol]这三种化合物是 SL 抗肿瘤作用的主要成分[218]。

(十一)石榴

石榴(*Punica granatum*),具有悠久的药用历史,这缘于其广谱的植物化学成分。石榴乳剂通过抑制环氧合酶 2(cyclooxygenase 2,COX-2)、HSP 90 和肿瘤内 ER(α 和 β)的表达,降低 ERα/ERβ,从而减少 DMBA 诱导的乳腺肿瘤发生。此外,它还阻止了 IkBα 的降解、NF-κB 从细胞质到细胞核的转位、β-catenin(一种 Wnt 信号转导通路的转录辅助因子)的细胞质积累和核转位,抑制了周期蛋白 D1(ER 和 Wnt/β-catenin 信号通路的下游靶点)的表达,并增加了 Nrf2 的表达。这些结果表明,抗炎、抗增殖和促凋亡机制参与了 PE 介导的大鼠乳腺肿瘤发生的预防过程[219,220][译者注:磷脂酰乙醇胺(PE)介导的细胞死亡是指 PE 介导的细胞死亡过程]。

石榴皮提取物(pomegranate peel extract,PPE)可增强细胞内黏附分子 1(intracellular adhesion molecule 1,ICAM1)和钙黏蛋白 E,而抑制细胞迁移相关蛋白,如 MMP-9、纤连蛋白、VEGF、波形蛋白、ZEB1 和 β-联蛋白。这体现了 PPE 治疗 TNBC 的抗转移的特效[221,222]。从石榴籽中分离出的石榴酸可诱导 MCF7 和 MDA-MB-231 细胞周期停滞在 G0/1 期。此外,它还能抑制 VEGF 和促炎性细胞因子的水平,如 IL-2、IL-6、IL-12、IL-17、IP-10、MIP-1α、MIP-1β、MCP-1 和 TNF-α[223]。

九、结论

乳腺癌是导致女性死亡的主要原因之一,但其治疗策略往往与不良反应相关,因此需要有效的替代疗法。药用植物是现代医学的基础,在当今生产的商业药物制剂中占有重要地位。全球约有 25% 的处方药来自植物。目前,人们对开发治疗乳腺癌的潜在药物越来越感兴趣,对药用植物及其生物活性成分开展多项研究来评估其疗效。然而,对于这些具有生物活性的天然产品的毒性、疗效和安全性进行严格评估尤为重要,以确保其不产生其他不良反应。

利益冲突

作者声明不存在利益冲突。

参 考 文 献

[1] Bray F, et al. Global cancer statistics 2018: GLOBOCAN estimates of incidence and mortality world-wide for 36 cancers in 185 countries. CA Cancer J Clin 2018;68(6):394-424.

[2] Chen JG, et al. Trends in the mortality of liver cancer in Qidong, China: an analysis of fifty years. Zhonghua Zhong Liu Za Zhi 2012;34(7):532-7.

[3] Torre LA, et al. Global cancer incidence and mortality rates and trends—an update. Cancer Epidemiol Biomarkers Prev 2016;25(1):16-27.

[4] Kamangar F, Dores GM, Anderson WF. Patterns of cancer incidence, mortality, and prevalence across five continents: defining priorities to reduce cancer disparities in different geographic regions of the world. J Clin Oncol 2006;24(14):2137-50.

[5] Parkin DM, et al. Global cancer statistics, 2002. CA Cancer J Clin 2005;55(2):74-108.

[6] Parkin DM, et al. Part Ⅰ: cancer in indigenous Africans—burden, distribution, and trends. Lancet Oncol 2008;9(7):683-92.

[7] Singh M, et al. Distinct breast cancer subtypes in women with early-onset disease across races. Am J Cancer Res 2014;4(4):337-52.

[8] Dogra A, et al. Clinicopathological characteristics of triple negative breast cancer at a tertiary care hospital in India. Asian Pac J Cancer Prev 2014;15(24):10577-83.

[9] Shetty P. India faces growing breast cancer epidemic. Lancet 2012;379(9820):992-3.

[10] Sen S, et al. A clinical and pathological study of triple negative breast carcinoma: experience of a tertiary care centre in eastern India. J Indian Med Assoc 2012;110(10):686-9 705.

[11] Kumar P, Aggarwal R. An overview of triple-negative breast cancer. Arch Gynecol Obstet 2016;293(2):247-69.

[12] Thummuri D, et al. Epigenetic regulation of protein tyrosine phosphatase PTPN12 in triple-negative breast cancer. Life Sci 2015;130:73-80.

[13] Lakshmaiah KC, et al. A study of triple negative breast cancer at a tertiary cancer care center in southern India. Ann Med Health Sci Res 2014;4(6):933-7.

[14] Zubeda S, et al. Her-2/neu status: a neglected marker of prognostication and management of breast cancer patients in India. Asian Pac J Cancer Prev 2013;14(4):2231-5.

[15] Nabi MG, et al. Clinicopathological comparison of triple negative breast cancers with non-triple negative breast cancers in a hospital in North India. Niger J Clin Pract 2015;18(3):381-6.

[16] Cherbal F, et al. Distribution of molecular breast cancer subtypes among Algerian women and correlation with clinical and tumor characteristics: a population-based study. Breast Dis 2015;35(2):95-102.

[17] Nigam JS, Yadav P, Sood N. A retrospective study of clinico-pathological spectrum of carcinoma breast in a West Delhi, India. South Asian J Cancer 2014;3(3):179-81.

[18] Singh R, et al. Evaluation of ER, PR and HER-2 receptor expression in breast cancer patients presenting to a semi urban cancer centre in Western India. J Cancer Res Ther 2014;10(1):26-8.

[19] Sood N, Nigam JS. Correlation of CK5 and EGFR with clinicopathological profile of triple-negative breast cancer. Patholog Res Int 2014;2014:141864.

[20] Lehmann BD, et al. Identification of human triple-negative breast cancer subtypes and preclinical models for selection of targeted therapies. J Clin Invest 2011;121(7):2750-67.

[21] Thomas DB. Factors that promote the development of human breast cancer. Environ Health Perspect 1983;50:209-18.

[22] Wu S, et al. Evaluating intrinsic and non-intrinsic cancer risk factors. Nat Commun 2018;9(1):3490.

[23] Kate RJ, Nadig R. Stage-specific predictive models for breast cancer survivability. Int J Med Inform 2017;97:304-11.

[24] Teshome M. Role of operative management in stage IV breast cancer. Surg Clin North Am 2018;98(4):859-68.

[25] Vuong D, et al. Molecular classification of breast cancer. Virchows Arch 2014;465(1):1-14.

[26] Maughan KL, Lutterbie MA, Ham PS. Treatment of breast cancer. Am Fam Physician 2010;81(11):1339-46.

[27] Saikolappan S, et al. Reactive oxygen species and cancer: a complex interaction. Cancer Lett 2019;452:132-43.

[28] Valko M, et al. Free radicals and antioxidants in normal physiological functions and human disease. Int J Biochem Cell Biol 2007;39(1):44-84.

[29] Liao Z, Chua D, Tan NS. Reactive oxygen species: a volatile driver of field cancerization

and metastasis. Mol Cancer 2019;18(1):65.

[30] Karar J, Maity A. PI3K/AKT/mTOR pathway in angiogenesis. Front Mol Neurosci 2011;4:51.

[31] Woo CC, et al. Thymoquinone inhibits tumor growth and induces apoptosis in a breast cancer xenograft mouse model: the role of p38 MAPK and ROS. PLoS One 2013;8(10)e75356.

[32] Hussain AR, et al. Thymoquinone suppresses growth and induces apoptosis via generation of reactive oxygen species in primary effusion lymphoma. Free Radic Biol Med 2011;50(8):978-87.

[33] Sosa V, et al. Oxidative stress and cancer: an overview. Ageing Res Rev 2013;12(1):376-90.

[34] Del Principe MI, et al. Apoptosis and immaturity in acute myeloid leukemia. Hematology 2005;10(1):25-34.

[35] Wong RSY. Apoptosis in cancer: from pathogenesis to treatment. J Exp Clin Cancer Res 2011;30(1):87.

[36] Kadam CY, Abhang SA. Chapter five: apoptosis markers in breast cancer therapy. In: Makowski GS, editor. Advances in clinical chemistry. Elsevier; 2016. p. 143-93.

[37] Schaeffer HJ, Weber MJ. Mitogen-activated protein kinases: specific messages from ubiquitous messengers. Mol Cell Biol 1999;19(4):2435-44.

[38] Hanahan D, Weinberg RA. The hallmarks of cancer. Cell 2000;100(1):57-70.

[39] Dhillon AS, et al. MAP kinase signalling pathways in cancer. Oncogene 2007;26(22):3279-90.

[40] Yue W, et al. Activation of the MAPK pathway enhances sensitivity of MCF-7 breast cancer cells to the mitogenic effect of estradiol. Endocrinology 2002;143(9):3221-9.

[41] Fresno Vara JA, et al. PI3K/Akt signalling pathway and cancer. Cancer Treat Rev 2004;30(2):193-204.

[42] Paplomata E, O'Regan R. The PI3K/AKT/mTOR pathway in breast cancer: targets, trials and biomarkers. Ther Adv Med Oncol 2014;6(4):154-66.

[43] Huang S, Houghton PJ. Targeting mTOR signaling for cancer therapy. Curr Opin Pharmacol 2003;3(4):371-7.

[44] Faivre S, Kroemer G, Raymond E. Current development of mTOR inhibitors as anticancer agents. Nat Rev Drug Discov 2006;5(8):671-88.

[45] Zhou BP, et al. HER-2/neu blocks tumor necrosis factor-induced apoptosis via the Akt/NF-kappaB pathway. J Biol Chem 2000;275(11):8027-31.

[46] Pópulo H, Lopes JM, Soares P. The mTOR signalling pathway in human cancer. Int J Mol Sci 2012;13(2):1886-918.

[47] Sharma VR, et al. PI3K/Akt/mTOR intracellular pathway and breast cancer: factors, mechanism and regulation. Curr Pharm Des 2017;23(11):1633-8.

[48] Malumbres M, Barbacid M. Cell cycle, CDKs and cancer: a changing paradigm. Nat Rev Cancer 2009;9(3):153-66.

[49] Abdullah C, Wang X, Becker D. Expression analysis and molecular targeting of cyclin-dependent kinases in advanced melanoma. Cell Cycle 2011;10(6):977-88.

[50] Georgieva J, Sinha P, Schadendorf D. Expression of cyclins and cyclin dependent kinases in human benign and malignant melanocytic lesions. J Clin Pathol 2001;54(3):229-35.

[51] Peyressatre M, et al. Targeting cyclin-dependent kinases in human cancers: from small molecules to peptide inhibitors. Cancer 2015;7(1):179-237.

[52] Husdal A, Bukholm G, Bukholm IRK. The prognostic value and overexpression of cyclin A is correlated with gene amplification of both cyclin A and cyclin E in breast cancer patient. Cell Oncol 2006;28(3):107-16.

[53] Ekberg J, et al. Expression of cyclin A1 and cell cycle proteins in hematopoietic cells and acute myeloid leukemia and links to patient outcome. Eur J Haematol 2005;75(2):106-15.

[54] Gillett C, et al. Amplification and overexpression of cyclin D1 in breast cancer detected by immunohistochemical staining. Cancer Res 1994;54(7):1812-7.

[55] Shaye A, et al. Cyclin E deregulation is an early event in the development of breast cancer. Breast Cancer Res Treat 2009;115(3):651-9.

[56] Wang M, et al. 8-Chloro-adenosine sensitizes a human hepatoma cell line to TRAIL-induced apoptosis by caspase-dependent and-independent pathways. Oncol Rep 2004;12(1):193-9.

[57] Morales J, et al. Review of poly (ADP-ribose) polymerase (PARP) mechanisms of action and rationale for targeting in cancer and other diseases. Crit Rev Eukaryot Gene Expr 2014;24(1):15-28.

[58] DiGiovanni J, Juchau MR. Biotransformation and bioactivation of 7,12-dimethylbenz[a]anthracene(7,12-DMBA). Drug Metab Rev 1980;11(1):61-101.

[59] Torre LA, et al. Global cancer statistics, 2012. CA Cancer J Clin 2015;65(2):87-108.

[60] Jazayeri SB, et al. Incidence of primary breast cancer in Iran: ten-year national cancer registry data report. Cancer Epidemiol 2015;39(4):519-27.

[61] Hamidinekoo A, et al. Deep learning in mammography and breast histology, an overview and future trends. Med Image Anal 2018;47:45-67.

[62] Gao J, et al. p53 and ATM/ATR regulate 7,12-dimethylbenz[a]anthracene-induced immunosuppression. Mol Pharmacol 2008;73(1):137-46.

[63] Nakatsugi S, et al. Chemoprevention by nimesulide, a selective cyclooxygenase-2 inhibitor, of 2-amino-1-methyl-6-phenylimidazo[4,5-b]pyridine (PhIP)-induced mammary gland carcinogenesis in rats. Jpn J Cancer Res 2000;91(9):886-92.

[64] Alfred LJ, et al. A chemical carcinogen, 3-methylcholanthrene, alters T-cell function and induces T-suppressor cells in a mouse model system. Immunology 1983;50(2):207-13.

[65] Lasfargues EY, Ozzello L. Cultivation of human breast carcinomas. J Natl Cancer Inst

1958;21(6):1131-47.

[66] Dai X, et al. Breast cancer cell line classification and its relevance with breast tumor subtyping. J Cancer 2017;8(16):3131-41.

[67] Gazdar AF, et al. Characterization of paired tumor and non-tumor cell lines established from patients with breast cancer. Int J Cancer 1998;78(6):766-74.

[68] Cailleau R, Olivé M, Cruciger QV. Long-term human breast carcinoma cell lines of metastatic origin: preliminary characterization. In Vitro 1978;14(11):911-5.

[69] Ghosh D. Chapter 64: Seed to patient in clinically proven natural medicines ** Partly adapted from Zangara and Ghosh (2014), with permission from CCR Press. In: Gupta RC, editor. Nutraceuticals. Boston: Academic Press; 2016. p. 925-31.

[70] Boadu AA, Asase A. Documentation of herbal medicines used for the treatment and management of human diseases by some Communities in Southern Ghana. Evid Based Complement Alternat Med 2017;2017:3043061.

[71] Sundarraj S, et al. γ-Sitosterol from *Acacia nilotica* L. induces G2/M cell cycle arrest and apoptosis through c-Myc suppression in MCF-7 and A549 cells. J Ethnopharmacol 2012;141(3):803-9.

[72] Rabi T, et al. Novel drug amooranin induces apoptosis through caspase activity in human breast carcinoma cell lines. Breast Cancer Res Treat 2003;80(3):321-30.

[73] Kumar S, et al. Andrographolide inhibits osteopontin expression and breast tumor growth through down regulation of PI3 kinase/Akt signaling pathway. Curr Mol Med 2012;12(8):952-66.

[74] Banerjee M, et al. Cytotoxicity and cell cycle arrest induced by andrographolide lead to programmed cell death of MDA-MB-231 breast cancer cell line. J Biomed Sci 2016;23:40.

[75] Mishra SK, et al. Andrographolide and analogues in cancer prevention. Front Biosci 2015;7:255-66.

[76] Menon V, Bhat S. Anticancer activity of andrographolide semisynthetic derivatives. Nat Prod Commun 2010;5(5):717-20.

[77] Roham PH, et al. Induction of mitochondria mediated apoptosis in human breast cancer cells (T-47D) by *Annona reticulata* L. Leaves methanolic extracts. Nutr Cancer 2016;68(2):305-11.

[78] Shafi G, et al. Artemisia absinthium (AA): a novel potential complementary and alternative medicine for breast cancer. Mol Biol Rep 2012;39(7):7373-9.

[79] Rautray S, et al. Anticancer activity of *Adiantum capillus* veneris and *Pteris quadriureta* L. in human breast cancer cell lines. Mol Biol Rep 2018;45(6):1897-911.

[80] Kamalanathan D, Natarajan D. Anticancer potential of leaf and leaf-derived callus extracts of *Aerva javanic* aagainst MCF-7 breast cancer cell line. J Cancer Res Ther 2018;14(2):321-7.

[81] Diab KAE, et al. In vitro anticancer activities of *Anogeissus latifolia*, *Terminalia belleri-*

ca, *Acacia catechu* and *Moringa oleiferna* indian plants. Asian Pac J Cancer Prev 2015;16 (15):6423-8.

[82] George VC, et al. Quantitative assessment of the relative antineoplastic potential of the n-butanolic leaf extract of *Annona muricata* Linn. in normal and immortalized human cell lines. Asian Pac J Cancer Prev 2012;13(2):699-704.

[83] Prabhakaran K, et al. Polyketide natural products, acetogenins from graviola (*Annona muricata* L.), its biochemical, cytotoxic activity and various analyses through computational and bio-programming methods. Curr Pharm Des 2016;22(34):5204-10.

[84] Bhagat J, et al. Cytotoxic potential of *Anisochilus carnosus* (L. f.) wall and estimation of luteolin content by HPLC. BMC Complement Altern Med 2014;14:421.

[85] Sahu N, et al. Extraction, fractionation and re-fractionation of *Artemisia nilagirica* for anticancer activity and HPLC-ESI-QTOF-MS/MS determination. J Ethnopharmacol 2018; 213:72-80.

[86] Kant K, Lal UR, Ghosh M. In silico prediction and wet lab validation of *Arisaema tortuosum* (Wall.) schott extracts as antioxidant and anti-breast cancer source: a comparative study. Pharmacogn Mag 2018;13(Suppl 4):S786-90.

[87] Khazaei S, et al. Cytotoxicity and proapoptotic effects of *Allium atroviolaceum* flower extract by modulating cell cycle arrest and caspase-dependent and p53-independent pathway in breast cancer cell lines. Evid Based Complement Alternat Med 2017;2017:1468957.

[88] Kaur V, et al. Inhibitory activities of butanol fraction from *Butea monosperma* (Lam.) Taub. Bark against free radicals, genotoxins and cancer cells. Chem Biodivers 2017;14 (6). https://doi.org/10.1002/cbdv.201600484.

[89] Kumar S, et al. Antiproliferative and apoptotic effects of black turtle bean extracts on human breast cancer cell line through extrinsic and intrinsic pathway. Chem Cent J 2017;11 (1):56.

[90] Johnson Inbaraj J, et al. Cytotoxicity, redox cycling and photodynamic action of two naturally occurring quinones. Biochim Biophys Acta 1999;1472(3):462-70.

[91] Bassan P, et al. Extraction, profiling and bioactivity analysis of volatile glucosinolates present in oil extract of *Brassica juncea* var. raya. Physiol Mol Biol Plants 2018;24(3): 399-409.

[92] Sreeja S, Sreeja S. An in vitro study on antiproliferative and antiestrogenic effects of *Boerhaavia diffusa* L. extracts. J Ethnopharmacol 2009;126(2):221-5.

[93] Thummuri D, et al. Boswellia ovalifoliolata abrogates ROS mediated NF-κB activation, causes apo ptosis and chemosensitization in triple negative breast cancer cells. Environ Toxicol Pharmacol 2014;38(1):58-70.

[94] Mishra T, et al. Isolation, characterization and anticancer potential of cytotoxic triterpenes from betula utilis bark. PLoS One 2016;11(7):e0159430.

[95] Park SE, et al. Induction of apoptosis in MDA-MB-231 human breast carcinoma cells with

an ethanol extract of *Cyperus rotundus* L. by activating caspases. Oncol Rep 2014;32(6):
2461-70.
[96] Mannarreddy P, et al. Cytotoxic effect of *Cyperus rotundus* rhizome extract on human cancer cell lines. Biomed Pharmacother 2017;95:1375-87.
[97] Wang F, et al. The treatment role of *Cyperus rotundus* L. to triple-negative breast cancer cells. Biosci Rep 2019;39(6)BSR20190502.
[98] Khoobchandani M, et al. Chenopodium album prevents progression of cell growth and enhances cell toxicity in human breast cancer cell lines. Oxid Med Cell Longev 2009;2(3):
160-5.
[99] Neethu PV, Suthindhiran K, Jayasri MA. Methanolic extract of costus pictus D. DON induces cytotoxicity in liver hepatocellular carcinoma cells mediated by histone deacetylase inhibition. Pharmacogn Mag 2017;13(Suppl 3):S533-8.
[100] Pitchai D, Roy A, Banu S. In vitro and in silico evaluation of NF-κB targeted costunolide action on estrogen receptor-negative breast cancer cells—a comparison with normal breast cells. Phytother Res 2014;28(10):1499-505.
[101] Prasanna R, et al. Anti-cancer effect of *Cassia auriculata* leaf extract in vitro through cell cycle arrest and induction of apoptosis in human breast and larynx cancer cell lines. Cell Biol Int 2009;33(2):127-34.
[102] Lambertini E, et al. Effects of extracts from Bangladeshi medicinal plants on in vitro proliferation of human breast cancer cell lines and expression of estrogen receptor alpha gene. Int J Oncol 2004;24(2):419-23.
[103] Looi CY, et al. Induction of apoptosis in human breast cancer cells via caspase pathway by vernodalin isolated from *Centratherum anthelminticum* (L.) seeds. PLoS One 2013;8(2) e56643.
[104] Ananda Sadagopan SK, et al. Forkhead Box Transcription Factor (FOXO3a) mediates the cytotoxic effect of vernodalin in vitro and inhibits the breast tumor growth in vivo. J Exp Clin Canc Res 2015;34:147.
[105] Arya A, et al. Chloroform fraction of *Centratherum anthelminticum* (L.) seed inhibits tumor necrosis factor alpha and exhibits pleotropic bioactivities: inhibitory role in human tumor cells. Evid Based Complement Alternat Med 2012;2012:627256.
[106] Moirangthem DS, et al. *Cephalotaxus griffithii* Hook. f. needle extract induces cell cycle arrest, apoptosis and suppression of hTERT and hTR expression on human breast cancer cells. BMC Complement Altern Med 2014;14:305.
[107] Chowdhury K, et al. Colocynth extracts prevent epithelial to mesenchymal transition and stemness of breast cancer cells. Front Pharmacol 2017;8:593.
[108] Naik Bukke A, et al. In vitro studies data on anticancer activity of *Caesalpinia sappan* L. heartwood and leaf extracts on MCF7 and A549 cell lines. Data Brief 2018;19:868-77.
[109] Masood Ur R, et al. Synthesis and biological evaluation of novel 3-O-tethered triazoles of

diosgenin as potent antiproliferative agents. Steroids 2017;118:1-8.

[110] Ghate NB, et al. Sundew plant, a potential source of anti-inflammatory agents, selectively induces G2/M arrest and apoptosis in MCF-7 cells through upregulation of p53 and Bax/Bcl-2 ratio. Cell Death Dis 2016;2:15062.

[111] Mohanakumara P, et al. *Dysoxylum binectariferum* Hook. f (Meliaceae), a rich source of rohitukine. Fitoterapia 2010;81(2):145-8.

[112] Shriram V, et al. Cytotoxic activity of 9,10-dihydro-2,5-dimethoxyphenanthrene-1,7-diol from *Eulophia nuda* against human cancer cells. J Ethnopharmacol 2010;128(1):251-3.

[113] Kumar S, Kashyap P. Antiproliferative activity and nitric oxide production of a methanolic extract of *Fraxinus micrantha* on Michigan cancer foundation-7 mammalian breast carcinoma cell line. J Intercult Ethnopharmacol 2015;4(2):109-13.

[114] Haneef J, et al. Bax translocation mediated mitochondrial apoptosis and caspase dependent photosensitizing effect of *Ficus religiosa* on cancer cells. PLoS One 2012; 7 (7):e40055.

[115] Sharma R, et al. Glycyrrhiza glabra extract and quercetin reverses cisplatin resistance in triple-negative MDA-MB-468 breast cancer cells via inhibition of cytochrome P450 1B1 enzyme. Bioorg Med Chem Lett 2017;27(24):5400-3.

[116] Sebastian KS, Thampan RV. Differential effects of soybean and fenugreek extracts on the growth of MCF-7 cells. Chem Biol Interact 2007;170(2):135-43.

[117] Jamila N, et al. In vivo carbon tetrachloride-induced hepatoprotective and in vitro cytotoxic activities of garcinia hombroniana (seashore mangosteen). Afr J Tradit Complement Altern Med 2017;14(2):374-82.

[118] Shoja MH, et al. *Glycosmis pentaphylla* (Retz.) DC arrests cell cycle and induces apoptosis via caspase-3/7 activation in breast cancer cells. J Ethnopharmacol 2015;168:50-60.

[119] Hasan TN, et al. Anti-proliferative effects of organic extracts from root bark of *Juglans Regia* L. (RBJR) on MDA-MB-231 human breast cancer cells: role of Bcl-2/Bax, caspases and Tp53. Asian Pac J Cancer Prev 2011;12(2):525-30.

[120] Mohanty SK, et al. Evaluation of antioxidant, in vitro cytotoxicity of micropropagated and naturally grown plants of *Leptadenia reticulata* (Retz.) Wight & Arn.-an endangered medicinal plant. Asian Pac J Trop Med 2014;7S1:S267-71.

[121] Rawat P, et al. Phytochemicals and cytotoxicity of launaea procumbens on human cancer cell lines. Pharmacogn Mag 2016;12(Suppl 4):S431-5.

[122] Ismail A, et al. Cytotoxicity and proteasome inhibition by alkaloid extract from *Murraya koenigii* leaves in breast cancer cells-molecular docking studies. J Med Food 2016; 19 (12):1155-65.

[123] Noolu B, et al. *Murraya koenigii* leaf extract inhibits proteasome activity and induces cell death in breast cancer cells. BMC Complement Altern Med 2013;13:7.

[124] Yeap SK, et al. Chemopreventive and immunomodulatory effects of *Murraya koenigii* a-

queous extract on 4T1 breast cancer cell-challenged mice. BMC Complement Altern Med 2015;15:306.

[125] Sharma K, et al. Anticancer effects of extracts from the fruit of *Morinda citrifolia* (noni) in breast cancer cell lines. Drug Res 2016;66(3):141-7.

[126] Sinha S, et al. *Mucuna pruriens* (L.) DC chemo sensitize human breast cancer cells via downregulation of prolactin-mediated JAK2/STAT5A signaling. J Ethnopharmacol 2018;217:23-35.

[127] Deepa M, Priya S. Purification and characterization of a novel anti-proliferative lectin from *Morus alba* L. leaves. Protein Pept Lett 2012;19(8):839-45.

[128] Deepa M, et al. Antioxidant rich Morus alba leaf extract induces apoptosis in human colon and breast cancer cells by the downregulation of nitric oxide produced by inducible nitric oxide synthase. Nutr Cancer 2013;65(2):305-10.

[129] Sodde VK, et al. Cytotoxic activity of *Macrosolen parasiticus* (L.) Danser on the growth of breast cancer cell line (MCF-7). Pharmacogn Mag 2015;11(Suppl 1):S156-60.

[130] Tiwary BK, et al. The in vitro cytotoxic activity of ethno-pharmacological important plants of Darjeeling district of West Bengal against different human cancer cell lines. BMC Complement Altern Med 2015;15:22.

[131] Ghosh P, et al. *Madhuca indica* inhibits breast cancer cell proliferation by modulating COX-2 expression. Curr Mol Med 2018;18(7):459-74.

[132] Chaudhary S, et al. Evaluation of antioxidant and anticancer activity of extract and fractions of *Nar dostachys jatamansi* DC in breast carcinoma. BMC Complement Altern Med 2015;15:50.

[133] Pandeti S, et al. Synthesis of novel anticancer iridoid derivatives and their cell cycle arrest and caspase dependent apoptosis. Phytomedicine 2014;21(3):333-9.

[134] Singh S, et al. Antiproliferative and antimicrobial efficacy of the compounds isolated from the roots of *Oenothera biennis* L. J Pharm Pharmacol 2017;69(9):1230-43.

[135] Singh MK, Dhongade H, Tripathi DK. *Orthosiphon pallidus*, a potential treatment for patients with breast cancer. J Pharm 2017;20(4):265-73.

[136] Naveen Kumar DR, et al. Cytotoxicity, apoptosis induction and anti-metastatic potential of *Oroxylum indicum* in human breast cancer cells. Asian Pac J Cancer Prev 2012;13(6):2729-34.

[137] Ghate NB, et al. An antioxidant extract of tropical lichen, *Parmotrema reticulatum*, induces cell cycle arrest and apoptosis in breast carcinoma cell line MCF-7. PLoS One 2013;8(12):e82293.

[138] Rajan V, et al. Mechanism of cytotoxicity by *Psoralea corylifolia* extract in human breast carcinoma cells. J Environ Pathol Toxicol Oncol 2014;33(3):265-77.

[139] Sharma M. Selective cytotoxicity and modulation of apoptotic signature of breast cancer cells by *Pithecellobium dulce* leaf extracts. Biotechnol Prog 2016;32(3):756-66.

[140] Vini R, Juberiya AM, Sreeja S. Evidence of pomegranate methanolic extract in antagonizing the endogenous SERM, 27-hydroxycholesterol. IUBMB Life 2016;68(2):116-21.

[141] Joseph MM, et al. Evaluation of antioxidant, antitumor and immunomodulatory properties of polysaccharide isolated from fruit rind of *Punica granatum*. Mol Med Rep 2012;5(2):489-96.

[142] Rajkumar V, Guha G, Kumar RA. Antioxidant and anti-neoplastic activities of *Picrorhiza kurroa* extracts. Food Chem Toxicol 2011;49(2):363-9.

[143] Ganie SA, et al. Long dose exposure of hydrogen peroxide (H_2O_2) in albino rats and effect of *Podophyllum hexandrum* on oxidative stress. Eur Rev Med Pharmacol Sci 2011;15(8):906-15.

[144] Kaur P, et al. Suppression of SOS response in *E. coli* PQ 37, antioxidant potential and antiproliferative action of methanolic extract of *Pteris vittata* L. on human MCF-7 breast cancer cells. Food Chem Toxicol 2014;74:326-33.

[145] Sharma R, et al. Furanoflavones pongapin and lanceolatin B blocks the cell cycle and induce senescence in CYP1A1-overexpressing breast cancer cells. Bioorg Med Chem 2018;26(23-24):6076-86.

[146] Kumar Singh S, Patra A. Evaluation of phenolic composition, antioxidant, anti-inflammatory and anticancer activities of *Polygonatum verticillatum* (L.). J Integr Med 2018;16(4):273-82.

[147] Suma HK, et al. *Pyrenacantha volubilis* Wight, (Icacinaceae) a rich source of camptothecine and its derivatives, from the Coromandel Coast forests of India. Fitoterapia 2014;97:105-10.

[148] Rajkumar V, Guha G, Kumar RA. Apoptosis induction in MDA-MB-435S, Hep3B and PC-3 cell lines by Rheum emodi rhizome extracts. Asian Pac J Cancer Prev 2011;12(5):1197-200.

[149] Dutta S, Khanna A. Aglycone rich extracts of phytoestrogens cause ROS-mediated DNA damage in breast carcinoma cells. Biomed Pharmacother 2016;84:1513-23.

[150] Mathivadhani P, Shanthi P, Sachdanandam P. Apoptotic effect of *Semecarpus anacardium* nut extract on T47D breast cancer cell line. Cell Biol Int 2007;31(10):1198-206.

[151] Chakraborty S, et al. Cytotoxic effect of root extract of *Tiliacora racemosa* and oil of *Semecarpus anacardium* nut in human tumour cells. Phytother Res 2004;18(8):595-600.

[152] Sowmyalakshmi S, et al. Investigation on *Semecarpus lehyam*—a Siddha medicine for breast cancer. Planta 2005;220(6):910-8.

[153] Dwivedi V, et al. Comparative anticancer potential of clove (*Syzygium aromaticum*)—an Indian spice—against cancer cell lines of various anatomical origin. Asian Pac J Cancer Prev 2011;12(8):1989-93.

[154] Yadav NK, et al. Saraca indica bark extract shows in vitro antioxidant, antibreast cancer activity and does not exhibit toxicological effects. Oxid Med Cell Longev 2015;

2015;205360.
[155] Musini A, Rao JP, Giri A. Phytochemicals of *Salacia oblonga* responsible for free radical scavenging and antiproliferative activity against breast cancer cell lines (MDA-MB-231). Physiol Mol Biol Plants 2015;21(4):583-90.
[156] Ansari JA, et al. ROS mediated pro-apoptotic effects of *Tinospora cordifolia* on breast cancer cells. Front Biosci 2017;9:89-100.
[157] Johnson Inbaraj J, Gandhidasan R, Murugesan R. Cytotoxicity and superoxide anion generation by some naturally occurring quinones. Free Radic Biol Med 1999;26(9-10):1072-8.
[158] Chattopadhyay SK, et al. Absolute configuration and anticancer activity of taxiresinol and related lignans of *Taxus wallichiana*. Bioorg Med Chem 2003;11(23):4945-8.
[159] Appadath Beeran A, et al. The enriched fraction of *Vernonia cinerea* L. induces apoptosis and inhibits multi-drug resistance transporters in human epithelial cancer cells. J Ethnopharmacol 2014;158(Pt A):33-42.
[160] Chakravarti B, et al. In vitro anti-breast cancer activity of ethanolic extract of *Wrightia tomentosa*: role of pro-apoptotic effects of oleanolic acid and urosolic acid. J Ethnopharmacol 2012;142(1):72-9.
[161] Dar PA, et al. An anti-cancerous protein fraction from *Withania somnifera* induces ROS-dependent mitochondria-mediated apoptosis in human MDA-MB-231 breast cancer cells. Int J Biol Macromol 2019;135:77-87.
[162] Vyry Wouatsa NA, et al. Zantholic acid, a new monoterpenoid from *Zanthoxylum zanthoxyloides*. Nat Prod Res 2013;27(21):1994-8.
[163] Mallick MN, et al. Exploring the cytotoxic potential of triterpenoids-enriched fraction of bacopa monnieri by implementing in vitro, in vivo, and in silico approaches. Pharmacogn Mag 2017;13(Suppl 3):S595-606.
[164] Karia P, Patel KV, Rathod SSP. Breast cancer amelioration by *Butea monosperma* in-vitro and in-vivo. J Ethnopharmacol 2018;217:54-62.
[165] Singh SK, et al. Chemically standardized isolates from *Cedrus deodara* stem wood having anticancer activity. Planta Med 2007;73(6):519-26.
[166] Choudhury B, et al. *Garcinia morella* fruit, a promising source of antioxidant and anti-inflammatory agents induces breast cancer cell death via triggering apoptotic pathway. Biomed Pharmacother 2018;103:562-73.
[167] Noolu B, et al. In vivo inhibition of proteasome activity and tumour growth by *Murraya koenigii* leaf extract in breast cancer xenografts and by its active flavonoids in breast cancer cells. Anticancer Agents Med Chem 2016;16(12):1605-14.
[168] Yuan C, et al. Inhibition on the growth of human MDA-MB-231 breast cancer cells in vitro and tumor growth in a mouse xenograft model by Se-containing polysaccharides from *Pyracantha fortuneana*. Nutr Res 2016;36(11):1243-54.

[169] Majumder M, et al. *Ricinus communis* L. fruit extract inhibits migration/invasion, induces apoptosis in breast cancer cells and arrests tumor progression in vivo. Sci Rep 2019;9(1):14493.

[170] Choi BY, Kim B-W. Withaferin-A inhibits colon cancer cell growth by blocking STAT3 transcriptional activity. J Cancer Prev 2015;20(3):185-92.

[171] Ray SD, Dewanjee S. Isolation of a new triterpene derivative and in vitro and in vivo anticancer activity of ethanolic extract from root bark of *Zizyphus nummularia* Aubrev. Nat Prod Res 2015;29(16):1529-36.

[172] Sareer O, Ahmad S, Umar S. *Andrographis paniculata*: a critical appraisal of extraction, isolation and quantification of andrographolide and other active constituents. Nat Prod Res 2014;28(23):2081-101.

[173] Akbar S. *Andrographis paniculata*: a review of pharmacological activities and clinical effects. Altern Med Rev 2011;16(1):66-77.

[174] Okhuarobo A, et al. Harnessing the medicinal properties of *Andrographis paniculata* for diseases and beyond: a review of its phytochemistry and pharmacology. Asian Pac J Trop Dis 2014;4(3):213-22.

[175] Islam MT, et al. Andrographolide, a diterpene lactone from *Andrographis paniculata* and its therapeutic promises in cancer. Cancer Lett 2018;420:129-45.

[176] Dar NJ, Hamid A, Ahmad M. Pharmacologic overview of *Withania somnifera*, the Indian Ginseng. Cell Mol Life Sci 2015;72(23):4445-60.

[177] Rai M, et al. Anticancer activities of *Withania somnifera*: current research, formulations, and future perspectives. Pharm Biol 2016;54(2):189-97.

[178] Dutta R, et al. *Withania Somnifera* (Ashwagandha) and Withaferin A: potential in integrative oncology. Int J Mol Sci 2019;20(21):5310.

[179] Dar PA, et al. Unique medicinal properties of *Withania somnifera*: phytochemical constituents and protein component. Curr Pharm Des 2016;22(5):535-40.

[180] Palliyaguru DL, Singh SV, Kensler TW. *Withania somnifera*: from prevention to treatment of cancer. Mol Nutr Food Res 2016;60(6):1342-53.

[181] Khazal KF, Hill DL. *Withania somnifera* extract reduces the invasiveness of MDA-MB-231 breast cancer and inhibits cytokines associated with metastasis. J Cancer Metastasis Treatment 2015;1(2):94-100.

[182] Ghosh K, et al. Withaferin A induced impaired autophagy and unfolded protein response in human breast cancer cell-lines MCF-7 and MDA-MB-231. Toxicol In Vitro 2017;44:330-8.

[183] Singh D, Chaudhuri PK. Chemistry and pharmacology of *Tinospora cordifolia*. Nat Prod Commun 2017;12(2):299-308.

[184] Sharma P, et al. The chemical constituents and diverse pharmacological importance of *Tinospora cordifolia*. Heliyon 2019;5(9)e02437.

[185] Rashmi KC, et al. A new pyrrole based small molecule from *Tinospora cordifolia* induces apoptosis in MDA-MB-231 breast cancer cells via ROS mediated mitochondrial damage and restoration of p53 activity. Chem Biol Interact 2019;299:120-30.

[186] Samanta SK, et al. Phytochemical portfolio and anticancer activity of *Murraya koenigii* and its primary active component, mahanine. Pharmacol Res 2018;129:227-36.

[187] Utaipan T, et al. Carbazole alkaloids from *Murraya koenigii* trigger apoptosis and autophagic flux inhibition in human oral squamous cell carcinoma cells. J Nat Med 2017;71(1):158-69.

[188] Iman V, et al. Anticancer and anti-inflammatory activities of girinimbine isolated from *Murraya koenigii*. Drug Des Devel Ther 2016;11:103-21.

[189] Kamala A, Middha SK, Karigar CS. Plants in traditional medicine with special reference to *Cyperus rotundus* L.: a review. 3 Biotech 2018;8(7):309.

[190] Pirzada AM, et al. *Cyperus rotundus* L.: traditional uses, phytochemistry, and pharmacological activities. J Ethnopharmacol 2015;174:540-60.

[191] Suryavanshi S, et al. A polyherbal formulation, HC9 regulated cell growth and expression of cell cycle and chromatin modulatory proteins in breast cancer cell lines. J Ethnopharmacol 2019;242:112022.

[192] Arya A, et al. Anti-diabetic effects of *Centratherum anthelminticum* seeds methanolic fraction on pancreatic cells, β-TC6 and its alleviating role in type 2 diabetic rats. J Ethnopharmacol 2012;144(1):22-32.

[193] Delaviz H, et al. A review study on phytochemistry and pharmacology applications of *Juglans regia* plant. Pharmacogn Rev 2017;11(22):145-52.

[194] Cosmulescu S. Seasonal variation of total phenols in leaves of walnut (*Juglans regia* L.). J Med Plant Res 2011;52:4938.

[195] Li Q, et al. Azacyclo-indoles and phenolics from the flowers of *Juglans regia*. J Nat Prod 2017;80(8):2189-98.

[196] Luo J-J, et al. Chemical constituents from the flower of *Juglans regia*. Zhong Yao Cai 2012;35(10):1614-6.

[197] Sun Z-L, Dong J-L, Wu J. Juglanin induces apoptosis and autophagy in human breast cancer progression via ROS/JNK promotion. Biomed Pharmacother 2017;85:303-12.

[198] Salimi M, et al. Anti-proliferative and apoptotic activities of constituents of chloroform extract of *Juglans regia* leaves. Cell Prolif 2014;47(2):172-9.

[199] Salimi M, et al. Cytotoxicity effects of various *Juglans regia* (walnut) leaf extracts in human cancer cell lines. Pharm Biol 2012;50(11):1416-22.

[200] Vanden Heuvel JP, et al. Mechanistic examination of walnuts in prevention of breast cancer. Nutr Cancer 2012;64(7):1078-86.

[201] Flower G, et al. Flax and breast cancer: a systematic review. Integr Cancer Ther 2014;13(3):181-92.

[202] Hu T, et al. Flaxseed extract induces apoptosis in human breast cancer MCF-7 cells. Food Chem Toxicol 2019;127:188-96.

[203] Mason JK, Thompson LU. Flaxseed and its lignan and oil components: can they play a role in reducing the risk of and improving the treatment of breast cancer? Appl Physiol Nutr Metab 2014;39(6):663-78.

[204] Di Y, et al. Flaxseed lignans enhance the cytotoxicity of chemotherapeutic agents against breast cancer cell lines MDA-MB-231 and SKBR3. Nutr Cancer 2018;70(2):306-15.

[205] Delman DM, et al. Effects of flaxseed lignan secoisolariciresinol diglucosideon preneoplastic biomarkers of cancer progression in a model of simultaneous breast and ovarian cancer development. Nutr Cancer 2015;67(5):857-64.

[206] Czemplik M, et al. Flavonoid C-glucosides derived from flax straw extracts reduce human breast cancer cell growth in vitro and induce apoptosis. Front Pharmacol 2016;7:282.

[207] Lee J, Cho K. Flaxseed sprouts induce apoptosis and inhibit growth in MCF-7 and MDA-MB-231 human breast cancer cells. In Vitro Cell Dev Biol Anim 2012;48(4):244-50.

[208] Kubatka P, et al. Antineoplastic effects of clove buds (*Syzygium aromaticum* L.) in the model of breast carcinoma. J Cell Mol Med 2017;21(11):2837-51.

[209] Yan X, et al. Eugenol inhibits oxidative phosphorylation and fatty acid oxidation via downregulation of c-Myc/PGC-1β/ERRα signaling pathway in MCF10A-ras cells. Sci Rep 2017;7(1):12920.

[210] Anita Y, et al. Structure-based design of eugenol analogs as potential estrogen receptor antagonists. Bioinformation 2012;8(19):901-6.

[211] Kumar PS, et al. Anticancer potential of *Syzygium aromaticum* L. in MCF-7 human breast cancer cell lines. Pharm Res 2014;6(4):350-4.

[212] Khan FA, et al. Extracts of clove (*Syzygium aromaticum*) potentiate FMSP-nanoparticles induced cell death in MCF-7 cells. Int J Biomater 2018;2018:8479439.

[213] Mathivadhani P, Shanthi P, Sachdanandam P. Effect of *Semecarpus anacardium* Linn. nut extract on mammary and hepatic expression of xenobiotic enzymes in DMBA-induced mammary carcinoma. Environ Toxicol Pharmacol 2007;23(3):328-34.

[214] Mathivadhani P, Shanthi P, Sachdanandam P. Hypoxia and its downstream targets in DMBA induced mammary carcinoma: protective role of *Semecarpus anacardium* nut extract. Chem Biol Interact 2007;167(1):31-40.

[215] Veena K, Shanthi P, Sachdanandam P. The biochemical alterations following administration of Kalpaamruthaa and *Semecarpus anacardium* in mammary carcinoma. Chem Biol Interact 2006;161(1):69-78.

[216] Sathish S, Shanthi P, Sachdanandam P. Mitigation of DMBA-induced mammary carcinoma in experimental rats by antiangiogenic property of Kalpaamruthaa. J Diet Suppl 2011;8(2):144-57.

[217] Veena K, Shanthi P, Sachdanandam P. Therapeutic efficacy of Kalpaamruthaa on reactive

oxygen/nitrogen species levels and antioxidative system in mammary carcinoma bearing rats. Mol Cell Biochem 2007;294(1-2):127-35.

[218] Zhao W, et al. Identification of urushiols as the major active principle of the Siddha herbal medicine *Semecarpus lehyam*: anti-tumor agents for the treatment of breast cancer. Pharm Biol 2009;47(9):886-93.

[219] Mandal A, Bhatia D, Bishayee A. Anti-inflammatory mechanism involved in pomegranate-mediated prevention of breast cancer: the role of NF-κB and Nrf2 signaling pathways. Nutrients 2017;9(5):436.

[220] Mandal A, Bishayee A. Mechanism of breast cancer preventive action of pomegranate: disruption of estrogen receptor and Wnt/β-catenin signaling pathways. Molecules 2015;20 (12):22315-28.

[221] Ahmadiankia N, Bagheri M, Fazli M. Gene expression changes in pomegranate peel extract-treated triple-negative breast cancer cells. Rep Biochem Mol Biol 2018;7(1):102-9.

[222] Bagheri M, et al. Pomegranate peel extract inhibits expression of β-catenin, epithelial mesenchymal transition, and metastasis in triple negative breast cancer cells. Cell Mol Biol 2018;64(7):86-91.

[223] Costantini S, et al. Potential anti-inflammatory effects of the hydrophilic fraction of pomegranate(*Punica granatum* L.) seed oil on breast cancer cell lines. Molecules 2014; 19(6):8644-60.

第 8 章
卡铂和紫杉醇在子宫内膜癌治疗中的作用

Sreedevi Muttathuveliyil Sivadasan, Pavan Kumar Kancharla, Neelakantan Arumugam

Department of Biotechnology, School of Life Sciences, Pondicherry University, Puducherry, India

摘要

子宫内膜癌是一种常见的妇科恶性肿瘤,是子宫恶性肿瘤中最常见的类型,起源于子宫内膜,常发生于绝经后。在过去十年里,其死亡率平均每年增加1.9%。根据病情的严重程度,子宫内膜癌可分为八期:ⅠA、ⅠB、Ⅱ、ⅢA、ⅢB、ⅢC、ⅣA和ⅣB。子宫内膜癌主要的危险因素包括肥胖、2型糖尿病、不孕、不育、因治疗乳腺癌而服用他莫昔芬、雌激素替代疗法、多囊卵巢综合征(polycystic ovarian syndrome, PCOS)、异常的代谢状态和家族病史等。治疗手段包括手术、放疗、激素治疗、化疗和靶向药物治疗。卡铂联合紫杉醇是最有效且毒性最小的化疗方案,这两种药物也因其独特的药理特性,在其他多种癌症治疗中得到广泛应用。卡铂是顺铂的衍生物,具有较低的毒性和更高的稳定性。该药能够通过烷基化作用产生活性铂复合物,进而损伤DNA。紫杉醇则通过与细胞微管相互作用,稳定微管,破坏细胞周期的正常进程,促使细胞凋亡。尽管单一药物治疗的总体反应率较低,但联合用药能显著提高疗效。此外,卡铂和紫杉醇与其他癌症治疗手段(如放疗、手术和激素治疗)的联合应用也显示出良好的治疗效果。

关键词

癌症,子宫内膜癌,卡铂,紫杉醇,化疗

缩略词

AI	芳香化酶抑制剂
AUC	曲线下面积
DNA	脱氧核糖核酸
EGCG	表没食子儿茶素没食子酸酯
LHRNa	促黄体素释放素激动剂

mTOR	哺乳动物雷帕霉素靶蛋白
NIH	美国国立卫生研究院
PLGA	聚(D,L-乳酸-共聚乙醇酸)
SEER	监测流行病学和最终结果计划

一、概述

子宫内膜癌(endometrial cancer,EC)是全球女性发病率第四的癌症类型。它起源于子宫内膜,故被称为子宫内膜癌。事实上,大约95%的子宫癌病例源自子宫内膜[1]。子宫肉瘤与EC不同,它发生在子宫肌层,因此"子宫体癌"这一术语不能与子宫内膜癌混淆。根据组织学特征,子宫内膜癌可分为6种类型,包括腺癌、子宫癌肉瘤、鳞状细胞癌、小细胞癌、移行细胞癌和浆液性癌。

根据2019年监测、流行病学和结局数据库(surveillance epidemiology and end result program,SEER)报告,子宫恶性肿瘤占所有新发癌症的3.5%。报告指出,2019年共有61 880例新发子宫恶性肿瘤病例,其中12 160人死亡。在过去十年中,新发病例数量以每年1%的速度增长,死亡率则以每年1.9%的速度上升。

EC的常见症状是月经异常、绝经后出血、与月经无关的出血、盆腔痛和性交疼痛。大多数情况下,EC是在绝经后确诊的。少数病例在绝经前确诊。研究表明,妊娠对抑制肿瘤生长有保护性作用,妊娠合并子宫内膜癌的情况罕见。由于缺乏临床试验数据,妊娠合并子宫内膜癌的治疗更加困难[2]。

二、子宫内膜癌的主要危险因素

EC的危险因素包括肥胖、2型糖尿病、PCOS、代谢综合征、子宫内膜癌家族史、林奇综合征等遗传性疾病和子宫内膜增生。早期研究已证实,接受雌激素治疗的患者发生EC的风险增加了4.5倍[3]。接受他莫昔芬治疗的乳腺癌患者也有发生EC的风险,这种药物通过雌激素途径影响子宫内膜细胞[4]。然而,也有研究表明,雌激素与孕激素联合治疗可降低患EC的风险[5]。

未生育过的女性患子宫内膜癌的风险更高。此外,月经初潮较早或绝经较晚也会增加子宫内膜暴露于雌激素的时间,从而增加患病风险[5]。高龄是另一个重要的危险因素,随着年龄的增长,患癌的风险也随之上升,这一规律适用于子宫内膜癌及其他类型的肿瘤[5]。

三、子宫内膜癌的治疗方案

EC治疗的选择取决于多种因素,包括患者的年龄、分期、类型、位置、整体健康状况及其他个人因素。手术是治疗子宫内膜癌的主要方法。然而,其他形式的治疗,特别是不同类型治疗的联合,可以实现更好的治疗效果。子宫内膜癌主要有五种标准治疗措施:包括手术治疗以及放疗、激素治疗、靶向治疗和化疗等术后治疗措施。

(一)手术治疗

手术切除肿瘤是治疗子宫内膜癌最常用的方法。手术方式的选择依赖于肿瘤的位置、大小和性质[6]。子宫全切术的范围包括切除子宫和子宫颈,而双附件切除术则包括切除双侧卵巢和输卵管。根治性子宫切除术则更为彻底,包括切除子宫、子宫颈、阴道、卵巢、输卵管和淋巴结,盆腔区域的淋巴结通常通过淋巴结清扫术来切除。

(二)放疗

放疗通过高能辐射照射肿瘤区域,诱导癌细胞死亡。辐射通常由外部设备发射,并集中照射于肿瘤组织上。另一种方法是将放射性物质放置于肿瘤组织附近。尽管放疗是治疗肿瘤的有效手段,但与其他治疗方法相比,肿瘤复发的风险更高[7,8]。

(三)激素治疗

EC的激素治疗包括:使用孕激素类似物来延缓子宫内膜癌的进展;还有一些药物被用于治疗乳腺癌,包括他莫昔芬(tamoxifen)、促黄体素释放素激动剂(luteinizing hormone-releasing hormone agonist,LHRHa),以及芳香化酶抑制剂(aromatase inhibitor,AI),这些药物可以降低体内的雌激素水平。激素治疗适用于激素受体阳性、低级别子宫内膜样肿瘤,以及有较长无瘤间隔期的患者。对于没有生命危险疾病的患者,激素治疗是一个理想的选择。首选治疗通常是孕激素,二线药物是他莫昔芬[9]。

(四)靶向治疗

靶向治疗旨在特异性地杀死癌细胞,同时不损害正常细胞。单克隆抗体、哺乳动物雷帕霉素靶蛋白(mechanistic target of rapamycin,mTOR)抑制剂和信号转导抑制剂等药物可能是 EC 靶向治疗的首选。可以制备并施用针对癌细胞特定表位的单克隆抗体，它们可以单独使用，也可以与化疗药物或放射治疗联合应用，以诱导癌细胞死亡。mTOR 抑制剂，如依维莫司和雷帕福莫司，能够阻止癌细胞中的细胞分裂和新血管的形成，从而可能防止癌症转移[6]。

(五) 化疗

化疗是指通过血液循环将能够杀死癌细胞的药物输送至全身，这是一种全身性治疗方法。药物也可直接施用于器官或体腔，这种方法称为局部化疗[6]。化疗适用于高级别肿瘤、无治疗间期短、浆液性或透明细胞肿瘤，以及激素受体水平阴性的患者；此外，对于一般状况差或无法接受激素治疗的患者，也可能是最有效的治疗选择[10]。

对于初次接受化疗的患者，其治疗反应率较之前接受过化疗的患者更高。因此，在复发病例中选择化疗方案时，必须考虑患者之前的治疗经历。现有多种化疗药物可用于子宫内膜癌的治疗，且可以单独或组合使用，以提高治疗效果。联合治疗的效率提高归因于所使用的单个药物作用方式的差异。根据年龄、整体健康状况、既往病史和现患疾病，药物的选择、治疗方法、剂量等治疗参数因患者而异。化疗药物的剂量通常根据称为曲线下面积（area under the curve，AUC）的参数来计算。它是血浆中药物浓度与时间的关系图。AUC 反映了服用指定剂量的药物后身体对药物的实际暴露量。AUC 实际上预示了药物在体内的消除速率。对于出现不良反应的患者，通常建议减少药物剂量。

紫杉醇是化疗中使用频率最高的单药之一[11,12]。在一项Ⅱ期临床试验中，对于未接受过化疗的患者，紫杉醇的缓解率达到了 77%；而在作为二线治疗药物的临床试验中，观察到的缓解率为 37%[13]。联合疗法涉及使用多种药物的组合，常用的药物包括紫杉醇、多柔比星和顺铂。尽管联合药物治疗的毒性较高[14]，但卡铂和紫杉醇的联合应用被认为是毒性最小的方案[13,15,16]。

大量研究评估了卡铂-紫杉醇联合化疗在不同分期的 EC 中的疗效和毒性。在手术分期为Ⅰ~Ⅱ期的浆液性子宫内膜癌患者中，阴道内放射治疗（intravaginal radiation therapy，IVRT）同步卡铂-紫杉醇化疗，能够在 5 年后达到 88% 的总生存率[17,18]。子宫浆液性乳头状癌（uterine papillary serous carcinoma，UPSC）相对罕见，Ⅱ期子宫浆液性乳头状癌发生盆腔外复发的风险较高。研究发现，紫杉醇-卡铂联合化疗能够降低这一风险，并改善无进展生存期。表 8-1 列出了使用卡铂-紫杉醇联合化疗治疗 EC 的不同研究，以及缓解率和不良反应。

表 8-1　使用卡铂和紫杉醇药物治疗子宫内膜癌的研究

癌症类型	化合物类型	缓解率	不良反应	参考文献
子宫浆液性乳头状癌	卡铂和紫杉醇	90%	非血液毒性	[18]
子宫内膜浆液性癌	卡铂和紫杉醇	88%	神经毒性,周围神经病变,耳鸣,嗅觉改变,疲劳,便秘,脱水,肌痛,膀胱毒性	[17]
子宫内膜癌	卡铂和紫杉醇	62%	骨髓毒性,中性粒细胞减少,血小板减少,贫血,神经病变	[19]
子宫内膜癌	卡铂和紫杉醇	60%—诊断 55%—复发	无	[20]
子宫内膜癌	紫杉醇和卡铂	56%	神经毒性,非危及生命的超敏反应	[21]
子宫内膜癌	卡铂和紫杉醇	87%	粒细胞减少,呕吐,神经病变,新皮质毒性,关节痛	[10]
子宫内膜癌	紫杉醇,卡铂和氨磷汀	40%	中性粒细胞减少	[16]
子宫内膜癌	紫杉醇	63%	无	[22]
子宫内膜癌	紫杉醇	27.3%	中性粒细胞减少,神经毒性,血小板减少,虚弱,胃肠疾病	[23]
子宫内膜癌	卡铂	13%	恶心,呕吐,白细胞(WBC)毒性(3级)	[24]
子宫内膜癌	紫杉醇和顺-二氯二氨络铂	67%	粒细胞减少,呕吐,神经毒性,贫血,肾毒性	[15]
子宫内膜癌	紫杉醇	23%	胃肠道毒性,耳毒性,神经毒性,粒细胞减少	[12]
子宫浆液腺癌	顺铂,表柔比星和紫杉醇	73%	中性粒细胞减少,周围神经病变,口炎,急性充血性心力衰竭	[25]
子宫内膜癌	紫杉醇	35.7%	白细胞减少,血小板减少,胃肠道毒性,神经毒性,贫血,心脏毒性,脱发	[11]
腺癌	紫杉醇	35%	中性粒细胞减少,血小板减少,贫血,脱发,恶心/呕吐,周围神经病变,肌痛,关节痛,腹泻,瘙痒	[13]
子宫内膜癌	卡铂	28%	恶心,呕吐,厌食,腹泻,脱发,肾毒性,感觉异常	[26]

Sovak 等[21]研究了Ⅲ期和Ⅳ期 EC 患者在肿瘤完全切除后接受卡铂和紫杉醇治疗的总生存期和无进展生存期。紫杉醇给药剂量为 175 mg/m²,卡铂给药剂量为 AUC 5~6,每 3~4 周进行一次药物组合的周期性治疗,共进行 6 个周期。研究结束时,3 年的总体生存率为 56%。结论是紫杉醇-卡铂联合治疗Ⅲ期和Ⅳ期 EC 的耐受性良好。在几项类似的研究中,复发性子宫内膜腺癌患者接受剂量为 135 mg/m² 的紫杉醇和 AUC 为 5 的卡铂治疗,每隔 21 天重复治疗 6 个周期,Ⅳ期癌症患者的总体缓解率约为 63%[19,22]。

卡铂和紫杉醇治疗晚期和复发性子宫癌肉瘤的缓解率为 60%。在这一治疗方案中卡铂的 AUC 为 5~6,紫杉醇的剂量为 175 mg/m²。这与异环磷酰胺联合方案的Ⅲ期临床试验具有相似的疗效。此外,卡铂-紫杉醇更便宜且更容易运输,这使其成为更合适的选择[20]。Michener 等[10]报道称,当卡铂和紫杉醇间隔 21 天给药(剂量为 4~6 AUC 和 135~175 mg/m²)时,晚期、转移性和复发性 EC 患者的总体缓解率高达 87%。尽管出现了血液毒性,但该治疗方案仍被认为是最有效且最安全的化疗方案。研究建议,这种治疗方法可以作为晚期或复发性 EC 患者的一线治疗选择。

手术后进行化疗、激素治疗或放疗是推荐的有效联合治疗方案。即使在使用这些组合中的任何一种进行一线治疗后,患者在随后的生命阶段仍有可能面临肿瘤复发。对于 EC 而言,复发率约为 13%[27],并且超过 50% 的复发是在 2 年内发生的,并且在复发后接受二线治疗取得良好疗效的可能性低于一线治疗。

四、卡铂的作用机制和化学特性

卡铂是一种小分子化合物,具有广谱抗肿瘤活性,属于顺铂衍生的有机金属化合物。与顺铂相比,卡铂的毒性较低且更为稳定。它是由 Creation Research (ICR)(译者注:勘误,应为 The Institute of Cancer Research,ICR)的科学家们发现的,在 20 世纪 70 年代,他们对大约 300 种顺铂衍生物进行了测试,旨在寻找一种更温和的抗肿瘤药物。这一过程中,卡铂被成功发现,它不仅是一种极为有效的抗肿瘤药物,而且不良反应明显减少。卡铂的分子量为 371.25 g/mol,分子式为 $C_6H_{12}N_2O_4Pt$。它由与两个氨基团和 1,1-环丁二甲酸残基络合的铂原子组成。除 EC 外,卡铂还用于治疗各种其他癌症,如宫颈癌、食管癌、头颈癌、晚期黑色素瘤、肺癌、肉瘤、视网膜母细胞瘤、卵巢癌、膀胱癌、睾丸癌等[28](图 8-1)。

卡铂作为一种烷化剂,可以将烷基添加到细胞中各种生物分子的电负性基团上,烷基的添加会增加 DNA 中碱基对的错配。此外,一旦它们进入细胞内,就会被水解作用激活,形成 1,1-环丁烷二羧酸酯和反应性带正电荷的铂络合物。这些

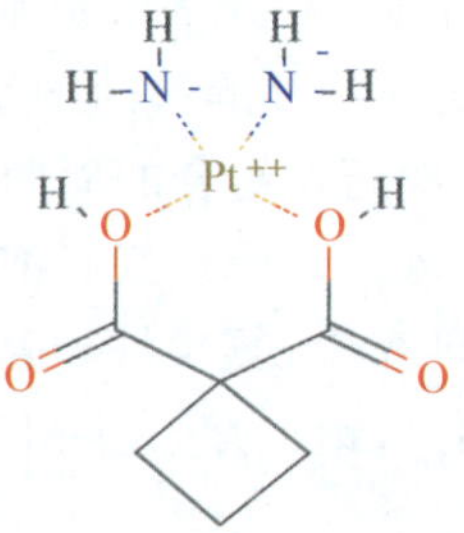

图 8-1　卡铂的化学结构(来源:PubChem)

反应性铂络合物可以稳定地结合到 DNA 富含 G-C 的区域。通过这种方式,卡铂直接攻击 DNA,形成 DNA 鸟嘌呤碱基的链内或链间交联,以及 DNA-蛋白质交联(图 8-2),可以防止 DNA 复制过程中 DNA 双螺旋的解旋,并干扰细胞分裂,最终导致细胞凋亡[29,30]。

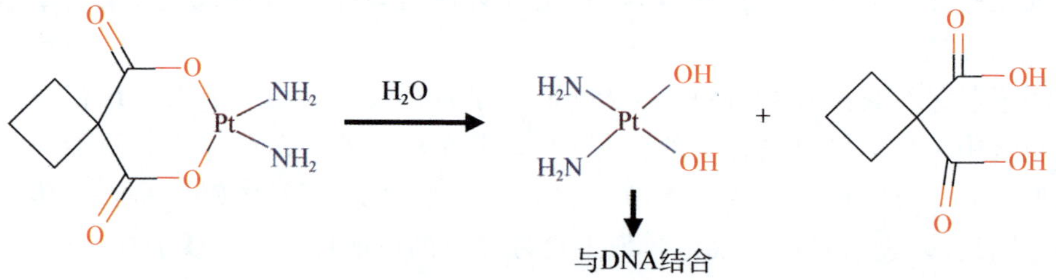

图 8-2　细胞内卡铂的水解

妊娠合并子宫内膜癌极为罕见。目前尚无关于卡铂对孕妇影响的人体试验数据。尽管如此,动物实验已经显示出卡铂可能导致诱变、胚胎毒性和致畸性。该药物对人类生殖能力的潜在影响尚不清楚。由于有明确的证据表明卡铂对胎儿存在风险,故不建议在妊娠期间使用卡铂。在母乳喂养的女性中,卡铂能够进入母乳,可能会导致潜在的不良反应,如骨髓抑制、过敏反应、肾毒性和喂养婴儿的神经毒性[31]。

卡铂的纳米封装

为了实现靶向药物递送,研究人员尝试将卡铂分子进行封装。体外试验表明基于磷脂的卡铂纳米胶囊在体外对癌细胞具有非常高的细胞毒性。这种细胞毒性的增强归因于癌细胞通过吞噬作用优先摄取这些纳米颗粒,导致细胞内铂的积累显著增加[32]。在 Karanam 等[33]的一项研究中,将卡铂装载至由生物可降解聚合物聚(ε-己内酯)构建的纳米颗粒中,在使用 U-87 MG 细胞系进行的体外试验中观察到药物呈现双相释放模式。结果发现,30%~40%的药物在第一个小时内释放,其余 70%~80%在 8~10 h 内释放。与游离药物相比,这种纳米封装的卡铂在杀伤癌细胞方面的效率提高了 3 倍。卡铂最重要的不良反应之一是溶血。研究发现,碳纳米管封装的卡铂在体外不会引起溶血,这表明它可能是游离药物的更好替代品。

此外,对封装在碳纳米管中的卡铂也进行了抗癌治疗有效性方面的测试。碳纳米管是通过卷制石墨烯薄片制成的。其独特的六边形网格结构可与细胞相互作用并引起急性炎症、活性氧的形成,以及自噬引起的细胞死亡。对卡铂填充的碳纳米管进行的细胞增殖和细胞毒性影响测试取得了积极的结果[34]。在另一项研究中,使用与透明质酸结合的封装在碳纳米管卡铂对小鼠肺癌细胞进行了测试,发现透明质酸被结合在碳纳米管的外侧。由于肿瘤细胞通常会过度表达透明质酸受体,这种结合使得纳米封装的卡铂更加特异性地定位于肿瘤细胞。与正常细胞相比,卡铂-透明质酸缀合碳纳米管被肿瘤细胞更大程度地内吞,因此,在肿瘤细胞中的细胞毒性仍然较高。肿瘤细胞还表现出代谢活性以剂量依赖性方式降低。当通过碳纳米管递送时,该药物的细胞毒性作用是单独递送卡铂的 2 倍[35]。

五、紫杉醇的作用机制及化学特性

紫杉醇是一种抗肿瘤药物,它于 1971 年首次从太平洋紫杉树的树皮中分离出来。该药物通过静脉注射给药,目前还没有紫杉醇的片剂或丸剂形式[36]。紫杉醇的分子式为 $C_{47}H_{51}NO_{14}$,分子量为 853.9 g/mol。其结构由二萜紫杉烷环与四元氧杂环丁烷环和 C-13 位的酯侧链组成。这种复杂的结构导致了其不寻常的特性[37,38]。

现在流行一种称为蛋白结合型紫杉醇的紫杉醇新配方,它含有与白蛋白结合的紫杉醇[39]。除抗肿瘤特性外,紫杉醇还是一种免疫抑制剂和骨髓抑制剂,除 EC 外,还用于治疗宫颈癌、头颈癌、食管癌、输卵管癌、肺癌、膀胱癌、乳腺癌、卵巢癌和睾丸癌[38](图 8-3)。

紫杉醇的细胞毒性作用在于其对细胞微管的干扰。与秋水仙碱等促使微管解聚的药物不同,紫杉醇通过增强微管的稳定性而发挥作用。体外研究显示,紫杉醇能够促进微管蛋白的聚合作用,形成更为稳定的微管结构。同时,紫杉醇与微管的相互作用还能阻止微管的解聚过程。这种作用是由于微管内存在着紫杉醇的高亲和力特异性结合位点。由于微管的动态平衡被破坏,细胞无法形成正常的有丝分裂结构,导致细胞周期在 G2/M 期停滞,细胞因此无法进行分裂而发生凋亡[38]。

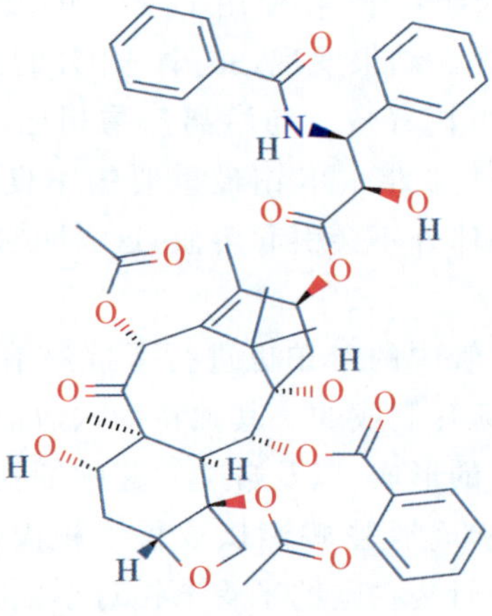

图 8-3　紫杉醇的化学结构（来源：PubChem）

动物研究表明，紫杉醇会引起胚胎毒性和胎儿毒性等不良反应。该药物可能导致人类胎儿畸形或其他不可逆的畸形。与卡铂类似，紫杉醇也被发现会大量分泌到母乳中。这种现象对母乳的正常微生物组和化学成分产生不利影响，并对婴儿造成骨髓抑制、过敏反应、肾毒性和神经毒性等不良反应[40]。

紫杉醇纳米胶囊化

紫杉醇是一种水溶性较差的药物。因此，为了提高其溶解度并提高其特异性和功效，建议将其纳米封装在聚乙基噁唑啉（poly-ethyl oxazoline，PEOX）中。纳米胶囊能够靶向肿瘤组织，避开正常健康组织。这种特异性来自增强渗透和保留（enhanced permeation and retention，EPR）效应。当运载紫杉醇的 PEOX 纳米颗粒接近肿瘤部位时，它会透过血管壁渗漏并在肿瘤部位释放药物。这种方法可以提高紫杉醇的肿瘤渗透性和疗效，同时最大限度地减少毒性[41]。紫杉醇和表没食子儿茶素没食子酸酯（epigallocatechin gallate，EGCG）的组合是一种多重信号转导抑制剂，封装在聚-L-丙交酯-co-乙醇酸（poly-L-lactide-co-glycolic，PLGA）-酪蛋白纳米颗粒中用于治疗乳腺癌。这种以纳米颗粒形式递送药物的方式有助于依次释放 EGCG 和紫杉醇。EGCG 的早期释放大大增加了紫杉醇对肿瘤细胞的敏感性，并使紫杉醇耐药细胞对紫杉醇敏感，从而诱导其凋亡。同时，紫杉醇诱导的 P-糖蛋白表达在转录和翻译水平上均被纳米组合抑制。这种组合对乳腺癌原代细胞产生了显著的细胞毒性反应[42]。

六、结论

卡铂和紫杉醇联合化疗是治疗 EC 最有效的化疗方案之一。尽管这 2 种药物单独使用时整体反应率较低,但一旦联合使用,疗效显著提升。这种联合疗法不仅提高了患者的生存率,而且相较于其他化疗药物,其毒副作用较小。此外,当卡铂和紫杉醇与其他癌症治疗手段(例如放射治疗、手术治疗和激素治疗)结合使用时,治疗效果更佳。考虑这种治疗方案相对较低的生存率优势,未来可以探索使用毒副作用更小的紫杉醇制剂与卡铂制剂的组合疗法,但这一方案仍需进一步的研究与验证。在治疗应用中,卡铂和紫杉醇的纳米胶囊化技术也展现出了积极的前景,尽管这一技术目前还处于早期发展阶段。通过将药物封装于特定的聚合物中,可以增强药物对肿瘤细胞的靶向性,并且药物的释放主要发生在肿瘤组织处。这种策略不仅减小了药物对正常组织的毒性影响,同时也提高了对肿瘤细胞的杀伤效果。鉴于此,纳米胶囊化技术在提高癌症治疗效率和效果方面具有巨大的潜力,值得进一步深入研究和开发。

参 考 文 献

[1] Endometrial Cancer Facts:Seattle Cancer Care Alliance. Retrieved 27 December 2019, from: https://www. seattlecca. org/diseases/endometrial-cancer/endometrial-cancer-facts; 2019.

[2] Skrzypczyk-Ostaszewicz A, Rubach M. Gynaecological cancers coexisting with pregnancy—a litera ture review. Contemp Oncol 2016;20(3):193.

[3] Smith DC, Prentice R, Thompson DJ, Herrmann WL. Association of exogenous estrogen and endometrial carcinoma. N Engl J Med 1975;293(23):1164-7.

[4] Hu R, Hilakivi-Clarke L, Clarke R. Molecular mechanisms of tamoxifen-associated endometrial cancer. Oncol Lett 2015;9(4):1495-501.

[5] Endometrial Cancer Risk Factors. Retrieved 27 December 2019, from: https://www. cancer. org/cancer/endometrial-cancer/causes-risks-prevention/risk-factors. html; 2019.

[6] Endometrial Cancer Treatment (PDQ®)-Patient Version. Retrieved 27 December 2019, from: https://www. cancer. gov/types/uterine/patient/endometrial-treatment-pdq; 2019.

[7] Lin LL, Grigsby PW, Powell MA, Mutch DG. Definitive radiotherapy in the management of isolated vaginal recurrences of endometrial cancer. Int J Radiat Oncol Biol Phys 2005;63(2):500-4.

[8] Tewari K, Cappuccini F, Brewster WR, DiSaia PJ, Berman ML, Manetta A, Puthawala A, Syed AN, Kohler MF. Interstitial brachytherapy for vaginal recurrences of endometrial

carcinoma. Gynecol Oncol 1999;74(3):416-22.

[9] Van Wijk FH, Van der Burg MEL, Burger CW, Vergote I, van Doorn HC. Management of recurrent endometrioid endometrial carcinoma: an overview. Int J Gynecol Cancer 2009; 19(3):314-20.

[10] Michener CM, Peterson G, Kulp B, Webster KD, Markman M. Carboplatin plus paclitaxel in the treatment of advanced or recurrent endometrial carcinoma. J Cancer Res Clin Oncol 2005;131(9):581-4.

[11] Ball HG, Blessing JA, Lentz SS, Mutch DG. A phase II trial of paclitaxel in patients with advanced or recurrent adenocarcinoma of the endometrium: a gynecologic oncology group study. Gynecol Oncol 1996;62(2):278-81.

[12] Ramondetta L, Burke TW, Levenback C, Bevers M, Bodurka-Bevers D, Gershenson DM. Treatment of uterine papillary serous carcinoma with paclitaxel. Gynecol Oncol 2001;82(1):156-61.

[13] Lissoni A, Zanetta G, Losa G, Gabriele A, Parma G, Mangioni C. Phase II study of paclitaxel as salvage treatment in advanced endometrial cancer. Ann Oncol 1996;7(8):861-3.

[14] Fleming GF, Brunetto VL, Cella D, Look KY, Reid GC, Munkarah AR, Kline R, Burger RA, Goodman A, Burks RT. Phase III trial of doxorubicin plus cisplatin with or without paclitaxel plus filgrastim in advanced endometrial carcinoma: a Gynecologic Oncology Group Study. J Clin Oncol 2004;22(11):2159-66.

[15] Dimopoulos MA, Papadimitriou CA, Georgoulias V, Moulopoulos LA, Aravantinos G, Gika D, Karpathios S, Stamatelopoulos S. Paclitaxel and cisplatin in advanced or recurrent carcinoma of the endometrium: long-term results of a phase II multicenter study. Gynecol Oncol 2000;78(1):52-7.

[16] Scudder SA, Liu PY, Wilczynski SP, Smith HO, Jiang C, Hallum III AV, Smith GB, Hannigan EV, Markman M, Alberts DS. Paclitaxel and carboplatin with amifostine in advanced, recurrent, or refractory endometrial adenocarcinoma: a phase II study of the Southwest Oncology Group. Gynecol Oncol 2005;96(3):610-5.

[17] Alektiar KM, Makker V, Abu-Rustum NR, Soslow RA, Chi DS, Barakat RR, Aghajanian CA. Concurrent carboplatin/paclitaxel and intravaginal radiation in surgical stage I-II serous endometrial cancer. Gynecol Oncol 2009;112(1):142-5.

[18] Kiess AP, Damast S, Makker V, Kollmeier MA, Gardner GJ, Aghajanian C, Abu-Rustum NR, Barakat RR, Alektiar KM. Five-year outcomes of adjuvant carboplatin/paclitaxel chemotherapy and intravaginal radiation for stage I-II papillary serous endometrial cancer. Gynecol Oncol 2012;127(2):321-5.

[19] Pectasides D, Xiros N, Papaxoinis G, Pectasides E, Sykiotis C, Koumarianou A, Psyrri A, Gaglia A, Kassanos D, Gouveris P, Panayiotidis J. Carboplatin and paclitaxel in advanced or metastatic endometrial cancer. Gynecol Oncol 2008;109(2):250-4.

[20] Hoskins PJ, Le N, Ellard S, Lee U, Martin LA, Swenerton KD, Tinker AV. Carboplatin

plus paclitaxel for advanced or recurrent uterine malignant mixed mullerian tumors. The British Columbia Cancer Agency experience. Gynecol Oncol 2008;108(1):58-62.

[21] Sovak MA, Hensley ML, Dupont J, Ishill N, Alektiar KM, Abu-Rustum N, Barakat R, Chi DS, Sabbatini P, Spriggs DR, Aghajanian C. Paclitaxel and carboplatin in the adjuvant treatment of patients with high-risk stage Ⅲ and Ⅳ endometrial cancer: a retrospective study. Gynecol Oncol 2006;103(2):451-7.

[22] Akram T, Maseelall P, Fanning J. Carboplatin and paclitaxel for the treatment of advanced or recurrent endometrial cancer. Am J Obstet Gynecol 2005;192(5):1365-7.

[23] Lincoln S, Blessing JA, Lee RB, Rocereto TF. Activity of paclitaxel as second-line chemotherapy in endometrial carcinoma: a Gynecologic Oncology Group Study. Gynecol Oncol 2003;88(3):277-81.

[24] Van Wijk FH, Lhomme C, Bolis G, Di Palumbo VS, Tumolo S, Nooij M, De Oliveira CF, Vermorken JB. Phase Ⅱ study of carboplatin in patients with advanced or recurrent endometrial carcinoma. A trial of the EORTC Gynaecological Cancer Group. Eur J Cancer 2003;39(1):78-85.

[25] Lissoni A, Gabriele A, Gorga G, Tumolo S, Landoni F, Mangioni C, Sessa C. Cisplatin-, epirubicin-and paclitaxel-containing chemotherapy in uterine adenocarcinoma. Ann Oncol 1997;8(10):969-72.

[26] Long HJ, Pfeifle DM, Wieand HS, Krook JE, Edmonson JH, Buckner JC. Phase Ⅱ evaluation of carboplatin in advanced endometrial carcinoma. J Natl Cancer Inst 1988;80(4): 276-8.

[27] Fung-Kee-Fung M, Dodge J, Elit L, Lukka H, Chambers A, Oliver T, Cancer Care Ontario Program in Evidence-based Care Gynecology Cancer Disease Site Group. Follow-up after primary therapy for endometrial cancer: a systematic review. Gynecol Oncol 2006; 101(3):520-9.

[28] Carboplatin—DrugBank. Retrieved 27 December 2019, from: https://www.drugbank.ca/drugs/DB00958; 2019.

[29] Gerson SL, Caimi PF, William BM, Creger RJ. Pharmacology and molecular mechanisms of antineoplastic agents for hematologic malignancies. In: Hematology. Elsevier; 2018. p. 849-912.

[30] Sousa GFD, Wlodarczyk SR, Monteiro G. Carboplatin: molecular mechanisms of action associated with chemoresistance. Braz J Pharm Sci 2014;50(4):693-701.

[31] Griffin SJ, Milla M, Baker TE, Liu T, Wang H, Hale TW. Transfer of carboplatin and paclitaxel into breast milk. J Hum Lact 2012;28(4):457-9.

[32] Hamelers IH, van Loenen E, Staffhorst RW, de Kruijff B, de Kroon AI. Carboplatin nanocapsules: a highly cytotoxic, phospholipid-based formulation of carboplatin. Mol Cancer Ther 2006;5(8):2007-12.

[33] Karanam V, Marslin G, Krishnamoorthy B, Chellan V, Siram K, Natarajan T, Bhaskar

B, Franklin G. Poly (ε-caprolactone) nanoparticles of carboplatin: preparation, characterization and in vitro cytotoxicity evaluation in U-87 MG cell lines. Colloids Surf B Biointerfaces 2015;130:48-52.

[34] Kumari A, Singla R, Guliani A, Yadav SK. Nanoencapsulation for drug delivery. EXCLI J 2014;13:265.

[35] Salas-Treviño D, Saucedo-Cárdenas O, Loera-Arias MDJ, Rodríguez-Rocha H, García-García A, Montes-de-Oca-Luna R, Piña-Mendoza EI, Contreras-Torres FF, García-Rivas G, Soto-Domínguez A. Hyaluronate functionalized Multi-Wall carbon nanotubes filled with carboplatin as a novel drug nanocarrier against murine lung cancer cells. Nanomaterials 2019;9(11):1572.

[36] Success Story: Taxol. Retrieved 27 December 2019, from: https://dtp.cancer.gov/timeline/flash/success_stories/S2_taxol.htm; 2019.

[37] Paclitaxel, 99+%. Retrieved 27 December 2019, from https://pubchem.ncbi.nlm.nih.gov/compound/133640187; 2019.

[38] Paclitaxel—DrugBank. Retrieved 27 December 2019, from: https://www.drugbank.ca/drugs/DB01229; 2019.

[39] Miele E, Spinelli GP, Miele E, Tomao F, Tomao S. Albumin-bound formulation of paclitaxel(Abraxane® ABI-007) in the treatment of breast cancer. Int J Nanomedicine 2009;4:99.

[40] Paclitaxel Use During Pregnancy. (n.d.). Retrieved 30 January 2020, from: https://www.drugs.com/pregnancy/paclitaxel.html

[41] Yin R, Pan J, Zhou B, Zhang Y, Dougherty J, Liu J, Riesenberger TA, Qin D, Vallejo YR. Evaluation of the toxicity and efficacy of paclitaxel nanoencapsulated with polyethyloxazoline polymers. J Clin Oncol 2013;31:e13538.

[42] Narayanan S, Mony U, Vijaykumar DK, Koyakutty M, Paul-Prasanth B, Menon D. Sequential release of epigallocatechin gallate and paclitaxel from PLGA-casein core/shell nanoparticles sensitizes drug-resistant breast cancer cells. Nanomedicine 2015;11(6):1399-406.

第 9 章
女性特异性肿瘤

P. S. Pradeep[a], D. Sivaraman[a], Jayshree Nellore[b], Sujatha Peela[c]

[a]Centre for Laboratory Animal Technology and Research, Sathyabama Institute of Science and Technology, Chennai, Tamil Nadu, India
[b]Department of Biotechnology, School of Bio and Chemical Engineering, Sathyabama Institute of Science and Technology, Chennai, Tamil Nadu, India
[c]Department of Biotechnology, Dr. BR Ambedkar University, Srikakulam, Andhra Pradesh, India

摘要

女性特异性肿瘤是女性最常见的肿瘤。其中的大多数仍然无法达到早期诊断,导致许多癌症在晚期才被发现。目前,针对女性特异性肿瘤的治疗方法包括手术、放疗和化疗。在此背景下,本章重点介绍女性特异性乳腺癌、腹膜恶性肿瘤、子宫恶性肿瘤和阴道恶性肿瘤。

女性特异性肿瘤			
乳腺癌	腹膜恶性肿瘤	子宫恶性肿瘤	阴道恶性肿瘤
导管癌	平滑肌肿瘤	间质肿瘤	上皮性肿瘤
小叶癌	间皮肿瘤	上皮性肿瘤	间质肿瘤
小管癌	上皮性肿瘤	混合上皮和间充质肿瘤	黑色素细胞瘤
黏液癌	肿瘤样病变	淋巴系及髓系肿瘤	淋巴系及髓系肿瘤
髓样癌	继发性肿瘤	继发性肿瘤	混合性上皮和间质肿瘤
乳头状肿瘤	其他原发性肿瘤	其他肿瘤	继发性肿瘤

关键词

乳腺癌,腹膜癌,子宫癌,阴道癌

缩略词

AMFB	血管成肌纤维细胞瘤
AML	急性髓系白血病
CNS	中枢神经系统
DCIS	导管原位癌
IARC	国际癌症研究机构
ILC	浸润性小叶癌
MMMT	恶性混合性米勒管肿瘤
MS	髓系肉瘤
US	超声

一、概述

女性特异性肿瘤,如乳腺或妇科恶性肿瘤(卵巢、阴道、子宫),治疗的难点在于此类肿瘤发生在女性身体的敏感部位,而治疗的手段可能会破坏这些部位的正常细胞。例如,乳腺癌是最常见的女性恶性肿瘤[1],在全球发达国家和发展中国家的女性恶性肿瘤中占比高达 30%[2]。早期诊断旨在控制晚期癌症的发病率。事实上,乳房 X 线检查的利弊在过去数十年中一直存在广泛的争论[3]。国际癌症研究机构(International Agency for Research on Cancer,IARC)在对乳房 X 线检查的益处和不良事件进行谨慎评估后,最新的研究表明对 50~74 岁的女性进行筛查是完全有益的。2018 年,全球有 200 万名女性确诊为乳腺癌,其中 62.7 万例因乳腺癌死亡[4]。而对于老年人来说,化疗药物安全性和有效性都是问题,必须进行更多更有针对性的临床试验。例如,在一项他莫昔芬和芳香化酶抑制剂的对比研究中发现,芳香化酶抑制剂可降低绝经后乳腺癌女性的慢性疾病风险[5]。早期乳腺癌试验者协作小组回顾分析了 91 项研究中 46 000 例乳腺癌治疗后 5 年内接受激素替代治疗的女性患者的数据,认为激素治疗后乳腺癌可能在 20 年后复发。研究者发现即使是最小的、侵袭性最小的肿瘤,在 20 年后也有 14% 的复发率,而病情更严重的癌症复发的可能性增加 47%,这表明 5 年的癌症治疗并不足够[6]。事实上,根据目前的数据得出的结论是,也许大多数的腹膜癌、子宫癌和阴道癌可能有一个共同的来源,即输卵管[7]。最常见的妇科恶性肿瘤是子宫恶性肿瘤,而乳腺癌在女性恶性肿瘤中是高度独立的。同时在多项流行病学研究中也发现,确诊为乳腺癌的女性患继发性子宫恶性肿瘤的可能性更大。在腹膜相关肿瘤组织活检中会发现大量新生血管形成,这种现象是基于血管生成是由癌细胞和肿瘤相关的间质上皮细胞一同触发的假设[8]。本章试图向读者介绍女性特有的癌症,包括乳腺癌、腹膜癌、子宫癌和阴道癌,同时讨论癌症治疗与预后结局之间的联系。

(一)乳腺癌

乳腺癌的症状可能包括乳房肿块、乳房变形、皮肤凹陷、乳头异常、红色或鳞状皮肤斑块,或乳头溢液。当某些乳腺细胞异常增殖时,乳腺癌就会发生。这些细胞比正常细胞分裂速度快,并不断积聚,形成肿块或团块[9]。乳腺癌通常始于产生乳汁的导管细胞(浸润性导管癌)。乳腺癌的症状包括乳房或腋下出现新发肿块,乳房局部炎症,乳房皮肤异常,乳头或乳房皮肤肿胀,乳头溢液(包括血液,非乳汁)。乳腺癌的种类包括浸润性导管癌、原位性导管癌、转移性乳腺癌和炎性乳腺癌[10]。

1. 乳腺导管癌 导管原位癌(ductal carcinoma in situ,DCIS)是一种非浸润性癌症。DCIS是最常见的乳腺癌类型,占所有乳腺癌的80%,其在乳腺导管内可以观察到癌细胞。DCIS是一种非常早期的癌症,是可以治愈的,但如果不及时诊断,它可能会在无明显症状的情况下扩散到邻近的乳腺组织。DCIS通常会引起乳房肿块和乳头出血等症状。DCIS高危因素包括年龄、乳腺疾病史、未孕、首次生育年龄超过30岁、绝经年龄超过55岁,以及乳腺癌高危基因变异(*BRCA1*和*BRCA2*)。DCIS的治疗成功率很高。对于部分病例来说,治疗方式是病灶去除和缩小复发灶[11]。对于另一部分病例来说,DCIS治疗方式为保乳手术(乳房肿瘤切除术)、放射治疗和乳房切除手术。

2. 乳腺小叶癌 浸润性小叶癌(invasive lobular carcinoma,ILC)是一种发生在乳腺泌乳腺(小叶)的乳腺癌。浸润性癌是指细胞从其起源的小叶扩散,有可能浸润淋巴结和其他软组织。早期乳腺癌患者生存率较晚期乳腺癌高。总的来说,随着药物的发展,小叶癌的诊断与导管癌的诊断密切相关。ILC通常不会形成肿块,而是以单排肿瘤的形式通过乳房脂肪组织扩散[12]。根据美国癌症协会研究,以下任何一个均可能是乳腺癌的首发征象:乳房的整体或局部炎症、皮肤刺激症状和乳房疼痛。当泌乳腺的细胞控制细胞增殖生长的DNA发生突变,导致细胞分裂和快速生长时,就会出现ILC。

3. 乳腺小管肿瘤 乳腺小管癌是浸润性导管癌的一个亚类(一种由导管内起源并向正常组织扩散的癌症)。虽然小管癌是一种浸润性乳腺癌,但它是一种恶性程度较低的类型,对治疗反应良好。小管腺瘤是乳腺腺瘤的一类,其特征是紧密排列的管状和腺泡(芽状)细胞结构。腺瘤是一种由多种腺、纤维和脂肪组织组成的肿瘤,可导致密度增加或假性损害。乳腺小管癌是浸润性导管型乳腺癌的一种,在所有乳腺癌中所占比例不到2%[13]。与其他形式的浸润性导管癌一样,乳腺小管癌先在导管内生长,然后扩散到整个乳腺腺体。肿瘤可以迅速繁殖,常在乳房自我触诊或医师检查时发现。小管腺瘤通常很小,直径在 1 cm 以下,难以发现。

4. 乳腺黏液癌 乳腺黏液癌,有时被称为胶样癌,是一种罕见的浸润性导管癌(一种发生在乳腺导管并从乳腺导管扩散到周围正常组织的癌症)。黏液癌是一种浸润性癌,可能全身转移。尽管如此,与许多其他浸润性癌相比,它的破坏性较小,而且通常对药物治疗反应良好[14]。乳腺黏液癌的生存率高于大多数其他类型的浸润性乳腺癌,其 5 年生存率为 87%。黏液性癌是卵巢上皮-间质细胞肿瘤的一个组成部分,占卵巢肿瘤总数的近 36%。单纯黏液性癌的遗传不确定性水平较低,混合型黏液性癌的基因组模式与单纯黏液性癌惊人相似。

5. 乳腺髓样癌 乳腺髓样癌是浸润性导管癌的一个亚型。这也是一种始于乳腺导管的乳腺癌。髓样癌很少转移到淋巴结,比常见的浸润性乳腺癌更容易治疗。它们在形态上非常像高度恶性肿瘤细胞,但在行为上却不像[15]。按分期比较,浸润性小叶癌的第一个 5 年总生存率明显高于导管癌。据报道 5 年生存率平均为 90%(77%~93%),乳腺髓样癌的诊断很有特点。有时诊断肿瘤的并非影像报告,而是女性自己的感觉。很多女性可能会遇到其他类似髓样癌的症状,包括乳房压痛、不适、肿胀、出血等。

6. 乳腺乳头状肿瘤 乳腺乳头状癌是一种罕见的浸润性乳腺导管癌,导管内乳头状瘤是一种发生在乳腺导管内的小的良性肿瘤。这种肿瘤由纤维组织、腺体和血管组成。这些肿瘤呈细长的结节状,很像"手指"。这种肿瘤由覆盖器官内壁的组织形成。乳头状肿瘤可以是良性的,也可以是恶性的,最常发生在膀胱、甲状腺和乳房,但也可能出现在人体的其他几个部位[16]。一般来说,浸润性乳头状癌由细的手指状突起组成,边界非常明确。与其他类型的浸润性导管癌一样,乳腺乳头状癌起源于乳腺导管。乳腺乳头状癌通常很小,雌激素和/或孕激素受体活跃(ER/PR 阳性),受体 HER2 不活跃。原发性乳头状瘤更容易单发,并引起乳头溢液出血[17]。在年轻女性中,多发病灶比单发更常见,因此更多为双侧、无症状、消融后持续存在。

(二)腹膜癌

腹膜癌是一种罕见的癌症。它生长在子宫周围的薄组织基质中,包括直肠和膀胱,由腹膜上皮细胞组成。它产生一种液体,使细胞能够有效地在腹部基质中移动[18]。如果不及时诊断,腹膜癌患者的平均寿命可能只有 6 周。如果给予适当的治疗,预期寿命可能会显著延长,但大多数患者发现时即诊断为难治的晚期腹膜癌。各种女性生殖系统癌症的 5 年生存率为 47%。晚期腹膜癌可能导致尿路或肠道完全性梗阻。随着肿瘤的进展,腹腔会产生一种水样液体(腹水),在化疗等治疗期间可被抑制。

1. 腹膜癌中的平滑肌肿瘤 子宫平滑肌肿瘤指的是良性平滑肌肌瘤到低危平滑肌肉瘤之间的一类肿瘤。有几种组织学亚型，包括普通（纺锤状）、上皮样和黏液样肿瘤。平滑肌肉瘤是平滑肌恶性肿瘤，可能起源于肌肉细胞。皮肤平滑肌肉瘤常在切除后复发，但很少发生转移。良性软组织肿瘤比良性骨肿瘤更常见。它们可以存在于所有部位，组织、肌肉、神经和血管[19]。这些肿瘤在行为模式和外观上有很大的不同。最常见的是被称为脂肪瘤的良性脂肪肿瘤。

2. 腹膜癌中的间皮瘤 间皮瘤可为良性（非癌性）或恶性（癌性）。间皮瘤是一种由吸入石棉纤维诱发的恶性肿瘤，起源于腹部、心脏或肺部的内壁。这类肿瘤的临床症状可能包括呼吸困难和胸痛[20]。大多数间皮瘤患者生存期为 12 个月。间皮细胞是一层特殊的路面状细胞，通常覆盖在体内的浆膜和重要器官上。它的主要作用是形成一个不黏附的、光滑的、保护性的表面。间皮瘤的主要危险因素是石棉的使用。

3. 腹膜癌中的上皮性肿瘤 卵巢上皮癌、输卵管癌和原发性腹膜癌是癌细胞在卵巢、输卵管或腹膜组织中发展的疾病[21]。腹膜是构成腹部内衬并包裹着腹部器官的组织。恶性组织学类型通常包括未分化癌、管状腺癌和乳头状腺癌。上皮-间质细胞肿瘤是一类卵巢良性或恶性肿瘤，这一类肿瘤被认为起源于卵巢表面的上皮（表面上皮）或异位子宫内膜或输卵管组织。卵巢透明细胞癌是卵巢癌的几种亚型之一；此外，卵巢上皮性癌和非上皮性癌也都是卵巢癌。良性上皮肿瘤存在多种类型，包括浆液性腺瘤、黏液性腺瘤和 Brenner 瘤。恶性上皮性肿瘤起源于卵巢上皮组织。

4. 腹膜癌中的肿瘤样病变 腹膜胶质瘤病可能形成于大部分浆膜表面。各种类型的反应性腹膜改变可引起轻微的肿瘤样病变。包括各种肉芽肿、化生、蜕膜病变和子宫内膜异位症。腹膜癌是一种罕见的癌症，生长在包括子宫、直肠和膀胱在内的腹部的薄组织层内。它会分泌一种液体，润滑器官。肿瘤和肿瘤样病变本质上是在超声（ultrasound，US）、计算机体层成像或磁共振成像报告中看起来相似的病变。腹膜转移包括已经进展或转移到腹腔的癌症。癌细胞从原发灶中分离，并种植转移到腹膜内的其他器官和组织中[22]。一旦肿瘤开始生长，患者可能会感到疼痛和疼痛相关症状。瘤样病变与肿瘤表现类似，但并非肿瘤。病变可以根据它们是否由癌症引起进行分类。例如硬币病灶是胸部 X 线片上一个类似硬币的圆形斑点。对于这些区域的透亮病变，包括标准的骨骺实体，如成软骨细胞瘤、巨细胞瘤和动脉瘤性骨囊肿。

5. 继发性腹膜肿瘤 继发性腹膜肿瘤往往起源于其他腹部器官，并向腹膜内扩散。这类肿瘤可能起源于妇科、泌尿生殖系统或胃肠道（胃、小肠、结肠、阑尾）。男性和女性都可能发病。截至 2019 年，患有各种类型的卵巢癌、输卵管癌和腹膜癌的女性 5 年生存率为 47%。65 岁以下女性的生存率更高(60%)，65 岁以上女性的 5 年生存率则较低(29%)。腹部肿瘤最常见的终末期表现就是腹膜癌。对于胃肠道外科医师和内科肿瘤学家来说这是一个令人担忧的情况，因为即使局限于腹膜表面，完全手术切除也是极其困难的，全身化疗也是无效的。腹膜转移包括已经进展到腹膜腔的肿瘤。有时癌细胞可能从原发性肿瘤中分离，并种植转移到腹膜内的其他器官和组织中[23]。当肿瘤逐渐长大，患者会经历疼痛和严重的并发症。腹膜癌的征象可能包括腹部肿胀或胀痛、消化不良、压痛、炎症、腹胀或痉挛、少量进食后饱腹感、呕吐或腹泻、便秘、尿频、食欲减退、体重异常增加或减轻，以及不规则阴道出血。

6. 腹膜的其他原发肿瘤　原发性肿瘤是指在肿瘤最初发生的部位形成的癌性肿块。许多肿瘤在原发部位生长，并扩散或转移到身体的其他部位，这类癌症被称为继发性肿瘤[24]。转移瘤也被称为继发性肿瘤。原发灶未知肿瘤是一种可能从身体任何其他部位转移(扩散)的疾病。它的起源部位，即原发部位是未知的。在美国，这类病例占确诊癌症的 2%～5%。

(三) 阴道癌

阴道癌是阴道恶性肿瘤细胞形成的一种疾病。阴道是从子宫颈(子宫开口)通向身体外部的通道。出生时，婴儿穿过阴道(也称为产道)出体外。阴道癌并不常见，在女性每年接受治疗的所有生殖器官癌症中，外阴癌和阴道癌加起来不到 7%。阴道癌罕见，且不会从其他部位转移而来。阴道癌的高危因素包括 60 岁以上，在母亲子宫内接触到己烯雌酚，人乳头状瘤病毒感染，有宫颈细胞异常或癌变的病史[25]。

1. 阴道上皮性肿瘤(译者注：原著该段标题与内容不符，译者未做修改)　上皮性卵巢癌是从构成卵巢外层的细胞中发生的。大多数卵巢上皮性肿瘤是良性的(非癌性的)。良性上皮性肿瘤种类繁多，如浆液性腺瘤、黏液性腺瘤、Brenner 瘤等。表面上皮-间质癌确实是一类卵巢良性或恶性肿瘤，这个群体中的肿瘤被认为起源于卵巢表面的上皮(修饰的腹膜)或异位子宫内膜或输卵管的组织[26]。癌是指恶性上皮性肿瘤。上皮性恶性肿瘤占所有癌症病例的 80%～90%。上皮性卵巢癌、输卵管癌和原发性腹膜癌是在覆盖卵巢或输卵管或腹膜的组织中形成恶性细胞(癌)的疾病。输卵管癌和原发性腹膜癌与卵巢上皮性癌相同，治疗方法相同。

2. 阴道间质肿瘤　女性下生殖道浅表性成肌纤维细胞瘤是一种罕见的间质肿瘤。间质组织的肿瘤是软组织肿瘤，通常被称为结缔组织肿瘤，在家畜中极为常见，在某些物种中发病率更高[27]。这些肿瘤可能发生在所有器官中，在特定组织中或多或少地发生。浅表性成肌纤维细胞瘤的发病机制尚不清楚。在一些特殊类型的软组织肿瘤中,病毒感染与间质肿瘤的相关性已经众所周知。间质肿瘤包含中胚层来源的前体细胞实体,可生长成为骨、软骨或其他结缔组织(如血管、脂肪组织、平滑肌或成纤维细胞),在中枢神经系统(central nervous system,CNS)中,它们更常发生在脑膜而不是实质[28]。血管成肌纤维细胞瘤(angiomyofibroblastoma,AMFB)是一种罕见的惰性间质肿瘤,最常见于绝经前女性生殖道,最常见于外阴和阴道。通常 AMFB 的直径小于 5 cm,有研究表明肿瘤直径最大可达 23 cm。肉瘤是一种间质(结缔组织)起源的肿瘤,由转化细胞发展而来。它与继发性(或转移性)结缔组织肿瘤相当,当肿瘤从身体其他部位(如肺、乳腺组织或前列腺)扩散到结缔组织时,就会形成这种肿瘤。

3. 阴道淋巴及髓系肿瘤 造血和淋巴组织肿瘤损害血液、骨髓、淋巴结和淋巴系统[29]。染色体易位是这些疾病的常见病因,但在实体瘤中很少见。髓系和淋巴系都参与了树突状细胞的产生。髓系细胞可包括血小板、单核细胞、中性粒细胞、巨噬细胞、红细胞、嗜碱性粒细胞、嗜酸性粒细胞和巨核细胞。淋巴细胞包括 B 细胞、T 细胞和自然杀伤细胞。髓系恶性肿瘤是祖细胞或造血干细胞的克隆性疾病,包括急性期[即急性髓系白血病(acute myeloid leukemia,AML)]和慢性期(即骨髓增殖性肿瘤、骨髓增生异常疾病、慢性粒单核细胞白血病)。淋巴瘤(也称为淋巴癌或淋巴细胞癌)是一种包含免疫细胞之一淋巴细胞的癌症。尽管 AML 是一种严重的疾病,化疗伴或不伴骨髓/干细胞移植是可以治愈的。

4. 阴道转移瘤 转移瘤在阴道内比原发阴道肿瘤更常见,这意味着肿瘤已经从其他器官扩散,比如子宫颈、子宫、外阴、肝脏、肠道,或者附近的其他器官[30]。阴道转移瘤的治疗方法与原发肿瘤不同。原发性肿瘤的治疗可能需要很长时间才能控制和缓解不良反应;而转移瘤的治疗方法为姑息治疗。阴道肿瘤的体征和症状包括与月经期无关的疼痛或异常阴道出血、盆腔疼痛、阴道肿块和排尿时疼痛。由于阴道癌罕见,它的生存率统计是一个大致范围。如果癌症在转移前被早期发现(Ⅰ期),5 年生存率为 75%～95%。如果肿瘤没有阴道外转移(Ⅱ期),5 年生存率为 50%～80%。

5. 阴道混合性上皮和间质肿瘤 癌肉瘤是一种具有高级别上皮和间质成分的双相恶性肿瘤,也称为恶性混合性米勒管肿瘤(malignant mixed Müllerian tumor,MMMT)。癌肉瘤是一类堵塞子宫腔的大息肉样肿块,伴有坏死和出血[31]。肿瘤与绝经后阴道出血有关。总的来说,目前关于 MMMT 起源的知识非常有限。MMMT 是一种包括两种类型细胞的肿瘤:癌和肉瘤细胞。这类肿瘤通常在女性生殖器组织中形成,预后较差。

(四)子宫体癌

子宫内膜癌是起源于子宫的一种恶性肿瘤。子宫是梨形的中空盆腔器官,胎儿在此发育。子宫内膜癌始于形成子宫内膜的细胞层（子宫内膜）。子宫内膜癌通常代表子宫恶性肿瘤[32]。子宫恶性肿瘤的早期预警症状是阴道非血性异常分泌物、排尿困难、盆腔疼痛和/或肿块，以及不明原因的体重减轻。对于患有子宫恶性肿瘤的女性，5年生存率为81%。不规则阴道出血是子宫内膜癌最常见的症状，包括阴道流液、血性分泌物增多或阴道出血增多。围绝经期和绝经后的阴道出血通常是一个征兆。子宫恶性肿瘤可以远处转移至直肠或膀胱。而其直接浸润的部位包括阴道、卵巢和输卵管。这种肿瘤生长缓慢，在扩散到身体更远的部位之前就能被发现，阴道检查、子宫内膜检查（宫腔镜）和组织取样（活检）是诊断子宫体癌的主要检查方法。巴氏涂片检查并不能用于诊断子宫体癌。全子宫双附件切除术是早期癌症最成功的治疗方法，即切除子宫、子宫颈、卵巢和输卵管[33]。患有晚期子宫内膜癌的患者通常会接受孕激素治疗以减缓肿瘤的进展。

1. 子宫间质肿瘤 子宫间质肿瘤在各个年龄组的女性中都可见。子宫间质肿瘤中最常见的肿瘤是子宫内膜平滑肌瘤。它们在月经初潮后出现，通常在育龄期发展，绝经后稳定或消退。肌瘤是在子宫内或子宫外发现的肿瘤，可以非常大，引起剧烈腹痛和月经不规律。子宫间质肿瘤发生于但又区别于中胚层相关组织肿瘤。一般情况下是向着子宫体内的子宫内膜间质细胞和子宫肌层平滑肌细胞分化的。子宫内膜间质肿瘤通常是一组异质性的肿瘤，因此对治疗有很大挑战。大量此类肿瘤（子宫平滑肌和子宫内膜间质）在中胚层组织中表现出同源分离。有时可以见到软骨、骨骼肌、骨等不同成分。良性和恶性间质肿瘤之间区别显著，要重视病理学家的意见（特别是在复杂的病例中）。在形态学评估后，上皮性和间质肿瘤主要根据其上皮和间质成分进行鉴别[34]。尽管免疫组织化学染色能够帮助确诊，但这类肿瘤的形态学特征是主要的诊断依据。本研究强调了子宫间质肿瘤诊断和鉴别所需的主要形态学特征，并简要总结了相关的免疫组化特征。

2. 子宫上皮性肿瘤 子宫内膜癌是发生在子宫内膜的上皮性肿瘤，通常伴有腺体分裂，具有穿透子宫内膜并向远处转移的能力[35]。良性子宫平滑肌瘤（子宫肌瘤）是迄今为止女性中最常见的盆腔肿瘤（终身发病风险为70%～80%）。一旦子宫内的正常细胞发生突变并扩散到正常范围之外，子宫内膜癌就会以肿块（肿瘤）的形式出现。子宫内膜癌一般会转移到直肠或膀胱。可能转移的区域还包括阴道、卵巢和输卵管。通常，这种类型的癌症倾向于局部生长，容易被早期发现。跟其他任何肿瘤一样，Ⅳ期患者很难治愈。Ⅳ期子宫内膜癌的治疗目标是减轻症状，延长生存期。接受现有标准治疗方案的病例很少能够痊愈。

3. 子宫体癌中混合性上皮和间质肿瘤 子宫混合性上皮和间质肿瘤代表了一个异质性的肿瘤群体，包括腺肌瘤、癌肉瘤、非典型息肉样腺肌瘤和腺纤维瘤等类别。子宫癌肉瘤MMMT是一种罕见的子宫肿瘤，通常发生在老年女性，可发生子宫肌层深浸润以及累及宫颈,占子宫肿瘤的比例不到5%[36]。混合性上皮和间质肿瘤包括腺纤维瘤、癌肉瘤、腺肉瘤、腺肌瘤和非典型息肉样腺肌瘤,后两种病变以平滑肌部分为主,混合了良性上皮和间质成分的肿瘤。

4. 子宫体癌中的淋巴系和髓系肿瘤 髓系肉瘤(myeloid sarcoma,MS)是一种罕见的肿瘤,其信息主要基于年代久远的临床研究和/或观察研究。在一项研究中,对92例具有可获得临床数据的髓系肉瘤进行了形态学和免疫组织化学检测。MS通常发生在皮肤、骨骼或淋巴结,也可以发生在全身任何部位[37]。淋巴细胞白血病由骨髓中的白细胞(淋巴细胞)演化而来。除淋巴细胞以外的白细胞、红细胞和血小板则会发生髓系白血病。髓系和淋巴系在树突状细胞的产生中都很重要。对成人而言,淋巴细胞和髓系细胞以及肿瘤细胞在一个特定器官中发育,最终分散并驻留在另一个器官中,这样的过程被称为归巢或转移。

5. 子宫转移瘤 子宫继发性肿瘤多由宫颈癌转移而来。冷冻手术、电刀或激光手术都可以治疗宫颈的癌前病变。早期宫颈癌和宫颈癌前病变的治愈率几乎可达100%。然而,即使接受了所有治疗,肿瘤仍可能会再次在盆腔或腹部出现,这就是所谓的复发性肿瘤[38]。子宫体癌在身体的其他部位生长的情况比较少见,这被称为转移瘤(继发性肿瘤)。转移性子宫体癌(子宫内膜癌)通常是指出现在子宫内膜并已扩散到身体远处的肿瘤。子宫内膜癌通常会转移到直肠或膀胱。它可能生长的特定部位包括阴道、卵巢和输卵管。根据加拿大的一项研究,高龄子宫内膜癌的患者以后患结肠癌的风险也可能增加。

6. 其他子宫恶性肿瘤 子宫内膜癌通常始于形成子宫内膜的细胞膜。子宫内膜癌有时也被称为子宫体癌。某些类型的癌症,如子宫肉瘤,也可以在子宫内产生,但它们的发病率远低于子宫内膜癌。子宫内膜癌可以生长于子宫内膜,这种类型的子宫癌分布最广,占子宫内膜癌患者的90%以上。对于患有子宫癌的女性来说,5年生存率为81%。如果癌症已经局部扩散,5年生存率约为69%。如果在癌症转移到身体其他部位后才确诊,存活率为16%。

二、结论

女性特异性肿瘤仍然是全球主要的健康问题。本章概述了乳腺癌、腹膜癌、子宫体癌和宫颈癌的概念和诊断方式,介绍了潜在有效的治疗方法。虽然癌症需要采取预防措施来降低死亡率,但获得更安全、更有效的抗肿瘤药物也同样迫在眉睫。

参 考 文 献

[1] Siegel RL, Miller KD, Jemal A. Cancer statistics, 2019. CA Cancer J Clin 2019;69(1):7-

34.

[2] Bray F, Ferlay J, Soerjomataram I, Siegel RL, Torre LA, Jemal A. Global cancer statistics 2018: GLOBOCAN estimates of incidence and mortality worldwide for 36 cancers in 185 countries. CA Cancer J Clin 2018;68:394e424.

[3] Lauby-Secretan B, Scoccianti C, Loomis D, BenbrahimTallaa L, Bouvard V, Bianchini F, et al. Breast-cancer screening-viewpoint of the IARC working group. N Engl J Med 2015;372:2353e8.

[4] Office for National Statistics. Cancer statistics regulations, England (Series MB1), http://www.ons.gov.uk/ons/rel/vsob1/cancerstatistics-registrationseenglandeseries-mb1-/index.html.

[5] The Breast International Group (BIG). A comparison on letrozole and tamoxifen in postmenopausal women with early breast cancer. N Engl J Med 2005;353:2747-57.

[6] Pan H, Gray R, Braybrooke J, Davies C, Taylor C, McGale P, Peto R, Pritchard KI, Bergh J, Dowsett M, Hayes DF, EBCTCG. 20-year risks of breast-cancer recurrence after stopping endocrine therapy at 5 years. N Engl J Med 2017;377(19):1836-46.

[7] Dahm-Kähler P, Borgfeldt C, Holmberg E, Staf C, Falconer H, Bjurberg M, Kjölhede P, Rosenberg P, Stålberg K, Hogberg T, Åvall-Lundqvist E. Population-based study of survival for women with serous cancer of the ovary, fallopian tube, peritoneum or undesignated origin-on behalf of the Swedish gynecological cancer group (SweGCG). Gynecol Oncol 2017;144(1):167-73.

[8] Sandoval P, et al. Carcinoma-associated fibroblasts derive from mesothelial cells via mesothelial-to-mesenchymal transition in peritoneal metastasis. J Pathol 2013;231(4):517-31.

[9] Barlow WE, Lehman CD, Zheng Y, Ballard-Barbash R, Yankaskas BC, Cutter GR, Carney PA, Geller BM, Rosenberg R, Kerlikowske K, Weaver DL. Performance of diagnostic mammography for women with signs or symptoms of breast cancer. J Natl Cancer Inst 2002;94(15):1151-9.

[10] Weigelt B, Reis-Filho JS. Histological and molecular types of breast cancer: is there a unifying taxonomy? Nat Rev Clin Oncol 2009;6(12):718.

[11] Fisher ER, Leeming R, Anderson S, Redmond C, Fisher B. Conservative management of intraductal carcinoma (DCIS) of the breast. J Surg Oncol 1991;47(3):139-47.

[12] Boelens MC, Nethe M, Klarenbeek S, de Ruiter JR, Schut E, Bonzanni N, Zeeman AL, Wientjens E, van der Burg E, Wessels L, van Amerongen R. PTEN loss in E-cadherin-deficient mouse mammary epithelial cells rescues apoptosis and results in development of classical invasive lobular carcinoma. Cell Rep 2016;16(8):2087-101.

[13] Steponavičienė L, Gudavičienė D, Meškauskas R. Rare types of breast carcinoma. Acta Med Lituanica 2012;19(2).

[14] Acs G. Serous and mucinous borderline (low malignant potential) tumors of the ovary. Pathol Patterns Rev 2005;123(Suppl_1):S13-57.

[15] Stelmach A, Ryś J, Mituś JW, Patla A, Skotnicki P, Reinfuss M, Pluta E, Walasek T, Sas-Korczyńska B. Typical medullary breast carcinoma: clinical outcomes and treatment results. Nowotwory J Oncol 2017;67(1):7-13.

[16] Rakha EA, Ellis IO. Diagnostic challenges in papillary lesions of the breast. Pathology 2018;50(1):100-10.

[17] Han Y, Li J, Han S, Jia S, Zhang Y, Zhang W. Diagnostic value of endoscopic appearance during ductoscopy in patients with pathological nipple discharge. BMC Cancer 2017;17(1):300.

[18] Salo SA, Ilonen I, Laaksonen S, Myllärniemi M, Salo JA, Rantanen T. Epidemiology of malignant peritoneal mesothelioma: a population-based study. Cancer Epidemiol 2017;51:81-6.

[19] Gadducci A, Zannoni GF. Uterine smooth muscle tumors of unknown malignant potential: a challenging question. Gynecol Oncol 2019;154(3):631-7.

[20] Røe OD, Stella GM. Malignant pleural mesothelioma: history, controversy, and future of a man-made epidemic. In: Asbestos and mesothelioma. Cham: Springer; 2017. p. 73-101.

[21] Berek JS, Friedlander ML, Bast Jr RC. Epithelial ovarian, fallopian tube, and peritoneal cancer. In: Holland-Frei cancer medicine; Wiley Online Library; 2016. p. 1-27.

[22] Ly T, Chan RC, Lau C. Peritoneal mesothelioma. Pathology 2018;50:S79-80.

[23] Mikuła-Pietrasik J, Uruski P, Tykarski A, Książek K. The peritoneal "soil" for a cancerous "seed": a comprehensive review of the pathogenesis of intraperitoneal cancer metastases. Cell Mol Life Sci 2018;75(3):509-25.

[24] Kotha NV, Baumgartner JM, Veerapong J, Cloyd JM, Ahmed A, Grotz TE, Leiting JL, Fournier K, Lee AJ, Dineen SP, Dessureault S. Primary tumor sidedness is predictive of survival in colon cancer patients treated with cytoreductive surgery with or without hyperthermic intraperitoneal chemotherapy: a US HIPEC collaborative study. Ann Surg Oncol 2019;26(7):2234-40.

[25] Hayes SC, Janda M, Ward LC, Reul-Hirche H, Steele ML, Carter J, Quinn M, Cornish B, Obermair A. Lymphedema following gynecological cancer: results from a prospective, longitudinal cohort study on prevalence, incidence and risk factors. Gynecol Oncol 2017;146(3):623-9.

[26] Deng S, Young B, Vilain R. Primary vaginal melanoma—report of 2 cases. Pathology 2018;50:S68-9.

[27] Fritchie KJ. Genital mesenchymal tumors. In: Soft tissue tumors of the skin. New York: Springer; 2019. p. 383-403.

[28] Prindull G, Zipori D. Environmental guidance of normal and tumor cell plasticity: epithelial mesenchymal transitions as a paradigm. Blood 2004;103(8):2892-9.

[29] Hernández JA, Navarro JT, Rozman M, Ribera JM, Rovira M, Bosch MA, Fantova MJ,

Mate JL, Millá F. Primary myeloid sarcoma of the gynecologic tract: a report of two cases progressing to acute myeloid leukemia. Leuk Lymphoma 2002;43(11):2151-3.

[30] Adams T, Denny L. Abnormal vaginal bleeding in women with gynaecological malignancies. Best Pract Res Clin Obstet Gynaecol 2017;40:134-47.

[31] McCluggage WG. A practical approach to the diagnosis of mixed epithelial and mesenchymal tumours of the uterus. Mod Pathol 2016;29(1):S78-91.

[32] Felix AS, Brinton LA. Cancer progress and priorities: uterine cancer. Cancer Epidemiol Biomarkers Prev 2018;27(9):985-94.

[33] Kruse AJ, ter Brugge HG, de Haan HH, Van Eyndhoven HW, Nijman HW. Vaginal hysterectomy with or without bilateral salpingo-oophorectomy may be an alternative treatment for endometrial cancer patients with medical co-morbidities precluding standard surgical procedures: a systematic review. Int J Gynecol Cancer 2019;29(2):299-304.

[34] Howitt BE, Nucci MR, Quade BJ. Uterine mesenchymal tumors. In: Diagnostic gynecologic and obstetric pathology. Elsevier; 2018. p. 652-715.

[35] Koh WJ, Greer BE, Abu-Rustum NR, Apte SM, Campos SM, Chan J, Cho KR, Cohn D, Crispens MA, DuPont N, Eifel PJ. Uterine neoplasms, version 1. 2014. J Natl Compr Canc Netw 2014;12(2):248-80.

[36] McCluggage WG. Mesenchymal and mixed epithelial-mesenchymal neoplasms of the cervix. In: Pathology of the cervix. Cham: Springer; 2017. p. 201-11.

[37] Cohen PR, Kurzrock R. Sarcoidosis and malignancy. Clin Dermatol 2007;25(3):326-33.

[38] Lee NK, Cheung MK, Shin JY, Husain A, Teng NN, Berek JS, Kapp DS, Osann K, Chan JK. Prognostic factors for uterine cancer in reproductive-aged women. Obstet Gynecol 2007;109(3):655-62.

第 10 章
宫颈癌的治疗方案

S. Shinde[a], N. K. Vishvakarma[a], A. K. Tiwari[b], V. Dixit[c], S. Saxena[d], D. Shukla[a]

[a] Department of Biotechnology, Guru Ghasidas Vishwavidyalaya, Bilaspur, Chhattisgarh, India
[b] Department of Zoology, Bhanwar Singh Porte Government Science College, Pendra, India
[c] Department of Botany, Guru Ghasidas Vishwavidyalaya, Bilaspur, Chhattisgarh, India
[d] Department of Medical Laboratory Sciences, Lovely Professional University, Phagwara, India

摘要

宫颈癌是全球癌症相关死亡的主要原因之一。与发达国家相比，发展中国家宫颈癌的发病率和死亡率更高。宫颈癌的主要风险因素包括人乳头状瘤病毒（human papillomavirus，HPV）感染和不良卫生习惯。在发展中国家，延误诊断是宫颈癌相关死亡的主要原因。其他风险因素包括吸烟、肥胖、缺乏运动以及感染或药物引起的免疫调节功能改变。这些因素间接促使人乳头状瘤病毒建立感染或调节免疫功能，从而增加宫颈癌的易感性。治疗策略主要取决于诊断的分期，包括手术、化疗、放疗及联合疗法。随着研究的深入，免疫疗法等新兴治疗方式已展现出对控制宫颈癌的效果。在过去几年中，HPV 疫苗接种等预防措施也成功地降低了宫颈癌的发病率。此外，提高认识、健康饮食、运动和早期诊断等其他预防措施可能有助于减少发展中国家 HPV 感染和宫颈癌的发生。

关键词

宫颈癌，人乳头状瘤病毒，化疗，免疫疗法

缩略词

AC	腺癌
AP-1	激活蛋白 1
CIN	宫颈上皮内瘤变
CLR	C 型凝集素受体
CRT	放化疗
DFS	无瘤生存期
FDA	美国食品药品监督管理局

FIGO	国际妇产科协会
HC2	二代杂交捕获法
HIV	人类免疫缺陷病毒
HPV	人乳头状瘤病毒
IFN	干扰素
IL	白介素
OS	总生存期
PAMP	病原体相关分子模式
PRR	模式识别受体
RH	根治性子宫切除术
RLR	RIG-I 样受体
RT	放射治疗
STAT	信号转换器和转录激活因子
STD	性传播疾病
TLR	Toll 样受体

一、概述

宫颈癌是全球女性死亡的主要原因之一。2018年,全球报告病例约为57万例,死亡31.1万例。此外,超过85%的宫颈癌死亡病例来自中低收入国家[1,2]。宫颈癌是女性最常确诊的癌症,每年导致27万人死亡,新增50万确诊病例[3]。宫颈癌年发病122 844例,死亡67 477例[4],在女性癌症中仅次于乳腺癌。在印度等大多数发展中国家,宫颈癌是15~44岁女性中最常见的肿瘤[4]。印度人口约占世界总人口的17%,但宫颈癌确诊人数却占全球的1/4以上。印度每5名女性中就有1名罹患宫颈癌。大多数确诊女性来自农村,这反映了印度的社会经济状况。印度农村地区宫颈癌发病率飙升的主要原因是人们对宫颈癌的症状和严重程度缺乏了解、卫生条件差、延误诊断及缺乏检测工具[5]。此外,笔者推测社会对此类生殖系统疾病(尤其是女性生殖系统疾病)的偏见也影响了及时诊断措施的实施。据报道,全球各地宫颈癌的发病率、传播和严重程度存在很大差异。在美国,实施巴氏涂片检查后,死亡人数减少了1/4,原因是通过该检查可以相对容易地进行早期诊断。这表明早期发现对疾病治疗意义重大,不及时治疗会导致宫颈癌患者预后不良。与其他恶性疾病不同,宫颈癌是有可能预防的。通过有效的筛查及早发现宫颈癌,就可以进行有效的治疗。致病性 HPV 感染是导致宫颈癌的主要原因之一[6]。此外,宫颈癌的病因还包括各种流行病学风险因素,如多个性伴侣、妊娠次数、生殖器卫生习惯不良、吸烟、营养不良、使用口服避孕药、认识不足或缺乏认识、初次性交年龄过早，以及因其他疾病［如人类免疫缺陷病毒（human immunodeficiency virus，HIV）感染、免疫抑制药物和器官移植］而导致免疫力低下等[7]。据世界卫生组织（Word Health Organization，WHO）估计，全球有 6.3 亿人感染 HPV，占世界人口的 9%～13%[8,9]。近期报告显示，男性 HPV 感染对男性（健康）造成了影响，特别是在生殖器上，表现为生殖器疣和阴茎癌[10]。HPV 是一种常见的性传播疾病，目前还没有特异性治疗方法。此外，HPV 在早期并无症状，症状出现较晚。许多研究表明，大多数宫颈癌都源于生殖器 HPV 感染[11]。印度的多项研究报告称，约 82.7% 的女性浸润性宫颈癌病例中存在 HPV 16 型或 18 型感染[12]。

通过 HPV 检查，可以检测出早期和晚期感染，以及与之相关的细胞变化，这些变化可以通过简单的细胞学检测（如巴氏涂片）或用醋酸目测发现。巴氏涂片检查结果可分为正常、良性病变和恶性病变。通过分子技术检测 HPV DNA 或 RNA 是组织活检和脱落细胞样本的常用方法。信号扩增杂交分析也可以实现准确的 HPV 检测[13]。此外，通过逆转录酶聚合酶链反应（reverse transcriptase polymerase chain reaction，RT-PCR）也能成功检测出 HPV 的 E6/E7 mRNA 和其他致癌基因[14,15]。其他基于核酸扩增的检测方法还有核酸序列依赖性扩增。除了经济有效的 HPV 筛查外，还可通过接种 HPV 疫苗的预防措施实现一级预防。美国食品药品监督管理局（Food and Drug Administration，FDA）已经批准了 3 种疫苗，可以预防致病的 HPV-16 型和 HPV-18 感染。包括印度在内的多个国家已批准加德西（Gardasil）、加德西 9（Gardasil 9）和希瑞适（Cervarix）的临床应用（NIH：国家癌症研究所）。然而，HPV 疫苗价格昂贵，并非所有潜在风险群体/个人都能负担得起。更重要的是，这些疫苗无法预防所有类型的具有潜在致病性的 HPV。因此，即使有疫苗可用，也有必要对女性进行宫颈癌常规筛查和随访。即便存在这些不足，疫苗也确实降低了感染已知 HPV 亚型的概率。

二、病理生理学

在大约 99.7% 的腺癌（adenocarcinomas，AC）和鳞状细胞癌中，都能检测到 HPV 感染[16]。宫颈癌通常始于宫颈鳞柱交界处。HPV 病毒利用鳞柱交界部作为活跃的转化区，高危 HPV 感染导致的大多数非典型性病变都发生在此处。女性体内的各种激素、生理和物理变化都会影响宫颈管内的转化区，导致无法经阴道肉眼检查发现 HPV 感染。此外，阴道内的酸性环境会破坏转化区的柱状细胞，导致鳞状上皮化生[17]。在过去数十年中，各个国家的宫颈腺癌发病率都有所上升。

大约25%的宫颈癌发生在子宫颈内的腺细胞中。由于这些腺细胞部位隐秘且分泌黏液,因此很难通过巴氏试验早期发现。许多调查显示,相比于其他癌症,宫颈腺癌的预后较差。此外,不容忽视的是,累积数据表明,早期筛查宫颈病变(包括癌症和癌前病变),降低了宫颈癌的发病率[18]。性行为频繁的成年人很有可能感染HPV;大约一半受感染的成年人年龄在20~24岁之间[19]。

三、风险因素

宫颈癌的发病受多种因素影响。其中一个主要风险因素是长期持续感染高危致病性HPV。其他风险因素有些会影响病毒的获得,另一些则会导致免疫功能紊乱,从而促进病毒的生长。研究表明,宿主的基因构成、接触诱变剂和激素因素也是宫颈癌的病因。其中一个显著的风险因素包括过早性行为和有多个性伴侣。被动或主动吸烟也是HPV感染导致宫颈癌的一个重要风险因素。接触其他性传播疾病(sexually transmitted diseases,STD)、感染HIV和使用免疫抑制剂也会增加女性患宫颈癌的风险。使用口服避孕药也与HPV感染和宫颈癌的高发相关,这可能是由于激素水平的改变所致。在经济欠发达国家,缺乏教育、卫生条件差、筛查服务有限也是宫颈癌的重要风险因素。

25岁以下女性的HPV感染率明显更高。在全球范围内,50%~80%的性活跃女性一生中至少会感染一次HPV。有趣的是,报告还显示,通常在45岁以后才会发现/检测出宫颈癌[20]。然而,其他因素,如长期使用激素类避孕药、吸烟、多次妊娠、HIV和/或STD感染(如沙眼衣原体或单纯疱疹病毒2型),以及某些营养缺乏也被认为是重要的辅助因素[21]。

(一)人乳头状瘤病毒

关于HPV感染与宫颈癌的发病和发展之间的因果关系,流行病学研究已经提供了充分的证据。在全球范围内,HPV相关疾病的发病率很高。据估计,超过5%的癌症都是由HPV引起的。在不同器官中,乳头状瘤病毒对鳞状上皮细胞的细胞嗜性非常明显,可导致良性、增生性病变,甚至浸润性癌。HPV的持续感染可导致宫颈上皮内瘤变(cervical intraepithelial neoplasia,CIN3)或宫颈癌[22]。HPV可分为30种类型,其中15种为高危(high risk,HR)类型,15种为低危(low risk,LR)类型。高危HPV(HPV-16、18、31、35、39、45、51、52、56、66、68、69和73)常与高级别病变和浸润性癌症病变相关。低危HPV包括HPV-6、11、40、42、43、44、54、61、70、72、81和CP6108。这些低危HPV多在皮肤疣、低级别病变中检测到,有时也在尖锐湿疣中检测到[23]。在所有 HPV 类型中,致癌性最强的是 HPV-16 和 HPV-18,几乎 70% 的宫颈癌病变中可以检测到这 2 种 HPV。

HPV 基因组由约 8000 bp 的单链环状 DNA 组成,可编码病毒生命周期中不同阶段表达的不同基因。这些基因分为 6 个早期基因($E1$、$E2$、$E4$、$E5$、$E6$ 和 $E7$)和 2 个晚期基因($L1$ 和 $L2$)[24]。其中,E6 和 E7 有许多细胞靶点,是 HPV 的主要癌蛋白。HPV 的 E6 与肿瘤抑制蛋白 p53 结合,阻止细胞凋亡[25];E7 则与 pRb 结合,使其相对无法接触 E2F 转录因子,从而取消细胞周期停滞[26]。E6 对 p53 的进一步下调稳定了缺氧诱导因子-1(hypoxia-inducing factor-1,HIF-1),有利于其下游基因的表达,如血管内皮生长因子(vascular endothelial growth factor,VEGF)、促红细胞生成素和葡萄糖转运蛋白。VEGF 负责增加血管生成,从而确保向正在发生转化的细胞提供营养,随后成为侵袭性癌细胞的通道。促红细胞生成素因其在增加红细胞形成中的作用而闻名,它能上调葡萄糖转运蛋白,导致葡萄糖摄取量增加。血管生成和代谢改变都被认为是癌症的标志[27]。这些因素和其他因素共同导致受感染的细胞转化为癌细胞,并且使这些肿瘤细胞适应代谢环境并存活,导致肿瘤形成。考虑到 E6 和 E7 蛋白在肿瘤形成和存活中的重要作用,它们目前正在成为治疗靶点。

1. HPV 的生命周期 HPV 诱发宫颈癌涉及一系列事件,可分为 4 个步骤,即传播、病毒持续感染、持续感染的细胞进展到癌前病变及浸润性癌阶段。宫颈上皮细胞中病毒持续感染,并发生转化。癌前病变细胞来自细胞学正常的轻度病变。然而,受 HPV 感染的细胞/组织不会被识别,这是因为几乎所有的初始病变都会保留病毒成分作为外显子,并在病毒基因组产物的调控下支持病毒复制[28]。细胞介导免疫可消除大多数宫颈 HPV 感染,在初次感染后 1~2 年内引起细胞学改变[29]。HPV 的传播和病毒持续感染上皮内部使病毒基因组进入受感染的宿主细胞。这一阶段是治疗的窗口期,可通过预防性治疗或接种疫苗来防止病毒载量在宫颈上皮中进一步扩散。在癌前病变阶段,低级别早期病变的细胞群具有同质性和遗传稳定性。这些细胞取代了全层的宫颈上皮。HPV 生命周期中最重要的步骤是将病毒基因组整合到人类宫颈细胞的基因组中。这就形成了高级别病变,其中的异质细胞具有遗传不稳定性,并表达病毒源性致癌蛋白。这种情况经常发生在 CIN3 或更高级别病变中。低级别病变或 CIN1 不属于癌前病变,经组织学研究证实,这类病变发展为宫颈癌的风险较低。病毒生命周期的最后一步是上调病毒癌基因的表达,从而维持癌细胞并使宫颈上皮分化。研究发现,宫颈上皮分化和其他相关细胞因素会加强 HPV 的病毒基因表达。目前已知宿主细胞来源的转录因子(AP-1、AP-2、KRF-1、NF-1、Oct-1、Sp1、STAT3、TEF-1、TEF-2、YY1 和糖皮质激素反应元件)间的相互作用,以及角化蛋白细胞特异性增强子存在于 HPV 基因的上游调控区。这确保了病毒和宿主细胞来源的基因根据感染细胞的分化阶段、特异性和HPV的组织嗜性进行表达[30]。

2. HPV的免疫调节作用 免疫系统在消除和稳定转化细胞方面对细胞转化的调节作用已得到充分证实。通常,癌症的特征之一是免疫逃逸[27];免疫系统的细胞会清除大多数最初的转化细胞。在HPV感染宫颈上皮细胞和转化过程中,免疫系统中的固有细胞负责清除初始阶段的宫颈上皮内癌。与其他来源的癌症一样,HPV诱导的宫颈癌细胞也会通过针对先天免疫系统的初始步骤(包括角化细胞)进行免疫逃逸,而角化细胞会吸收表面的Toll样受体(toll-like receptors,TLR)并释放细胞因子,从而削弱针对侵入性病原体的免疫反应[31]。免疫细胞的模式识别受体(pattern recognition receptors,PRR),如TLR、CLR、RLR和XLR,具有识别微生物病原体或损伤信号的能力。这些PRR识别病原体的机制是与病原体上或损伤相关状态中存在的病原相关分子模式(pathogen-associated molecular patterns,PAMP)或损伤相关分子模式(damage-associated molecular patterns,DAMP)相互作用。当PRR与PAMP或DAMP接触时,它们会通过合成和分泌细胞因子促进免疫反应[32]。对抗病毒免疫至关重要的PRR受体包括TLR,以及在病毒复制过程中检测核酸的核苷酸结合寡聚结构域样受体[33]。TLR3、TLR7、TLR8和TLR9可识别病毒核酸,这些TLR表达的增加与HPV清除有关,可作为受感染女性HPV-16清除的预测标志物[34]。然而,高危HPV的某些结构能够降低TLR表达,核因子κB(nuclear factor-kappaB,NF-κB)和干扰素调节因子3(interferon regulatory factor 3,IRF3)的活化/核转位,帮助病毒的免疫逃避和持续存在[35,36]。那些对病毒感染做出免疫反应的基因,其多态性往往和感染的结局或进展有关。与白介素(interleukin,IL)-1β、IL-18、NLR1和NLR3等先天免疫基因相关的基因多态性与HPV感染和持续存在有关。然而,DNA传感器TLR9的多态性与病毒清除或持续存在无关[37]。HPV可通过多种机制逃避免疫反应。其中一种机制是调节细胞因子和趋化因子,以及下调干扰素(interferon,IFN)通路。抗原递呈障碍和各种细胞黏附分子(尤其是细胞间黏附分子1)表达的减少也会影响免疫逃避。这些实现免疫逃逸的调节主要由源自HPV的E6和E7肿瘤蛋白介导[38]。IFN介导的免疫系统逃避是病毒肿瘤蛋白采取的另一种机制,它通过干扰素调节因子(interferon regulatory factors,IRF)使IFN的中间产物磷酸化,从而减少角化细胞的IFN分泌。IRF1在宫颈组织中的表达减少。HPV感染的高风险也与IRF3的磷酸化减少有关[39]。炎性成分和IL-1β网络中PRR的表达下调与高危HPV相关。这影响了由IL-1β介导的先天免疫和适应性免疫反应[40]。HPV感染也会影响抗原呈递细胞(antigen-presenting cells,APC)、巨噬细胞和自然杀伤细胞(natural killer,NK)的功能。树突细胞(dendritic cells,

DC)在 CIN 中减少[41]。此外,肿瘤细胞过度表达程序性死亡受体配体 1(programmed death-ligand 1,PD-L1),该配体通过与 T 细胞上表达的 PD-1 受体相互作用,使免疫系统细胞失活。据报道,与高危 HPV 阴性宫颈癌树突状细胞相比,高危 HPV 阳性宫颈癌树突状细胞也过度表达 PD-L1[42]。

(二)吸烟

吸烟与许多疾病有关,尤其是支气管肺功能障碍相关的疾病。然而,吸烟对其他器官的病理生理表现的影响也不容忽视。在 HPV 诱发的宫颈癌中,持续感染,尤其是高危 HPV 持续感染是首要威胁之一。然而,疾病发展和恶化的各种诱因也需要配合其他因素。2004 年,国际癌症研究机构(International Agency for Research on Cancer,IARC)将吸烟列为宫颈癌的致病因素[43]。尽管吸烟与宫颈癌并无直接关系,但吸烟会干扰 HPV 的感染和发展,因此与宫颈癌的发病率相关。此外,烟草对宫颈癌的影响还体现在其直接的局部致癌作用和一定程度上的全身致癌作用,以及免疫抑制作用。研究结果还表明,吸烟可影响全身免疫、避孕和营养吸收/消化。这些由吸烟引起的变化会导致宫颈癌的发生,尤其是 HPV 感染人群。

(三)体重

肥胖(体重指数＞30)与癌症发病率之间存在密切关系。研究表明,肥胖会通过影响免疫抑制而增加罹患各种癌症的风险,包括白血病、淋巴瘤、多发性骨髓瘤、肝癌和胆囊癌[44]。肥胖还会影响诊断的敏感性。调查显示,肥胖女性患宫颈癌的风险更高[45]。

(四)运动

经常运动对健康有许多益处,其中之一就是降低患癌风险。运动会影响人体生化、代谢、炎症和表观遗传变化,从而诱导不同的抗癌途径,进而改善整体健康状态[46]。其中一些重要的途径包括促细胞凋亡生长因子的表达、抗氧化途径的激活、端粒长度的维持、炎症、热休克蛋白等。多项研究表明,运动可能会影响女性罹患卵巢癌和乳腺癌的风险程度。在一项病例对照研究中,Szender 等[47]证实,缺乏运动会增加女性罹患宫颈癌的风险。

(五)饮食

健康饮食是降低癌症发病率和进展的重要因素之一。营养过剩会导致肥胖,从而增加罹患各种癌症的风险。营养不良与癌症的发生并无直接关系,但营养不良导致的免疫力下降可能会导致癌症进展[48]。然而,营养不良通常发生在社会经济地位较低的患者身上,他们的卫生条件也很差,因此,容易感染 HPV 和患宫颈癌[49]。研究还表明,西式饮食与更高的 HPV 感染风险有关[48]。

(六)感染

高危 HPV 感染是女性患宫颈癌的首要原因。生殖道和生殖器的其他感染,如 HIV、衣原体等,也会间接影响宫颈癌的发病风险。HPV 以外的感染会导致宿主免疫功能低下,原因是感染引起的免疫抑制(如 HIV)或药物的免疫抑制作用[50]。此外,感染还为继发感染的入侵和建立铺平道路。据报道,感染 HIV 或其他 STD 与 HPV 的合并感染会增加女性罹患宫颈癌的风险。降低其他感染率可以减少 HPV 感染的概率,这一点已得到公认,同时也有助于降低宫颈癌的发病率。然而,性传播也是 HPV 的一种传播方式。在性生活中采取避孕用品等预防措施可以减少 HPV 的传播,以降低宫颈癌的发病率。

四、治疗策略

宫颈癌的临床表现多种多样,包括难以察觉的微浸润性病变和巨块型肿瘤。通过分子生物标志物的检测,宫颈癌的早期发现和筛查率得到提高。在国际妇产科联合会(the International Federation of Gynecology and Obstetrics,FIGO)的宫颈癌分期系统中,Ⅰ期肿瘤被分为两类,包括ⅠA 期(微浸润)和ⅠB 期(巨大肿瘤)。宫颈癌的治疗选择主要取决于被诊断时的分期。宫颈癌的早期发现可提供多种治疗方案,治愈的可能性很大。根治性子宫切除术(radical hysterectomy,RH)加盆腔淋巴结切除术是女性早期宫颈癌的标准治疗选择。然而,这种手术会导致无法生育。对于希望保持生育能力的患者而言,根治型子宫颈切除术加盆腔淋巴结切除术也是一种可行的选择[51]。根据严重程度,晚期宫颈癌患者可能需要手术治疗、放疗和/或化疗或综合治疗。随着诊断和治疗措施的进步,目前正在开发更具针对性的策略,包括免疫疗法和预防疫苗接种。表 10-1 总结了各阶段的治疗方案及其疗效。

表 10-1 不同分期宫颈癌的治疗策略

分期	癌特征	治疗策略	生存率/疗效	参考文献
Ⅰ	癌仅存在于子宫颈(微浸润)			
ⅠA	浸润性癌,最大浸润深度<5 mm			

续表

分期	癌特征	治疗策略	生存率/疗效	参考文献
ⅠA$_1$	测得的间质浸润深度＜3 mm	子宫切除术和希望保留生育能力的患者（锥切，手术切缘阴性）	在早期腺癌中保留卵巢是安全的，不会增加总体死亡风险，存活率为100%	[52]
ⅠA$_2$	测得的间质浸润深度＞3 mm且＜5 mm	淋巴管间隙、淋巴结转移——根治性子宫切除术和盆腔淋巴结切除术		[51]
ⅠB	浸润性癌，最大浸润深度＞5 mm，病变仅存在于子宫颈	根治性子宫切除术，包括盆腔淋巴结切除术	5年OS＝88.2%，无放疗生存率＝83.8%、90.7%(FIGO)	[53]
ⅠB$_1$	间质侵犯深度＞5 mm，最大径线＜2 cm	根治性子宫切除术或放疗		
ⅠB$_2$	最大径线＞2 cm且＜4 cm	放疗、化疗		
ⅠB$_3$	最大径线＞4 cm			
Ⅱ	癌扩展至子宫以外，但未扩展至阴道下1/3处和盆壁			
ⅡA	受累范围仅限于阴道上2/3处，无子宫旁侵犯	根治性手术、放疗	5年OS＝87%～92%，FIGO＝82.8%	[54]
ⅡA$_1$	浸润性癌最大径线＜4 cm			
ⅡA$_2$	浸润性癌最大径线＞4 cm			
ⅡB	宫旁侵犯，盆侧壁无扩散		FIGO＝55.6%	
Ⅲ	癌扩展至盆壁、肾脏、盆腔或主动脉旁淋巴结			
ⅢA	癌累及阴道下1/3处，未扩展至盆壁	单独化疗或先化疗	3年（CRT）OS＝63.2%或OS＝67.7%。(CRT后行RH)是一种有效方法	[55]

续表

分期	癌特征	治疗策略	生存率/疗效	参考文献
ⅢB	扩展至盆壁,导致肾盂积水或肾功能衰失	然后行根治性子宫切除术 顺铂联合(chemoradiotherapy, CRT)或单独(radiotherapy, RT)治疗子宫颈鳞状细胞癌	顺铂(CRT) 5年 DFS = 52.3%,OS=54%,RT 5年 DFS = 43.8%,OS=46%;CRT 的 DFS 和 OS 更好	[56]
ⅢC	盆腔和主动脉旁淋巴结受累			
ⅢC₁	盆腔淋巴结转移	辅助放疗和化疗	仅有一个转移性结节的患者 OS 良好,而有两个或更多转移性结节的患者 OS 结果较差	[57]
ⅢC₁r	通过诊断影像学识别/定性			
ⅢC₁p	通过组织学/细胞病理学识别/定性			
ⅢC₂	主动脉旁淋巴结转移			
Ⅳ	扩展至真骨盆以外,累及膀胱或直肠黏膜			
ⅣA	扩散到邻近器官	近距离放疗、化疗		
ⅣB	扩散到远处器官	放疗、联合疗法(紫杉醇+顺铂)、丝裂霉素、伊立替康		[58]

注:OS. 总生存期;CRT. 放化疗;RT. 放疗;DFS. 无病生存期。

常规治疗

大多数宫颈癌都是由 HPV 感染导致的细胞转化引起的,故在治疗时应同时采用抗癌和抗病毒疗法。治疗策略的首选目标是清除病灶,而不是消除 HPV 感染。然而,传统治疗策略并不能检测和清除微小病变,也无法消除 HPV 感染。对于癌前病变细胞,应根据要求对 CIN 的整个转化区进行治疗。子宫切除术需要全身麻醉,在 20 世纪 70 年代之前,大多数 CIN3 病变都建议采用这种方法。宫颈冷刀锥切也可用于切除受影响区域的延伸组织[59]。大多数 CIN 病变不会发展到癌症浸润阶段。因此，在 CIN 期，子宫切除术可以作为一种预防手段。在许多国家，宫颈癌前病变的治疗方案不包括子宫切除术。局部麻醉下的宫颈冷刀锥切和冷冻疗法是治疗宫颈上皮内病变的首选方法。

在门诊采用大环状切除术或环形电切术切除病毒转化区，对受影响的宫颈部分进行锥形切除[60]。现在已经证实，越来越少的宫颈癌前病变女性患者需要接受手术治疗。世界卫生组织也建议将消融术作为宫颈上皮内病变（CIN1/CIN2）的首选治疗方法。20 世纪 90 年代，一种使用二氧化碳和一氧化二氮的冷冻消融技术问世。冷却后的探针作用于宫颈组织，诱导靶细胞坏死并将其摧毁。这是一种低成本的治疗方法，用于治疗可触及的良性增生癌前病变。不过，冷冻消融术的恢复时间较长，需要数周时间。另外，也可以采用热凝疗法，其中采用加热探针代替冷探针。然而，热探针并没有像冷探针那样得到广泛认可。

浸润性宫颈癌治疗的一项重要进展是对Ⅰ期宫颈癌进行根治性子宫切除术（radical hysterectomy，RH）治疗。在过去数年中，RH 已成为肿瘤较小的女性患者的首选治疗方法。此外，接受根治性阴道子宫颈切除术和腹腔镜盆腔淋巴结切除术的女性，其生育能力也不会受到影响，这种手术还是相对安全的。Plante 等[61]报道称，在 72 例接受该治疗方法的患者中，有 31 例（43%）怀孕。

1. 放疗 放疗（radiotherapy，RT）是对早期诊断出宫颈癌的女性进行手术治疗后的一种治疗方法。一项研究表明，与不进行补充治疗相比，放疗可减少宫颈癌的进展。尽管如此，ⅠB 期宫颈癌术后总生存期（overall survival，OS）的改善并不明显[62]。此外，一项针对 401 例ⅠA_2～ⅡA 早期宫颈癌女性患者的 Cochrane 研究发现，术后接受化疗的女性患者死亡率降低[63]。这表明放化疗联合治疗是有效的。放化疗通常是局部晚期宫颈癌患者的首选治疗方法。用于癌症治疗的有机金属化合物也可用于 HPV 引起的宫颈癌。铂类联合治疗方案已取得了显著的成功。放疗采用外照射，治疗宫颈癌时，将密封放射源置于靠近病变组织的位置[64]。

2. 化疗 化疗通常用于治疗晚期转移性癌症，包括宫颈癌。对于复发/晚期宫颈癌的治疗，顺铂是首选的化疗药物之一，它能改善患者 OS[65]。然而，化疗耐药性阻碍了顺铂在临床实践中的应用。贝伐珠单抗等更具针对性的药物是一种针对 VEGF 的抗体，可抑制肿瘤血管生成，最终使宫颈肿瘤缩小，且毒性较低。有研究进行了口服帕唑帕尼（VEGF 抑制剂）和拉帕替尼（Her2/neu 抑制剂）的临床试验[66]。结果发现，与拉帕替尼相比，帕唑帕尼的毒性更低，无进展生存期也更长。在一项随机双盲安慰剂对照Ⅱ期试验中，另一种药物"西地尼布"（一种有效的 VEGF 1-3 酪氨酸激酶抑制剂）与标准化疗药物卡铂和紫杉醇联合用于治疗转移性/复发性宫颈癌患者。研究显示,西地尼布与卡铂联合治疗有疗效,但毒性反应增加[67]。这些结果表明,联合治疗比单一治疗更具优势。如果能控制联合治疗的毒性,就能取得更好的治疗效果,这可能需要应用生物信息学的计算机模拟预测工具。表10-2列出了药物的详细信息、作用机制和对患者的疗效。

表 10-2 宫颈癌药物及其靶点

药物	作用机制	患者/结果	参考文献
贝伐珠单抗	识别 VEGF,防止其与内皮细胞表面的受体(Flt-1 和 KDR)相互作用	转移性、顽固性、复发性宫颈癌;宫颈肿瘤缩小,毒性低	[68]
帕唑帕尼	抑制 VEGFR、PDGFR 和 c-kit 的酪氨酸激酶活性	ⅣB 期,宫颈腺癌	[66]
西地尼布+卡铂	抑制 VEGF 1、2 和 3 的酪氨酸激酶活性	转移性/复发性宫颈癌;患者毒性增加	[67]

3. 联合治疗 随着对宫颈癌分子改变的了解不断深入,新的治疗方法正通过临床试验不断被开发出来,如免疫调节剂、治疗型疫苗和单克隆抗体治疗。目前的研究重点是通过靶向多种分子来限制癌细胞的生长,即所谓的联合疗法。各种临床试验表明,与单一疗法相比,联合疗法对转移性、顽固性/复发性宫颈癌患者更有效,并能提高 OS。例如,通过比较顺铂与顺铂/紫杉醇、顺铂/拓扑替康和吉西他滨/长春瑞滨的联合疗法,确定了治疗晚期宫颈癌患者的最佳铂类细胞毒性治疗方案。顺铂/紫杉醇的疗效较好[66]。针对顺铂耐药的宫颈癌进行了进一步研究,开发出了新的治疗策略来识别和靶向宫颈癌生长的关键分子通路。卡铂和紫杉醇联合疗法已被批准作为转移性宫颈癌的一线疗法。贝伐珠单抗是一种抗 VEGF 单克隆抗体,它的作用靶点是限制血管生成,因此可以限制肿瘤生长所需的营养和氧气供应。研究发现,贝伐珠单抗与卡铂-紫杉醇的联合疗法对治疗晚期转移性宫颈癌也有效。至于另一种联合用药拓扑替康-紫杉醇-贝伐珠单抗,虽然对有铂过敏史或肾功能不全的患者有益,但 OS 并没有发生变化[69]。

五、先进疗法

早期宫颈癌患者一般采用手术治疗,唯一获准用于转移性、顽固性/复发性宫颈癌的化疗药物是贝伐珠单抗联合化疗。然而,由于缺乏有效的二线治疗方法,经过一线治疗后病情进展的患者死亡率很高[70]。因此,目前正在考虑新的先进治疗方案，如免疫疗法。细胞免疫的调控既有激活信号（如共刺激分子），也有抑制信号（如免疫检查点）[71]。在正常情况下，免疫检查点可维持自我耐受，防止自身免疫，并在感染时保护正常细胞免受免疫攻击。癌细胞通过改变肿瘤微环境来逃避这种免疫监视。因此，免疫检查点抑制可能是增强宫颈癌抗肿瘤免疫力的潜在方法之一。细胞毒性 T 淋巴细胞相关抗原 4（cytotoxic T lymphocyte-associated antigen 4，CTLA-4）是宫颈癌免疫疗法的重要靶点之一。淋巴结中的 T 细胞活化后，CTLA-4 开始表达并下调活化的 T 细胞[72]。因此，次级淋巴器官内的 T 细胞活化也会受到抑制[73]。另一个潜在靶点是在外周组织效应 T 细胞上表达的 PD-1。PD-1 与表达在 DC、TAF 或肿瘤细胞上的 PD-L1 结合，阻止 T 细胞攻击癌症细胞[74]。正常情况下，IFN-γ 诱导的 PD-L1 可保护 DC 免受 T 细胞介导的细胞毒性。在肿瘤组织中，可以观察到表达 PD-1 的 $CD8^+$ T 细胞比例升高。目前，FDA 仅批准了 CTLA-4 和 PD-1/PD-L1 抑制剂[75]。在 CTLA-4 的帮助下，表达在 APC 表面的 B7-1 和 B7-2 共刺激分子也得以整合[76]。此外，很明显，通过阻断淋巴结内初始 T 细胞表面的 CTLA-4 表达和效应 T 细胞上的 PD-1 表达，可以成为潜在的治疗靶点。表 10-3 列出了免疫疗法药物的详细信息。

表 10-3 宫颈癌免疫疗法药物

单克隆抗体	研究	显著性水平（译者注：研究结果）	参考文献
抗 CTLA-4			
伊匹木单抗（经 FDA 批准）	转移性或复发性 HPV 相关宫颈癌女性患者	药物可耐受，但活性不明显	[77,78]
抗 PD-1			
西米普利单抗	REGN2810	与放疗结合使用时，响应率更高，这表明会产生远端效应	[79]
帕博利珠单抗	Keynote-028 Trial	未发现死亡病例，药物具有抗肿瘤活性和安全性	[80]
纳武利尤单抗	Checkmate358	宫颈癌患者持久反应	[81]

六、治疗性 HPV 疫苗

预防宫颈癌的重要治疗措施之一是接种 HPV 疫苗，临床证明接种该疫苗可预防前期病变和高级别 CIN 的形成。经证实，为女孩（11 或 12 岁左右）接种疫苗可有效保护她们免受日后可能导致宫颈癌的主要类型 HPV 感染[82]。通过对男孩进行免疫接种,综合传播率和 HPV 相关癌症的风险也有可能降低[83]。乙型肝炎疫苗可降低肝癌风险,预计全球范围内越来越多地使用 HPV 疫苗也会带来类似的益处[84]。此外,患者死亡率也因宫颈癌筛查和治疗方案成功开展而有所下降。鉴于高危 HPV 与宫颈癌之间明确的致病关系,HPV 疫苗能够利用病毒样颗粒产生抗体反应。FDA 批准了 3 种 HPV 疫苗(加德西、加德西 9 和希瑞适),目前已在市场上销售。加德西可预防导致生殖器疣的 HPV-6 和 HPV-11;加德西 9 可作用于更多的 HPV 株系,预计可将宫颈癌的预防率提高到 90%[85];希瑞适使用铝和一种 LPS 衍生物作为佐剂,可刺激先天免疫系统,从而激活 TLR4,通过激活 DC 和 NK 细胞促进 HPV 感染细胞的死亡[85],该疫苗还能抵御导致 70% 宫颈癌的 HPV-16 和 HPV-18。

七、宫颈癌预防措施

过去 200 年的研究中发现,接触环境或饮食中的诱导剂会导致癌症,这也是发达国家和欠发达国家癌症发病率和死亡率上升的原因。然而,过去 50 年的研究表明,可以采取不同的预防措施来降低癌症发病率。其中一项措施就是改变生活方式,通过调节免疫系统在癌症的发展过程中发挥重要作用。其他措施包括避免接触环境中的致癌物质、健康饮食和保持良好的卫生习惯,这些都有助于预防癌症。宫颈癌是一种可以预防的疾病,因此,提高公众对可能致癌原因的认识可以减轻宫颈癌负担。

参 考 文 献

[1] Balasubramaniam SD, et al. Key molecular events in cervical cancer development. Medicina (Kaunas) 2019;55(7):384.

[2] World Health Organization. WHO guidelines for screening and treatment of precancerous lesions for cervical cancer prevention: supplemental material: GRADE evidence-to-recommendation tables and evidence profiles for each recommendation. World Health Organization; 2013.

[3] Bray F, et al. Global cancer statistics 2018: GLOBOCAN estimates of incidence and mortality worldwide for 36 cancers in 185 countries. CA Cancer J Clin 2018;68(6):394-424.

[4] Sreedevi A, Javed R, Dinesh A. Epidemiology of cervical cancer with special focus on India. Int J Womens Health 2015;7:405-14.

[5] Tripathi N, et al. Barriers for early detection of cancer amongst Indian rural women. South Asian J Cancer 2014;3(2):122.

[6] Faridi R, et al. Oncogenic potential of human papillomavirus (HPV) and its relation with

cervical cancer. Virol J 2011;8(1):269.

[7] Opoku CA, et al. Perception and risk factors for cervical cancer among women in northern Ghana. Ghana Med J 2016;50(2):84-9.

[8] Pandhi D, Sonthalia S. Human papilloma virus vaccines: current scenario. Indian J Sex Transm Dis 2011;32(2):75.

[9] World Health Organization. WHO guidelines for screening and treatment of precancerous lesions for cervical cancer prevention. World Health Organization; 2013.

[10] Sichero L, Giuliano AR, Villa LL. Human papillomavirus and genital disease in men: what we have learned from the HIM study. Acta Cytol 2019;63(2):109-17.

[11] Wardak S. Human papillomavirus (HPV) and cervical cancer. Med Dosw Mikrobiol 2016; 68(1):73-84.

[12] Bosch FX, de Sanjosé S. Chapter 1: Human papillomavirus and cervical cancer—burden and assessment of causality. J Natl Cancer Inst Monogr 2003;2003(31):3-13.

[13] Zaravinos A, et al. Molecular detection methods of human papillomavirus (HPV). Int J Biol Markers 2009;24(4):215-22.

[14] Smits HL, et al. Application of the NASBA nucleic acid amplification method for the detection of human papillomavirus type 16 E6-E7 transcripts. J Virol Methods 1995;54(1): 75-81.

[15] Sotlar K, et al. Detection of high-risk human papillomavirus E6 and E7 oncogene transcripts in cervical scrapes by nested RT-polymerase chain reaction. J Med Virol 2004;74 (1):107-16.

[16] Böhmer G, et al. No confirmed case of human papillomavirus DNA-negative cervical intraepithelial neoplasia grade 3 or invasive primary cancer of the uterine cervix among 511 patients. Am J Obstet Gynecol 2003;189(1):118-20.

[17] Jacobson D, et al. Cervical ectopy and the transformation zone measured by computerized planimetry in adolescents. Int J Gynaecol Obstet 1999;66(1):7-17.

[18] Sankaranarayanan R, Budukh AM, Rajkumar R. Effective screening programmes for cervical cancer in low-and middle-income developing countries. Bull World Health Organ 2001;79:954-62.

[19] Satterwhite CL, et al. Sexually transmitted infections among US women and men: prevalence and incidence estimates, 2008. Sex Transm Dis 2013;40(3):187-93.

[20] Das BC, et al. Prospects and prejudices of human papillomavirus vaccines in India. Vaccine 2008; 26(22):2669-79.

[21] Munoz N, et al. Chapter 1: HPV in the etiology of human cancer. Vaccine 2006;24(Suppl 3) S3/1-10.

[22] Rodríguez AC, et al. Longitudinal study of human papillomavirus persistence and cervical intraepithelial neoplasia grade 2/3: critical role of duration of infection. J Natl Cancer Inst 2010;102(5):315-24.

[23] Bharti AC, et al. Human papillomavirus and control of cervical cancer in India. Expert Rev Obstet Gynecol 2010;5(3):329-46.

[24] Doorbar JJCS. Molecular biology of human papillomavirus infection and cervical cancer. Clin Sci(Lond) 2006;110(5):525-41.

[25] Mantovani F, Banks L. The human papillomavirus E6 protein and its contribution to malignant progression. Oncogene 2001;20(54):7874-87.

[26] Munger K, et al. Biological activities and molecular targets of the human papillomavirus E7 oncoprotein. Oncogene 2001;20(54):7888-98.

[27] Hanahan D, Weinberg RA. Hallmarks of cancer: the next generation. Cell 2011;144(5):646-74.

[28] Bharti AC, et al. Anti-human papillomavirus therapeutics: facts & future. Indian J Med Res 2009;130(3):296.

[29] Stanley M. Immune responses to human papillomavirus. Vaccine 2006;24(Suppl 1):S16-22.

[30] Thierry F. Transcriptional regulation of the papillomavirus oncogenes by cellular and viral transcription factors in cervical carcinoma. Virology 2009;384(2):375-9.

[31] Grabowska AK, Riemer AB. The invisible enemy—how human papillomaviruses avoid recognition and clearance by the host immune system. Open Virol J 2012;6:249-56.

[32] Medzhitov R, Janeway Jr. CA. Innate immunity: impact on the adaptive immune response. Curr Opin Immunol 1997;9(1):4-9.

[33] Jo EK, et al. Molecular mechanisms regulating NLRP3 inflammasome activation. Cell Mol Immunol 2016;13(2):148-59.

[34] Daud II, et al. Association between toll-like receptor expression and human papillomavirus type 16 persistence. Int J Cancer 2011;128(4):879-86.

[35] Hasan UA, et al. TLR9 expression and function is abolished by the cervical cancer-associated human papillomavirus type 16. J Immunol 2007;178(5):3186-97.

[36] Tummers B, et al. The interferon-related developmental regulator 1 is used by human papillomavirus to suppress NFκB activation. Nat Commun 2015;6:6537.

[37] Oliveira LB, et al. Polymorphism in the promoter region of the Toll-like receptor 9 gene and cervical human papillomavirus infection. J Gen Virol 2013;94(Pt 8):1858-64.

[38] Kanodia S, Fahey LM, Kast WM. Mechanisms used by human papillomaviruses to escape the host immune response. Curr Cancer Drug Targets 2007;7(1):79-89.

[39] Um SJ, et al. Abrogation of IRF-1 response by high-risk HPV E7 protein in vivo. Cancer Lett 2002;179(2):205-12.

[40] Karim R, et al. Human papillomavirus deregulates the response of a cellular network comprising of chemotactic and proinflammatory genes. PLoS One 2011;6(3):e17848.

[41] Mota F, et al. The antigen-presenting environment in normal and human papillomavirus (HPV)-related premalignant cervical epithelium. Clin Exp Immunol 1999;116(1):33-40.

[42] Nunes RAL, et al. Innate immunity and HPV: friends or foes. Clinics (Sao Paulo) 2018; 73(Suppl 1): e549s.

[43] Fonseca-Moutinho JA. Smoking and cervical cancer. ISRN Obstet Gynecol 2011; 2011:847684.

[44] Lichtman MA. Obesity and the risk for a hematological malignancy: leukemia, lymphoma, or myeloma. Oncologist 2010;15(10):1083-101.

[45] Clarke MA, et al. Epidemiologic evidence that excess body weight increases risk of cervical cancer by decreased detection of precancer. J Clin Oncol 2018;36(12):1184-91.

[46] Thomas RJ, Kenfield SA, Jimenez A. Exercise-induced biochemical changes and their potential influence on cancer: a scientific review. Br J Sports Med 2017;51(8):640-4.

[47] Szender JB, et al. Impact of physical inactivity on risk of developing cancer of the uterine cervix: a case-control study. J Low Genit Tract Dis 2016;20(3):230-3.

[48] Barchitta M, et al. The association of dietary patterns with high-risk human papillomavirus infection and cervical cancer: a cross-sectional study in Italy. Nutrients 2018;10(4):469.

[49] Lee JK, et al. Mild obesity, physical activity, calorie intake, and the risks of cervical intraepithelial neoplasia and cervical cancer. PLoS One 2013;8(6):e66555.

[50] Reusser NM, et al. HPV carcinomas in immunocompromised patients. J Clin Med 2015;4(2):260-81.

[51] Ramirez PT, et al. Management of low-risk early-stage cervical cancer: should conization, simple trachelectomy, or simple hysterectomy replace radical surgery as the new standard of care? Gynecol Oncol 2014;132(1):254-9.

[52] Hu J, et al. Should ovaries be removed or not in early-stage cervical adenocarcinoma: a multicenter retrospective study of 105 patients. J Obstet Gynaecol 2017;37(8):1065-9.

[53] Zhou J, et al. Postoperative clinicopathological factors affecting cervical adenocarcinoma: stages Ⅰ-ⅡB. Medicine 2018;97(2):e9323.

[54] Gray HJ. Primary management of early stage cervical cancer (ⅠA1-ⅠB) and appropriate selection of adjuvant therapy. J Natl Compr Canc Netw 2008;6(1):47-52.

[55] Fanfani F, et al. Radical hysterectomy after chemoradiation in FIGO stage Ⅲ cervical cancer patients versus chemoradiation and brachytherapy: complications and 3-years survival. Eur J Surg Oncol 2016;42(10):1519-25.

[56] Shrivastava S, et al. Cisplatin chemoradiotherapy vs radiotherapy in FIGO stage ⅢB squamous cell carcinoma of the uterine cervix: a randomized clinical trial. JAMA Oncol 2018;4(4):506-13.

[57] Bogani G, et al. The role of human papillomavirus vaccines in cervical cancer: prevention and treatment. Crit Rev Oncol Hematol 2018;122:92-7.

[58] Colombo N, et al. Cervical cancer: ESMO Clinical Practice Guidelines for diagnosis, treatment and follow-up. Ann Oncol 2012;23(Suppl_7):vii27-32.

[59] Melnikow J, et al. Cervical intraepithelial neoplasia outcomes after treatment: long-term

follow-up from the British Columbia Cohort Study. J Natl Cancer Inst 2009;101(10):721-8.

[60] Prendiville W, Cullimore J, Norman S. Large loop excision of the transformation zone (LLETZ). A new method of management for women with cervical intraepithelial neoplasia. BJOG 1989;96(9):1054-60.

[61] Plante M, et al. Vaginal radical trachelectomy: a valuable fertility-preserving option in the management of early-stage cervical cancer. A series of 50 pregnancies and review of the literature. Gynecol Oncol 2005;98(1):3-10.

[62] Rogers L, et al. Radiotherapy and chemoradiation after surgery for early cervical cancer. Cochrane Database Syst Rev 2012;2012(5)Cd007583.

[63] Falcetta FS, et al. Adjuvant platinum-based chemotherapy for early stage cervical cancer. Cochrane Database Syst Rev 2016;11:Cd005342.

[64] Liu Y, et al. PD-1/PD-L1 inhibitors in cervical cancer. Front Pharmacol 2019;10:65.

[65] Lorusso D, et al. A systematic review comparing cisplatin and carboplatin plus paclitaxel-based chemotherapy for recurrent or metastatic cervical cancer. Gynecol Oncol 2014;133(1):117-23.

[66] Monk BJ, et al. Phase II, open-label study of pazopanib or lapatinib monotherapy compared with pazopanib plus lapatinib combination therapy in patients with advanced and recurrent cervical cancer. J Clin Oncol 2010;28(22):3562-9.

[67] Symonds RP, et al. Cediranib combined with carboplatin and paclitaxel in patients with metastatic or recurrent cervical cancer (CIRCCa): a randomised, double-blind, placebo-controlled phase 2 trial. Lancet Oncol 2015;16(15):1515-24.

[68] Tewari KS, et al. Bevacizumab for advanced cervical cancer: final overall survival and adverse event analysis of a randomised, controlled, open-label, phase 3 trial (Gynecologic Oncology Group 240). Lancet 2017;390(10103):1654-63.

[69] Krill LS, Tewari KS. Integration of bevacizumab with chemotherapy doublets for advanced cervical cancer. Expert Opin Pharmacother 2015;16(5):675-83.

[70] Minion LE, Tewari KS. Cervical cancer—state of the science: from angiogenesis blockade to checkpoint inhibition. Gynecol Oncol 2018;148(3):609-21.

[71] Pardoll DM. The blockade of immune checkpoints in cancer immunotherapy. Nat Rev Cancer 2012;12(4):252-64.

[72] Hodi FS, et al. Improved survival with ipilimumab in patients with metastatic melanoma. N Engl J Med 2010;363(8):711-23.

[73] Kurup SP, et al. Regulatory T cells impede acute and long-term immunity to blood-stage malaria through CTLA-4. Nat Med 2017;23(10):1220-5.

[74] Ribas A. Tumor immunotherapy directed at PD-1. N Engl J Med 2012;366(26):2517-9.

[75] Bagcchi S. Pembrolizumab for treatment of refractory melanoma. Lancet Oncol 2014;15(10):e419.

[76] Fife BT, Bluestone JA. Control of peripheral T-cell tolerance and autoimmunity via the CTLA-4 and PD-1 pathways. Immunol Rev 2008;224:166-82.

[77] Ku GY, et al. Single-institution experience with ipilimumab in advanced melanoma patients in the compassionate use setting: lymphocyte count after 2 doses correlates with survival. Cancer 2010;116(7):1767-75.

[78] Lheureux S, et al. Association of Ipilimumab with Safety and Antitumor Activity in women with metastatic or recurrent human papillomavirus-related cervical carcinoma. JAMA Oncol 2018;4(7):e173776.

[79] Papadopoulos KP, et al. A first-in-human study of REGN2810, a monoclonal, fully human antibody to programmed death-1 (PD-1), in combination with immunomodulators including hypofractionated radiotherapy (hfRT). J Clin Oncol 2016;34:3024.

[80] Frenel J-S, et al. Safety and efficacy of pembrolizumab in advanced, programmed death ligand 1-positive cervical cancer: results from the phase Ⅰb KEYNOTE-028 trial. J Clin Oncol 2017;35(36):4035-41.

[81] Hollebecque A, et al. An open-label, multicohort, phase Ⅰ/Ⅱ study of nivolumab in patients with virus-associated tumors (CheckMate 358): efficacy and safety in recurrent or metastatic (R/M) cervical, vaginal, and vulvar cancers. J Clin Oncol 2017;35:5504.

[82] GlaxoSmithKline Vaccine HPV-007 Study Group, et al. Sustained efficacy and immunogenicity of the human papillomavirus (HPV)-16/18 AS04-adjuvanted vaccine: analysis of a randomised placebo-controlled trial up to 6.4 years. Lancet 2009;374(9706):1975-85.

[83] Kim JJ. Focus on research: weighing the benefits and costs of HPV vaccination of young men. N Engl J Med 2011;364(5):393-5.

[84] Lavanchy D. Worldwide epidemiology of HBV infection, disease burden, and vaccine prevention. J Clin Virol 2005;34:S1-3.

[85] Van Damme P, et al. Use of the nonavalent HPV vaccine in individuals previously fully or partially vaccinated with bivalent or quadrivalent HPV vaccines. Vaccine 2016;34(6):757-61.

第 11 章
通过计算方法识别宫颈癌靶分子

Manoj Kumar Gupta, Vadde Ramakrishna

Department of Biotechnology and Bioinformatics, Yogi Vemana University, Kadapa, Andhra Pradesh, India

摘要

宫颈癌是成年女性癌症死亡的第二大原因。放疗、手术和激素化疗（译者注：译者认为此处应为化学治疗）是宫颈癌最广泛使用的3种技术。最近，研究者利用传统和高通量技术确定了一些生物标志物。高通量技术会产生海量数据，这反过来又要求开发强大的计算方法，以更全面的方式分析这些大数据。这就对更好地了解包括宫颈癌在内的许多疾病相关机制提出了要求。考虑到这一点，笔者在本章中介绍了用于检测与宫颈癌相关的目标分子的不同计算方法。目前，尽管只进行了有限的计算研究，但已经确定了多个宫颈癌相关的关键枢纽基因（如 *BTD*、*PEG3*、*RPLP2* 和 *SPON1*）、长非编码 RNA（如 GOLGA2P5、EMX2OS、FLJ10038、FAM66C、ACVR2B-AS1、AMZ2P1、LINC00341、ZNF876P、MIR9-3HG 和 ILF3-AS1）和 miRNA（如 Hsa-mir-1273g、Hsa-mir-5095、Hsa-mir-5096 和 Hsa-mir-1273f），它们在宫颈癌发展中发挥着关键作用。由于对宫颈癌数据集进行计算的研究为数不多，开发更强大的软件、算法和分析宫颈癌数据集仍有很大的空间。预计在不久的将来，本章所提供的信息将对癌症生物学家和免疫学家在治疗宫颈癌方面提供很大的帮助。

关键词

宫颈癌，计算方法，关键基因，药物

缩略词

circRNA	环状 RNA
GWAS	全基因组相关研究
HPV	人乳头状瘤病毒
lncRNA	长链非编码 RNA
miRNA	微小 RNA

一、概述

宫颈癌是年轻成年女性癌症死亡的第二大原因。宫颈癌对不同国家女性的影响各不相同。高收入国家女性的宫颈癌发病率低于中低收入国家[1]。这主要是因为发达国家增加了对女性的筛查和人乳头状瘤病毒（human papillomavirus，HPV）疫苗的接种[2]。尽管如此，2018年，全球报告了新增宫颈癌病例570 000例，新增死亡病例311 000例[3]。在印度，每年有122 000名女性诊断为宫颈癌，67 000例患者死于宫颈癌[4]。因此，迫切需要更有效的宫颈癌治疗手段。迄今为止，根据疾病状态、肿瘤的组织病理学类型、肿瘤分化程度、患者年龄和转移能力等因素，宫颈癌的治疗方法有多种。放疗、手术和激素化疗（译者注：译者认为此处应为化学治疗）是使用最广泛的3种技术。手术是唯一能有效治疗浸润前和微浸润期（Ⅰa期）宫颈癌的方法。放疗被广泛用于Ⅱb、Ⅲa、Ⅲb和Ⅳa期宫颈癌的治疗。放疗和手术结合用于治疗Ⅰb和Ⅱa期宫颈癌[5]。此外，最近已利用经典和高通量技术发现了多个生物标志物，例如，肿瘤甲基化抑制基因和型别特异性病毒载量。这些生物标志物被广泛用于宫颈癌的早期检测和预防[5]。在大多数情况下，HPV是宫颈癌的主要致病原因[6]。

早期的候选基因研究已经确定了多种与宫颈癌相关的基因，如 IRF3、DMC1、EXO1、TLR2、FANCA、XRCC1、CYBA、ERAP1、EVER1/2、TP53、TAP2、IL17、TERT、LMP7、GTF2H4、DUT、SULF1、OAS3 和 IFNG[7-12]。在一项全基因组相关研究（genome-wide association study，GWAS）中，作者报道称，敲除 ARRDC3 基因会减慢细胞的增长，从而阻止 HPV16 假病毒颗粒的感染。这证实了 ARRDC3 基因在 HPV 感染过程中起关键作用[13]。其他数项 GWAS 研究也确定了宫颈癌与亚洲和欧洲人群中不同的 HLA Ⅱ 等位基因之间的关系[14-17]。多态性 rs9277535（DPB1）、rs3077（DPA1）、rs3117027（DPB2）和 rs4282438（DPB2），也与宫颈癌有关[18]。还有报告其他核苷酸多态性，如 TNF-α-238G＞A 和 TNF-α-308G＞A，分别降低和增加了宫颈癌的易感性[19]。据报道，HLA-B * 0702-DRB1 * 1501/HLADQB1 * 0602 和 HLA-B * 1501/HLA-DRB1 * 1301/HLA-DQA1 * 0103/HLA-DQB1 * 0603 单倍型也会分别增加和降低宫颈癌的风险[12]。2016年，Martínez-Nava 等发现3个多态性，即 p21（rs1801270）和 BRIP1（rs11079454 和 rs2048718），可以降低女性患宫颈癌的风险[20]。

近年来，高通量技术的发展产生了海量数据，这要求研究者开发强大的计算方法，以更全面的方式分析大数据。这将更好地了解包括宫颈癌在内的许多疾病的相关机制[21-24]。然而，通过实验检测蛋白-蛋白相互作用和关键基因需要大量资金和时间。计算方法为短时间内以较低成本解决这些问题提供了一种独特的途径。考虑到这一点，笔者的实验室之前采用了不同的计算方法来了解与胆管狭窄[25]、日本脑炎[26]、糖尿病[27]、阿尔茨海默病[24]，以及水稻植物中生物和非生物作用的相关的机制[28-30]。在本章中，笔者将介绍通过计算方法发现的各种宫颈癌相关靶向分子信息。在不久的将来，这些靶向分子可能会成为早期检测和预防女性宫颈癌的生物标志物。

二、靶分子的鉴定

迄今为止，研究者们已经开发了多种计算方法来识别与宫颈癌相关的多种靶分子（表11-1）。

表 11-1　通过计算方法鉴定的与宫颈癌相关的靶分子

靶分子	基因/微小 RNA/长非编码 RNA/环状 RNA	参考文献
基因	$MMP1$, VIM, $CDC45$, CAT, BTD, $PEG3$, $RPLP2$, $SPON1$, $SLC5A3$, $PRDX3$, $LSM3$, $AS1B$, $COPB2$, $PCNA$, $CDK1$, CC-$NB1$, $BIRC5$, $MAD2L1$, $TOP2A$, $TSPO$, FOS, $CCND1$, $MCM2$, $PCNA$ & $RNASEH2A$, $TNNI3$, $CCDC136$, $ABCG2$, $CYP26A1$, $TMEM233S$, $YT13$, $FOXC2$, $CXCL5$, $RRB1$, $ARRB2$, $CAV1$, $CFTR$, $EP300$, $ERBB3$, $HIF1A$, $INSR$, $JAK2$, JUN, LYN, PML, RET, $SMAD3$, SR, $RACGAP1$, $CHEK1$, $KIF11$, $KIF23$, $RRM2$, $CEP55$, and $ATAD2$	[31-37]
微 RNA	miR-194-1, miR-204, miR-150, miR-193b-3p, miR-215-5p and miR-192-5p, miR-548d-5p, miR-5095, miR-548c-5p, miR-133a-3p, miR-215-5p, miR-944, miR-31-3p, miR-548d-5p, miR-11-3p, miR-491-3p, miR-107, miR-133a-5p, miR-133b, Hsa-mir-1273g, Hsa-mir-5095, Hsa-mir-5096, and Hsa-mir-1273f	[38-42]
长链非编码 RNA	EPB41L4A-AS1, LINC00649, HCP5, SNHG12, GOLGA2P10, ACVR2B-AS1, ATP1A1-AS1, LOH12CR2, A2M-AS1, FTX, MST1P2, GOLGA2P5, EMX2OS, FLJ10038, FAM66C, ACVR2B-AS1, AMZ2P1, LINC00341, ZNF876P, MIR9-3HG, ILF3-AS1, GOLGA2P5, MIR9-3HG ILF3-AS1, FAM66C, LINC00312, MIR9-3HG, SYS1-DBNDD2, and DDX12P	[43, 44]
环状 RNA	hsa_circRNA_103519, hsa_circRNA_101958, hsa_circRNA_000596, hsa_circRNA_400068, hsa_circRNA_104315, hsa_circ_0031027, hsa_circ_0070190, hsa_circ_0084927, hsa_circ_0043280, hsa_circ_0000745, and hsa_circ_0065898 and hsa_circ_0000077	[37, 45]

(一)关键基因和蛋白质

Zhang 等进行了致病网络分析,确定了 4 个与宫颈癌相关的基因,即 $MMP1$、VIM、$CDC45$ 和 CAT[31]。Tan 等通过 21 个基因表达数据集的功能分析发现了与宫颈癌相关的基因,包括 4 个上调基因(BTD、$PEG3$、$RPLP2$ 和 $SPON1$)和 5 个下调基因($SLC5A3$、$PRDX3$、$LSM3$、$AS1B$ 和 $COPB2$)[32]。Cheng 等通过基因调控分析表明,DNA 聚合酶(PLOA1/E2/E3/Q)和复制性 DNA 螺旋酶蛋白(MCM6、MCM4、MCM2、MCM10 和 MCM5)在宫颈癌中增加了 DNA 复制过程[46]。他们发现一组转录因子、激酶和细胞周期蛋白,如 CCNB2、CDK1、TFDP2 和 CCNA2,可增强细胞周期从 G1 期向 S 期和从 G2 期向 M 期的转换。此外,还发现一组运动蛋白,如 KIF4A、KIF11 和 KIF14,以及 PRC1,可在宫颈癌进展过程中调节细胞分裂过程[46]。另一项计算分析发现与宫颈癌相关的基因,包括 6 个上调基因($PCNA$、$CDK1$、$CCNB1$、$BIRC5$、$MAD2L1$ 和 $TOP2A$)和 3 个下调基因($TSPO$、FOS 和 $CCND1$),这 9 个关键基因主要与 DNA 复制、p53 信号通路、卵母细胞成熟分裂和细胞周期相关[33]。2016 年,Deng 等使用生物信息学方法发现了 143 个与宫颈癌相关的差异表达基因[47]。Li 等报道,$MCM2$、$PCNA$ 和 $RNASEH2A$ 3 个关键基因及 DNA 复制在宫颈癌中起重要作用[34]。另一组研究人员对癌症基因组图谱数据库(https://portal.gdc.cancer.gov)进行了生物信息学分析,报告了 4 个高甲基化基因($TNNI3$、$CCDC136$、$ABCG2$ 和 $CYP26A1$)和 4 个低甲基化基因($TMEM233S$、$YT13$、$FOXC2$ 和 $CXCL5$),分别与宫颈癌患者的总体生存率呈正相关和负相关[35]。Hindumathi 等通过基因本体论和图论方法确定了 15 个与宫颈癌相关的关键基因,即 $RRB1$、$ARRB2$、$CAV1$、$CFTR$、$EP300$、$ERBB3$、$HIF1A$、$INSR$、$JAK2$、JUN、LYN、PML、RET、$SMAD3$ 和 SRC[36]。Yi 等发现 7 个基因 $RACGAP1$、$CHEK1$、$KIF11$、$KIF23$、$RRM2$、$CEP55$ 和 $ATAD2$ 在宫颈癌发展中起关键作用[37]。

(二)微 RNA

微 RNA(micro RNA,miRNA)是长约 22 个核苷酸的非编码 RNA,在自然界中高度保守。miRNA 与众多生物学过程有关,包括癌症的发生。迄今为止,已确认几种 miRNA 存在于 HPV 的附近整合位点[48]。Liu 等研究发现 3 种与宫颈癌相关的 miRNA,即 miR-194-1、miR-204 和 miR-150[38]。2018 年,Kori 等利用生物信息学方法鉴定出多种宫颈癌生物标志物,包括代谢产物(花生四烯酸)、肾上腺素受体(EPHB2、EPHA4 和 EPHA5)、内皮素受体(EDNRB 和 EDNRA)、核受体(NR2C1、NR2C2 和 NCOA3)、miRNA(miR-193b-3p、miR-215-5p 和 miR-192-

5p)、转录因子(ETS1、CUTL1 和 E2F4)和蛋白(CDK1、WNK1、GSK3B、CRYAB、KAT2B 和 PARP1)[39]。2018 年,Rampogu 等利用计算方法鉴定出 272 种与宫颈癌相关的 miRNA,他们还报道了 3 种 miRNA(miR-548d-5p、miR-5095 和 miR-548c-5p)及多种基因可调节细胞周期,其中有 10 种 miRNA 是高度保守的,包括 miR-133a-3p、miR-215-5p、miR-944、miR-31-3p、miR-548d-5p、miR-11-3p、miR-491-3p、miR-107、miR-133a-5p 和 miR-133b。另一项计算研究发现,在宫颈癌中 miR-21 上调而 miR-29a 下调[40]。另一项计算研究发现,miR-21 在宫颈癌患者中上调[49]。2011 年,Reshmi 等检测到 4 种新的 miRNA,即 Hsa-mir-1273g、Hsa-mir-5095、Hsa-mir-5096 和 Hsa-mir-1273f,这些 miRNA 主要位于宿主基因的启动子区域,如 $SCP2$ 和 $BMP2K$[41]。

(三)长链非编码 RNA

长链非编码 RNA(long noncoding RNA,lncRNA)是功能性 RNA 分子。它们的长度通常长于 200 个核苷酸,缺乏编码蛋白的能力[50]。它们可以调节转录因子活性和染色质结构[51]。最近,He 等利用计算方法鉴定出 4 种与宫颈癌相关的 lncRNA,包括 EPB41L4A-AS1、LINC00649、HCP5 和 SNHG12。这 4 种 lncRNA 主要与液泡转运、细胞周期阻滞和组蛋白修饰相关[43]。另一项研究鉴定出在不同病理阶段表达水平不同的 5 种 lncRNA(GOLGA2P10、ACVR2B-AS1、ATP1A1-AS1、LOH12CR2 和 A2M-AS1),2 种与宫颈癌患者不同种族相关的 lncRNA(FTX 和 MST1P2)、10 种基于肿瘤分期表达的 lncRNA(GOLGA2P5、EMX2OS、FLJ10038、FAM66C、ACVR2B-AS1、AMZ2P1、LINC00341、ZNF876P、MIR9-3HG 和 ILF3-AS1)、4 种基于患者预后评估异常表达的 lncRNA(GOLGA2P5、MIR9-3HG、ILF3-AS1 和 FAM66C),以及 4 种基于 HPV 感染程度不同表达的 lncRNA(LINC00312、MIR9-3HG、SYS1-DBNDD2 和 DDX12P)[44]。2018 年,Zhang 等利用机器学习方法鉴定出 lncRNA NNT-AS1。这些 lncRNA 可通过 Wnt/β-catenin 信号通路启动宫颈癌细胞增殖和侵袭[52]。

(四)环状 RNA

环状 RNA(circular RNA,circRNA)是存在于真核生物中的共价闭环内源性生物分子。其生物合成过程由特定的反式转录因子和顺式作用元件调控。它们高度保守,与多种生物学过程和疾病有关,包括癌症的发生[53]。早期的一些研究表明,circRNA 可以解除 miRNA 的活性,并调控转录过程。也有报道少数 circRNA 可翻译成蛋白质,这暗示 circRNA 可能在不同水平上与基因的表达有关[54]。Yi 等利用计算方法鉴定出 5 种与宫颈癌相关的 circRNA,包括 hsa_circRNA_

103519、hsa_circRNA_101958、hsa_circRNA_000596、hsa_circRNA_400068 和 hsa_circRNA_104315[37]。另一项计算研究鉴定出 7 种与宫颈癌相关的 circRNA，包括 hsa_circ_0031027、hsa_circ_0070190、hsa_circ_0084927、hsa_circ_0043280、hsa_circ_0000745、hsa_circ_0065898 和 hsa_circ_0000077[45]。这些已鉴定的分子，尤其是蛋白质，也被确定为抗宫颈癌的最佳药物。

三、药物鉴定

2018 年，Rampogu 等采用"药理引导的分子建模方法"，鉴定出 51 种化合物，这些化合物可在 HeLa 细胞中剂量依赖性地下调 $NOS2$、$PP2B$ 和 $IL-6$ 基因，并且在宫颈癌中与凋亡基因 caspase-3、Bax 和 Bcl2 的表达有关[42]。其他一些计算研究发现，莱索克里巴丁 7 (lissoclibadin 7)、莱托酸Ⅱ (litospermic Ⅱ acid) 和柚皮素 3-鼠李糖苷 (kaempferol 3-ramnoglucoside) 分别与 3 种宫颈癌相关蛋白 HDAC4、HDAC5 和 HDAC10 具有较好的结合亲和力[55]。Ricci-López 等发现了 3 种针对 HPV E6 蛋白的潜在药物，分别是 ZINC111606147、ZINC96096545 和 ZINC362643639[56]。Ramnath 等报道了松脂酸可能是一种治疗宫颈癌和阿尔茨海默病的潜在药物[57]。本芘醇与半合酶 caspase 3 的结合亲和力低于喜树碱 (camptothecin)，低于表没食子儿茶素 (epigallocatechin)，低于槲皮素 (quercetin)[58]；西瑞香素 (daphnoretin)[59] 和 ZINC14761180[60] 也被报道对 E6 蛋白具有最佳抑制活性。巴西莱因 (Brazilein) 对 p53 和半胱酶 caspase9 的结合亲和力更好[61]。查尔酮 3 (Chalcone 3) 对 HeLa 细胞系具有更好的细胞毒性效果[62]。另一种药物 5-{(1-[(1-苯基-1H-1,2,3-三唑-4-基) 甲基]-1H-吲哚-3-基) 亚甲基} 嘧啶-2,4,6-(1H,3H,5H) 三酮衍生物 (5e) 也表现出更好的抗癌特性[63]。因此，计算方法可用于鉴定与宫颈癌相关的生物标志物和药物。

四、结论

综上所述，宫颈癌是女性最致命的癌症之一。尽管放疗、手术和激素治疗被广泛用于宫颈癌的治疗，患者的存活率仍然较低。近年来，高通量测序技术的进步使癌症的早期检测和预防成为可能。然而，这些技术产生了大量数据，需要研究者开发出强大的计算方法以更全面地分析这些大数据。这些计算方法为人们提供了一种独特的方式，让人们能在短时间内利用公开的基因组和蛋白质组数据集，以较低的成本找出关键基因和药物。迄今为止，仅有少数研究使用这些计算方法鉴定出了许多与宫颈癌相关的基因、miRNA 和蛋白质，它们可作为开发抗宫颈癌药物的生物标志物。因此,开发更强大的软件/算法并分析宫颈癌数据集仍有很大空间。预计在不久的将来,本章所提供的信息将对癌症生物学家和免疫学家在治疗宫颈癌方面提供极大的帮助。

利益冲突

无。

参 考 文 献

[1] Siegel RL, Miller KD, Jemal A. Cancer statistics, 2019. CA Cancer J Clin 2019;69:7-34. https://doi.org/10.3322/caac.21551.

[2] Lin M, Ye M, Zhou J, Wang ZP, Zhu X. Recent advances on the molecular mechanism of cervical carcinogenesis based on systems biology technologies. Comput Struct Biotechnol J 2019;17:241-50. https://doi.org/10.1016/j.csbj.2019.02.001.

[3] Bray F, Ferlay J, Soerjomataram I, Siegel RL, Torre LA, Jemal A. Global cancer statistics 2018: GLOBOCAN estimates of incidence and mortality worldwide for 36 cancers in 185 countries. CA Cancer J Clin 2018;68:394-424. https://doi.org/10.3322/caac.21492.

[4] Sreedevi A, Javed R, Dinesh A. Epidemiology of cervical cancer with special focus on India. Int J Womens Health 2015;7:405-14. https://doi.org/10.2147/IJWH.S50001.

[5] Šarenac T, Mikov M. Cervical cancer, different treatments and importance of bile acids as therapeutic agents in this disease. Front Pharmacol 2019;10: https://doi.org/10.3389/fphar.2019.00484.

[6] Chan CK, Aimagambetova G, Ukybassova T, Kongrtay K, Azizan A. Human papillomavirus infection and cervical cancer: epidemiology, screening, and vaccination—review of current perspectives. J Oncol 2019; https://doi.org/10.1155/2019/3257939.

[7] Wang SS, Bratti MC, Rodríguez AC, Herrero R, Burk RD, Porras C, et al. Common variants in immune and DNA repair genes and risk for human papillomavirus persistence and progression to cervical cancer. J Infect Dis 2009;199:20-30. https://doi.org/10.1086/595563.

[8] Klug SJ, Ressing M, Koenig J, Abba MC, Agorastos T, Brenna SM, et al. TP53 codon 72 polymorphism and cervical cancer: a pooled analysis of individual data from 49 studies. Lancet Oncol 2009;10:772-84. https://doi.org/10.1016/S1470-2045(09)70187-1.

[9] Mehta AM, Jordanova ES, van Wezel T, Uh H-W, Corver WE, Kwappenberg KMC, et al. Genetic variation of antigen processing machinery components and association with cervical carcinoma. Genes Chromosomes Cancer 2007;46:577-86. https://doi.org/10.1002/gcc.20441.

[10] Rafnar T, Sulem P, Stacey SN, Geller F, Gudmundsson J, Sigurdsson A, et al. Sequence

variants at the TERT-CLPTM1L locus associate with many cancer types. Nat Genet 2009; 41:221-7. https://doi.org/10.1038/ng.296.

[11] Hardikar S, Johnson LG, Malkki M, Petersdorf EW, Galloway DA, Schwartz SM, et al. A population-based case-control study of genetic variation in cytokine genes associated with risk of cervical and vulvar cancers. Gynecol Oncol 2015;139:90-6. https://doi.org/10.1016/j.ygyno.2015.07.110.

[12] Leo PJ, Madeleine MM, Wang S, Schwartz SM, Newell F, Pettersson-Kymmer U, et al. Defining the genetic susceptibility to cervical neoplasia—a genome-wide association study. PLoS Genet 2017;13: https://doi.org/10.1371/journal.pgen.1006866.

[13] Takeuchi F, Kukimoto I, Li Z, Li S, Li N, Hu Z, et al. Genome-wide association study of cervical cancer suggests a role for ARRDC3 gene in human papillomavirus infection. Hum Mol Genet 2019;28:341-8. https://doi.org/10.1093/hmg/ddy390.

[14] Lehoux M, D'Abramo CM, Archambault J. Molecular mechanisms of human papillomavirus-induced carcinogenesis. Public Health Genomics 2009; 12: 268-80. https://doi.org/10.1159/000214918.

[15] Burk RD, Harari A, Chen Z. Human papillomavirus genome variants. Virology 2013; 445:232-43. https://doi.org/10.1016/j.virol.2013.07.018.

[16] Skinner SR, Wheeler CM, Romanowski B, Castellsagué X, Lazcano-Ponce E, Rosario-Raymundo MRD, et al. Progression of HPV infection to detectable cervical lesions or clearance in adult women: analysis of the control arm of the VIVIANE study. Int J Cancer 2016;138:2428-38. https://doi.org/10.1002/ijc.29971.

[17] Mirabello L, Clarke MA, Nelson CW, Dean M, Wentzensen N, Yeager M, et al. The intersection of HPV epidemiology. Genomics and mechanistic studies of HPV-mediated carcinogenesis. Viruses 2018;10:80. https://doi.org/10.3390/v10020080.

[18] Cheng L, Guo Y, Zhan S, Xia P. Association between HLA-DP gene polymorphisms and cervical cancer risk: a meta-analysis. Biomed Res Int 2018; https://doi.org/10.1155/2018/7301595.

[19] Pan F, Tian J, Ji C-S, He Y-F, Han X-H, Wang Y, et al. Association of TNF-α-308 and-238 polymorphisms with risk of cervical cancer: a meta-analysis. Asian Pac J Cancer Prev 2012;13:5777-83. https://doi.org/10.7314/apjcp.2012.13.11.5777.

[20] Martínez-Nava GA, Fernández-Niño JA, Madrid-Marina V, Torres-Poveda K. Cervical cancer genetic susceptibility: a systematic review and meta-analyses of recent evidence. PLoS One 2016;11: https://doi.org/10.1371/journal.pone.0157344.

[21] Gupta MK, Sarojamma V, Reddy MR, Shaik JB, Vadde R. Computational biology: toward early detection of pancreatic cancer. Crit Rev Oncog 2019;24: https://doi.org/10.1615/CritRevOncog.2019031335.

[22] Gupta MK, Donde R, Gouda G, Vadde R, Behera L. De novo assembly and characterization of transcriptome towards understanding molecular mechanism associated with

MYMIV-resistance in Vigna mungo-a computational study. BioRxiv 2019; 844639: https://doi.org/10.1101/844639.

[23] Gupta MK, Vadde R. Insights into the structure-function relationship of both wild and mutant zinc transporter ZnT8 in human: a computational structural biology approach. J Biomol Struct Dyn 2019;1-22. https://doi.org/10.1080/07391102.2019.1567391.

[24] Gupta MK, Vadde R. In silico identification of natural product inhibitors for γ-secretase activating protein, a therapeutic target for Alzheimer's disease. J Cell Biochem 2018; https://doi.org/10.1002/jcb.28316.

[25] Gupta MK, Behara SK, Vadde R. In silico analysis of differential gene expressions in biliary stricture and hepatic carcinoma. Gene 2017;597:49-58.

[26] Gupta MK, Behera SK, Dehury B, Mahapatra N. Identification and characterization of differentially expressed genes from human microglial cell samples infected with Japanese encephalitis virus. J Vector Borne Dis 2017;54:131-8.

[27] Gupta MK, Vadde R. Identification and characterization of differentially expressed genes in type 2 diabetes using in silico approach. Comput Biol Chem 2019; https://doi.org/10.1016/j.compbiolchem.2019.01.010.

[28] Gupta MK, Vadde R, Donde R, Gouda G, Kumar J, Nayak S, et al. Insights into the structure-function relationship of brown plant hopper resistance protein, Bph14 of rice plant: a computational structural biology approach. J Biomol Struct Dyn 2018;1-17. https://doi.org/10.1080/07391102.2018.1462737.

[29] Donde R, Gupta MK, Gouda G, Kumar J, Vadde R, Sahoo KK, et al. Computational characterization of structural and functional roles of DREB1A, DREB1B and DREB1C in enhancing cold tolerance in rice plant. Amino Acids 2019;51:839-53. https://doi.org/10.1007/s00726-019-02727-0.

[30] Gupta MK, Vadde R, Gouda G, Donde R, Kumar J, Behera L. Computational approach to understand molecular mechanism involved in BPH resistance in Bt-rice plant. J Mol Graph Model 2019;88:209-20. https://doi.org/10.1016/j.jmgm.2019.01.018.

[31] Zhang Y-X, Zhao Y-L. Pathogenic network analysis predicts candidate genes for cervical cancer. Comput Math Methods Med 2016; https://doi.org/10.1155/2016/3186051.

[32] Tan MS, Chang S-W, Cheah PL, Yap HJ. Integrative machine learning analysis of multiple gene expression profiles in cervical cancer. Peer J 2018;6:e5285 https://doi.org/10.7717/peerj.5285.

[33] Wu X, Peng L, Zhang Y, Chen S, Lei Q, Li G, et al. Identification of key genes and pathways in cervical cancer by bioinformatics analysis. Int J Med Sci 2019;16:800-12. https://doi.org/10.7150/ijms.34172.

[34] Li X, Tian R, Gao H, Yan F, Ying L, Yang Y, et al. Identification of significant gene signatures and prognostic biomarkers for patients with cervical cancer by integrated bioinformatic methods. Technol Cancer Res Treat 2018; https://doi.org/10.1177/1533033818767455.

[35] Xie F, Dong D, Du N, Guo L, Ni W, Yuan H, et al. An 8-gene signature predicts the prognosis of cervical cancer following radiotherapy. Mol Med Rep 2019;20:2990-3002. https://doi.org/10.3892/mmr.2019.10535.

[36] Hindumathi V, Kranthi T, Rao SB, Manimaran P. The prediction of candidate genes for cervix related cancer through gene ontology and graph theoretical approach. Mol Biosyst 2014;10:1450-60. https://doi.org/10.1039/C4MB00004H.

[37] Yi Y, Liu Y, Wu W, Wu K, Zhang W. Reconstruction and analysis of circRNA-miRNA-mRNA network in the pathology of cervical cancer. Oncol Rep 2019;41:2209-25. https://doi.org/10.3892/or.2019.7028.

[38] Liu H, Liu L, Zhu H. The role of significantly deregulated microRNAs in recurrent cervical cancer based on bioinformatic analysis of the cancer genome atlas data. J Comput Biol 2019;26:387-95. https://doi.org/10.1089/cmb.2018.0241.

[39] Kori M, Arga KY. Potential biomarkers and therapeutic targets in cervical cancer: insights from the meta-analysis of transcriptomics data within network biomedicine perspective. PLoS One 2018;13: e0200717 https://doi.org/10.1371/journal.pone.0200717.

[40] Pardini B, De Maria D, Francavilla A, Di Gaetano C, Ronco G, Naccarati A. MicroRNAs as markers of progression in cervical cancer: a systematic review. BMC Cancer 2018;18:696. https://doi.org/10.1186/s12885-018-4590-4.

[41] Reshmi G, Chandra SSV, Babu VJM, Babu PSS, Santhi WS, Ramachandran S, et al. Identification and analysis of novel microRNAs from fragile sites of human cervical cancer: computational and experimental approach. Genomics 2011;97:333-40. https://doi.org/10.1016/j.ygeno.2011.02.010.

[42] Rampogu S, Ravinder D, Pawar SC, Lee KW. Natural compound modulates the cervical cancer microenvironment—a pharmacophore guided molecular modelling approaches. J Clin Med 2018;7: https://doi.org/10.3390/jcm7120551.

[43] He M, Lin Y, Xu Y. Identification of prognostic biomarkers in colorectal cancer using a long non-coding RNA-mediated competitive endogenous RNA network. Oncol Lett 2019;17:2687-94. https://doi.org/10.3892/ol.2019.9936.

[44] Wu W-J, Shen Y, Sui J, Li C-Y, Yang S, Xu S-Y, et al. Integrated analysis of long non-coding RNA competing interactions revealed potential biomarkers in cervical cancer: based on a public database. Mol Med Rep 2018;17:7845-58. https://doi.org/10.3892/mmr.2018.8846.

[45] Gong J, Jiang H, Shu C, Hu M, Huang Y, Liu Q, et al. Integrated analysis of circular RNA-associated ceRNA network in cervical cancer: observational study. Medicine (Baltimore) 2019;98:e16922 https://doi.org/10.1097/MD.0000000000016922.

[46] Cheng J, Lu X, Wang J, Zhang H, Duan P, Li C. Interactome analysis of gene expression profiles of cervical cancer reveals dysregulated mitotic gene clusters. Am J Transl Res 2017;9:3048-59.

[47] Deng S-P, Zhu L, Huang D-S. Predicting hub genes associated with cervical cancer through gene co-expression networks. IEEE/ACM Trans Comput Biol Bioinform 2016;13: 27-35. https://doi.org/10.1109/TCBB.2015.2476790.

[48] Guerrero Flórez M, Guerrero Gómez OA, Mena Huertas J, Yepez Chamorro MC. Mapping of micro-RNAs related to cervical cancer in Latin American human genomic variants. F1000Research 2018;6:946. https://doi.org/10.12688/f1000research.10138.2.

[49] Liolios T, Kastora SL, Colombo G. MicroRNAs in female malignancies. Cancer Inform 2019;18: https://doi.org/10.1177/1176935119828746 1176935119828746.

[50] Cao H, Wahlestedt C, Kapranov P. Strategies to annotate and characterize long noncoding RNAs: advantages and pitfalls. Trends Genet 2018;34:704-21. https://doi.org/10.1016/j.tig.2018.06.002.

[51] Guglas K, Bogaczyńska M, Kolenda T, Ryś M, Teresiak A, Bliźniak R, et al. lncRNA in HNSCC: challenges and potential. Contemp Oncol 2017;21:259-66. https://doi.org/10.5114/wo.2017.72382.

[52] Zhang X, Wang J, Li J, Chen W, Liu C. CRlncRC: a machine learning-based method for cancer-related long noncoding RNA identification using integrated features. BMC Med Genomics 2018;11:120. https://doi.org/10.1186/s12920-018-0436-9.

[53] Kristensen LS, Andersen MS, Stagsted LVW, Ebbesen KK, Hansen TB, Kjems J. The biogenesis, biology and characterization of circular RNAs. Nat Rev Genet 2019;20:675-91. https://doi.org/10.1038/s41576-019-0158-7.

[54] Bach D-H, Lee SK, Sood AK. Circular RNAs in cancer. Mol Ther Nucleic Acids 2019;16:118-29. https://doi.org/10.1016/j.omtn.2019.02.005.

[55] Tambunan USF, Parikesit AA, Nasution MAF, Hapsari A, Kerami D. Exposing the molecular screening method of Indonesian natural products derivate as drug candidates for cervical cancer. Iran J Pharm Res 2017;16:1113-27.

[56] Ricci-López J, Vidal-Limon A, Zunñiga M, Jimènez VA, Alderete JB, Brizuela CA, et al. Molecular modeling simulation studies reveal new potential inhibitors against HPV E6 protein. PLoS One 2019;14:e0213028 https://doi.org/10.1371/journal.pone.0213028.

[57] Ramnath MG, Thirugnanasampandan R, NagaSundaram N, Bhuvaneswari G. Molecular docking and dynamic simulation studies of terpenoids of I. wightii (Bentham) H. Hara against acetylcholinesterase and histone deacetylase3 receptors. Curr Comput Aided Drug Des 2018;14:234-45. https://doi.org/10.2174/1573409914666180321111925.

[58] Ashwini S, Varkey SP, Shantaram M. In silico docking of polyphenolic compounds against caspase 3-HeLa cell line protein. Int J Drug Dev Res 2017;9:28-32.

[59] Mamgain S, Sharma P, Pathak RK, Baunthiyal M. Computer aided screening of natural compounds targeting the E6 protein of HPV using molecular docking. Bioinformation 2015;11:236. https://doi.org/10.6026/97320630011236.

[60] Kumar A, Rathi E, Kini SG. E-pharmacophore modelling, virtual screening, molecular

dynamics simulations and in-silico ADME analysis for identification of potential E6 inhibitors against cervical cancer. J Mol Struct 2019; 1189: 299-306. https://doi.org/10.1016/j.molstruc.2019.04.023.

[61] Laksmiani NPL, Astuti NMW, Arisanti CIS, Paramita NLPV. Ethyl acetate fraction of secang as anti cervical cancer by inducing p53 and caspase 9. IOP Conf Ser Earth Environ Sci 2018;207:012065. https://doi.org/10.1088/1755-1315/207/1/012065.

[62] Tantawy MA, Sroor FM, Mohamed MF, El-Naggar ME, Saleh FM, Hassaneen HM, et al. Molecular docking study, cytotoxicity, cell cycle arrest and apoptotic induction of novel chalcones incorporating thiadiazolyl isoquinoline in cervical cancer. Anticancer Agents Med Chem 2019; https://doi.org/10.2174/1871520619666191024121116.

[63] Kumar A, Sathish Kumar B, Sreenivas E, Subbaiah T. Synthesis, biological evaluation, and molecular docking studies of novel 1,2,3-triazole tagged 5-[(1H-Indol-3-yl)methylene] pyrimidine-2,4,6(1H,3H,5H)trione derivatives. Russ J Gen Chem 2018;88:587-95. https://doi.org/10.1134/S1070363218030313.

第 12 章
宫颈癌代谢：代谢途径和细胞能量产生的主要重编程

K. Vijaya Rachel, Nagarjuna Sivaraj

Department of Biochemistry and Bioinformatics, GITAM Deemed to be University, Visakhapatnam, Andhra Pradesh, India

摘要

肿瘤细胞生物能量学的重要变化主要包括糖酵解增强、谷氨酰胺分解通量增加、氨基酸上调和脂质代谢、线粒体生物合成出现、磷酸戊糖途径（pentose phosphate pathway，PPP）的激活，以及大分子的生物合成等。也有研究发现，宫颈癌（cervical cancer，CC）细胞对细胞代谢途径进行了重编程。己糖激酶 2 表达的增加为癌细胞的生长提供了代谢物，为三羧酸提供了中间体，在葡萄糖缺乏时协助自噬，并与电压依赖性阴离子通道相结合，使癌细胞受益。研究发现，人乳头状瘤病毒（human papillomavirus，HPV）E6/E7 可靶向激活雷帕霉素蛋白激酶 B 等相关致癌信号通路，并可抑制 p53 和 pRb 等抑癌通路，这表明 HPV E6/E7 可调节宫颈癌细胞葡萄糖的分解。癌细胞代谢的变化与癌基因（c-Myc）和转录因子（缺氧诱导因子 1a）的过度表达有关。目前正在研究 6-磷酸甘油醛脱氢酶的表达和 PPP 活性与 c-MET 磷酸化的关系。此外，已知在某些条件下，宫颈癌细胞可以产生脂蛋白 A。代谢重编程也有助于治疗干预。对于宫颈癌和其他癌症而言，最大标准化摄取值与淋巴结分级、癌症分期和肿瘤大小一样，都是重要的预后指标。

关键词

宫颈癌，己糖激酶 2，HPV E6/E7，磷酸戊糖途径，脂蛋白 A，SUV_{max}。

缩略词

5-FU	氟尿嘧啶
ADC	表观扩散系数
ADP	二磷酸腺苷
ATP	三磷酸腺苷
CC	宫颈癌

G. P. Nagaraju, R. R. Malla (eds.)
A Theranostic and Precision Medicine Approach for Female-Specific Cancers
ISBN 978-0-12-822009-2
https://doi.org/10.1016/B978-0-12-822009-2.00012-1

© 2021 Elsevier Inc.
All rights reserved.

c-Myc	细胞质原癌基因调节器
DWI	弥散加权成像
HGF	肝细胞生长因子
HPV	人乳头状瘤病毒
IL-2	白介素-2
LPA	脂蛋白 A
MCF7	密歇根癌症基金会-7
Met	二甲双胍
MRS	磁共振波谱学
NADPH	烟酰胺腺嘌呤二核苷酸磷酸氢
p53	肿瘤蛋白 53
PMA	12-棕榈酸 13-醋酸酯
PPP	磷酸戊糖途径
pRB	视网膜母细胞瘤蛋白
SUV_{max}	最大标准摄取值
TCA	三羧酸循环
VDAC	电压依赖性阳离子通道

一、概述

宫颈癌(cervical cancer,CC)是女性特有的一种癌症[1],与其他癌症一样,CC 也是子宫颈或任何终末器官细胞无限增殖的结果[2]。据报道,2018 年共有近 57 万例 CC 患者,其中 31.1 万例患者不幸去世。CC 是女性第四大最常见的癌症,仅次于乳腺癌、结直肠癌和肺癌(分别有 210 万例、80 万例和 70 万例)。在全球范围内,CC 的年龄标准化发病率在每 10 万名女性中为 13.1 例;而在西部、东部、中部和南非国家,CC 是导致女性死亡的主要原因。约有 6.5% 的女性在 75 岁之前会被诊断出患有 CC。据估计,发病率最高的国家是斯威士兰。中国和印度共占全球 CC 发病率的 1/3 以上,分别有近 10.6 万例和 9.7 万例 CC 患者,并分别导致 4.8 万人和 6 万人死亡。在全球范围内,CC 患者的平均诊断年龄为 53 岁,平均诊断年龄最小的是瓦努阿图(44 岁),最大的是新加坡(68 岁)。对于 CC 的平均死亡年龄而言,全球平均为 59 岁,最小的是瓦努阿图(45 岁),最大的是马提尼克岛(76 岁)。在对 185 个国家进行的评估中发现,146 个国家(79%)的女性罹患宫颈癌的年龄小于 45 岁[3]。在全球范围内,CC 是女性中第三高发病率的癌症。据 2008 年的数据显示,有 275 000 人死于 CC,其中 88% 发生在发展中国家,仅在亚洲就有

159 800人[4]。尽管筛查和疫苗接种的普及已使宫颈癌的发病率逐步下降，但在包括印度在内的发展中国家，宫颈癌仍然具有巨大的影响[5]。大多数CC由人乳头状瘤病毒（human papillomavirus，HPV）引起，其他危险因素包括多个性伴侣、长期服用避孕药和吸烟等[6]。癌症是一种与许多因素相关的多因素疾病。癌细胞对能量代谢进行了重编程，导致能量介质升高，从而使细胞增长，有利于细胞的存活、转移、迁移，以及抵抗化疗和放疗[7-9]。肿瘤细胞生物能的一些重要变化，其中包括糖酵解增强、谷氨酰胺分解通量增加、氨基酸上调和脂质代谢、线粒体生物合成出现、磷酸戊糖途径（pentose phosphate pathway，PPP）的激活，以及大分子的生物合成[1-9]。

二、糖酵解

即使有了HPV疫苗，宫颈癌仍是世界范围内女性死亡的主要原因。目前，用于化疗的细胞抑制药物主要是顺铂[顺式二氯二胺铂（Ⅱ）]。尽管顺铂特异性较差且对患者具有明显毒性，但其仍是目前较为常用的治疗方法[10]。有氧糖酵解是癌细胞特有的代谢过程。

早在20世纪70年代，就有研究报道了宫颈癌细胞具有活性，并且与正常宫颈上皮相比，已糖激酶2的表达量有所增加。最近的免疫组化分析显示，正常宫颈组织的已糖激酶2信号很低或没有信号，而近60%的CC标本（$n=197$）中已糖激酶2染色呈阳性（译者注：原文未标明197个样本的出处）。已糖激酶2的过度表达可能与临床相关，因为许多实体瘤的不良预后都与其表达增加有关。研究发现，高水平的已糖激酶2与放射治疗的耐受性有关，这与糖酵解增强可使癌细胞产生放射耐受性的观点一致。鉴于已糖激酶2在许多肿瘤中的高表达，以及其潜在的促肿瘤作用，已糖激酶2被认为是癌症治疗的一个新靶点。

一些研究表明，癌细胞可以通过不同方式从已糖激酶2的表达增加中获益。在有氧状态下，已糖激酶2可以为肿瘤细胞生长提供能量和必要的代谢物。此外，已糖激酶2还参与提供三羧酸（tricarboxylic acid，TCA）循环的中间产物，利用谷氨酰胺衍生的碳，在葡萄糖缺乏情况下，已糖激酶2通过协助细胞自噬来维持细胞能量稳态。此外，已糖激酶2能够与电压依赖性阴离子通道（voltage-dependent anion channel，VDAC）结合，VDAC是一种位于线粒体外膜上的成孔膜蛋白。VDAC与已糖激酶2的相互作用至关重要，因为它将糖酵解与氧化磷酸化结合在一起。此外，已糖激酶2与VDAC的相互作用可阻止以线粒体外膜为目标的促凋亡蛋白，进而干扰线粒体通透性转换孔的形成，抑制细胞凋亡。近期报道证实，E6/E7有可能刺激已糖激酶2的表达，这为HPV致癌基因与癌细胞中负责代谢重编程和抵抗凋亡的关键细胞酶的表达之间提供了直接联系。这种情况伴随着治疗敏感性的降低和致癌能力的增强[11]。

癌细胞新陈代谢的变化与癌基因(c-myc)和转录因子(低氧诱导因子1a)的过度表达有关,它们有助于使癌细胞远离活性氧诱导的细胞凋亡。有多项研究探讨了二甲双胍(metformin,Met)对宫颈转移性肿瘤细胞代谢的影响。这些研究通过调节癌基因及其下游蛋白的表达,记录了二甲双胍通过抑制糖酵解表型而诱使暴发性CC细胞凋亡的过程。在这些研究中,Met同步了线粒体代谢,特别是通过在TCA循环中补充$C_3H_4O_3$(酮酸丙酮酸)和$C_5H_{10}N_2O_3$-谷氨酰胺。当Met靶向肿瘤细胞的上皮细胞和间充质细胞标志物时,会增加CC细胞的持久性特征[12-14]。

三、磷酸戊糖途径

合成代谢所需的代谢物主要由PPP供应,且与糖酵解和其他代谢途径相关联。因此,PPP在肿瘤细胞生成过程中具有明确的作用[15]。PPP利用葡萄糖-6-磷酸作为该途径的序列氧化和非氧化环节的底物。氧化型PPP会产生核酮糖-5-磷酸,每利用一分子葡萄糖-6-磷酸,产生1个CO_2、3个质子和2个烟酰胺腺嘌呤二核苷酸磷酸氢(nicotinamide adenine dinucleotide phosphate hydrogen,NADPH),二氧化碳和质子有助于肿瘤酸化[16-18],而NADPH是谷胱甘肽过氧化物酶和脂肪酸合成所必需的辅助因子。在PPP的非氧化环节中,核酮糖-5-磷酸被用于合成核酸。许多研究人员已经发现,PPP促使肿瘤细胞的生长脱离监视[19,20]。糖酵解和PPP的联系由丙酮酸激酶M界定,丙酮酸激酶M是糖酵解途径中的一种酶,它可将磷酸烯醇丙酮酸和二磷酸腺苷转化为丙酮酸和三磷酸腺苷。肿瘤细胞主要表达通过交替剪接所产生的丙酮酸激酶肌同工酶M2,而分化细胞主要表达丙酮酸激酶肌同工酶M1。特定核糖核蛋白的表达受丙酮酸激酶肌同工酶和丙酮酸激酶肌同工酶2的诱导,而后者分别受HIF1和c-Myc的调控[21]。虽然现在已对PPP与失巢凋亡(译者注:一种特殊的细胞程序死亡,由于细胞与细胞外基质或相邻细胞脱离接触而诱发)的冲突有很好的理解,但其如何影响肿瘤细胞的迁移和侵袭,直到最近才得以充分证实。一些研究结果表明,静默PPP的第3种酶是6-磷酸葡萄糖酸脱氢酶,其能够减少肺癌细胞在肝细胞生长因子(hepatocyte growth factor,HGF)刺激下的体外转移[22]。这种现象背后的机制是酪氨酸磷酸化减少,以及HGF受体c-MET的激活,其分子机制目前仍有待确认,需要进一步研究6-磷酸甘油醛脱氢酶的表达和PPP活性与c-MET磷酸化之间的关联。

四、脂肪酸氧化

Shen 等的研究表明[22]，在特定条件下，卵巢癌细胞和宫颈癌细胞能够产生脂蛋白 A(lipoprotein A，LPA)，并且证实了恶性肿瘤细胞的 LPA 分泌[23]。实验数据显示，卵巢癌细胞会分泌 LPA，而乳腺癌[(转移性乳腺癌安德森和密歇根癌症基金会(Michigan Cancer Foundation-7，MCF7)]和白血病(Jurkat 和 K562)细胞不会分泌 LPA。通过抑制剂研究发现，胞质磷脂酶 A2 或非 Ca^{2+} 依赖性的磷脂酶 A2 在宫颈癌和卵巢癌中会升高，但并没有参与调节肿瘤细胞分泌 LPA 可能相关联的分泌型磷脂酶 A。在不同条件下，白血病和乳腺癌细胞可能会向培养基中分泌 LPA。另一项研究指出，白血病细胞和乳腺细胞不分泌 LPA 并不是因为这些细胞对佛波肉豆蔻醋酸(phorbol 12-myristate 13-acetate，PMA)(译者注：一种广泛用于体内外实验的佛波酯类 PKC 激活剂，PMA 可抑制 Fas 诱导的细胞凋亡，同时又可诱导 HL-60 细胞的凋亡发生。并且 PMA 是一种强效的肿瘤促进剂，能够诱导小鼠皮肤瘤生成)不敏感。例如，Jurkat 细胞在 PMA 刺激下会增殖并产生白介素-2(interleukin-2，IL-2)[24]，而 K562 细胞在 PMA 刺激下会发生分化[25,26]。此外，PMA 还能促进 MCF7 细胞中芳香化酶的活性[27]。也有研究表明，在 231 个细胞中，PMA 可以促进前列腺素 E2 的产生、抑制细胞生长，并在细胞中激发芳香化酶的作用[28,29]。然而，导致这些差异的刺激因素仍然未知。体外研究表明，各种恶性细胞展现出相似的特异性，并且血浆 LPA 的计量结果也证实了这一点[30]。研究结果表明，卵巢上皮细胞的癌变可能是卵巢癌患者检测到高 LPA 水平的重要基础[31]。据报道，一旦生长因子耗尽，卵巢癌细胞体外分泌 LPA 的现象会停止。生长因子、细胞因子、转化生长因子 β、表皮生长因子、两性胰岛素、胰岛素样生长因子、IL-1、碱性成纤维细胞生长因子和肿瘤坏死因子 α 等因子都可作为体外触发器，引发细胞系中磷脂酶 2 的作用[32-34]，而卵巢癌细胞在生理和病理情况下也不例外[35-37]。目前，研究人员正在对卵巢癌细胞受到的各种生理刺激下产生 LPA 的分类进行研究。在病理和生理条件下的研究中，动物模型对于支持肿瘤组织/原发肿瘤培养分泌的血浆 LPA 升高的来源至关重要(图 12-1)。

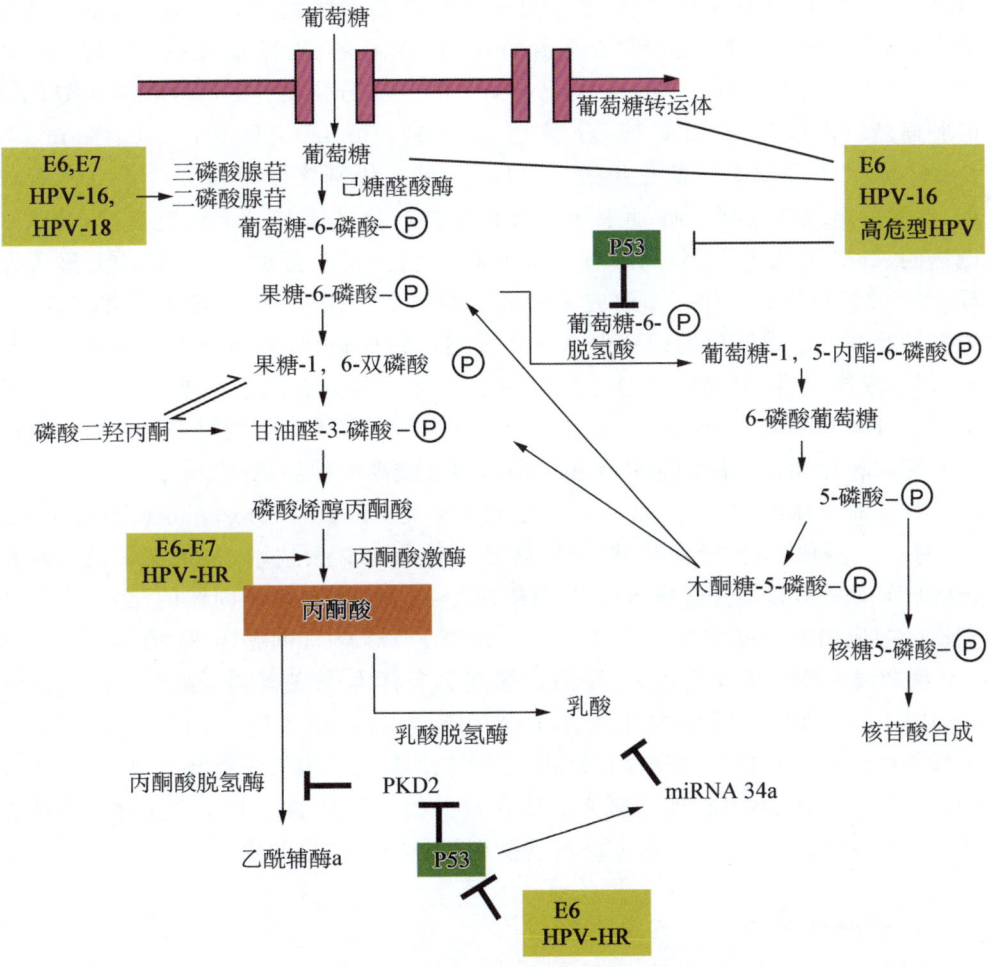

图 12-1 宫颈癌中的代谢重编程

注：HPV. 人乳头瘤病毒；miRNA. 微 RNA。

五、癌症代谢和诊断成像

(一) 磁共振成像与磁共振波谱成像的结合

宫颈恶性组织显示扩散受限，与正常组织对比，表现出较低的表观弥散系数（apparent diffusion coefficient，ADC）数值。弥散加权成像（diffusion-weighted imaging，DWI）和 ADC 图对宫颈的良恶性区域识别具有很高的敏感度和特异度。

研究表明,ADC 值有助于区分宫颈组织的不同类型和级别[38]。Payne 团队在其研究中发现,正常宫颈组织和宫颈癌的 ADC 值存在显著差异(分别为 1.7×10^{-3} mm^2/s 和 1.1×10^{-3} mm^2/s;$P < 0.001$)[39]。分化良好的肿瘤相对于分化差的肿瘤显示出较高的 ADC 值(分别为 1.2×10^{-3} mm^2/s 和 1.1×10^{-3} mm^2/s;$P = 0.01$)。其他研究团队也报道了 ADC 与肿瘤级别之间的相关性[40]。尽管如此,在区分组织学亚型方面,此种差异性仍然是经验之谈[41]。有研究发现,鳞状细胞癌的 ADC 值低于腺癌;另一项研究则称不同组织学亚型之间 ADC 无显著差异[42]。此领域仍需要进一步研究来验证这些结果。此外,已有信息表明,DWI 在原发肿瘤和淋巴结转移的识别中具有高敏感性和准确性,其性能优于或者至少与 T2 加权成像相当,但尚未经过系统评估。尽管大部分着眼于早期肿瘤成像的研究,其 ADC 值为 $0.86 \times 10^{-3} \sim 1.38 \times 10^{-3}$ mm^2/s,但大范围的浸润性肿瘤很可能因肿瘤内坏死和相应的细胞外体积增加而伴有较高的平均 ADC 值。

目前对于体内和/或高磁场离体磁共振波谱(magnetic resonance spectroscopy,MRS)/魔角旋转[译者注:魔角旋转是一种核磁共振技术,包括交叉极化魔角旋转(CP-MAS)和高分辨魔角旋转(HR-MAS)2 项,主要用于固体的测定]在宫颈癌诊断中应用的研究较少。Delikatny[43]评估了 159 例宫颈癌样本(40 例浸润性和 119 例非浸润性),结果显示,在浸润性癌症患者样本中观察到了高分辨率的脂质峰(1.3 ppm),而未浸润的样本中几乎没有脂质谱,但在 3.8~4.2 ppm 之间有一个较强的未被解析的共振谱段。Mahon 及其团队[44,45]用组织病理学评估了 MRS 和相关离体光谱的性能,他们研究了体内重要的同相甘油三酯在恶性肿瘤诊断方面的潜在应用。然而,该分析有时可能受到相外脂质信号的限制。

(二)治疗意义

根据 Kidd 等的研究[45],一般生存期是宫颈癌的关键终点策略。通常肿瘤分期被用作一般生存期的预测指标。最新研究证实,CC 中淋巴结的受累是一种可靠的预后因素,可显示癌症处于 Ⅱ 期。其他研究显示,最大标准化摄取值(SUV_{max})作为持久性而非肿瘤分期的额外预后指标。一项研究使用 SUV_{max} 将患者分为 3 个不同的预后组,结果表明,对于宫颈癌和其他癌症,SUV_{max} 是比淋巴结分级、癌症分期或肿瘤大小更重要的预后结果,而原发性肿瘤的 SUV_{max} 在预测早期标准的结果方面有所提高。这一标准有助于将 SUV_{max} 描述为预测性的反应衡量指标。在补充研究内容时,建议根据 SUV_{max} 对患者预后进行分组分析。SUV_{max} 可作为一种定量的生物标志物,在开始治疗前预测标志物对特定患者的影响。因此,原发性肿瘤 SUV_{max} 可作为对 CC 治疗反应性的可测量生物标志物。

(三)抑制 E6/E7 介导的糖酵解可使 5-FU 耐受的细胞增敏

大多数证据表明,癌细胞依赖无氧糖酵解作为能量来源和其他代谢中间产物来促进肿瘤发展[46-49]。研究发现,乳酸脱氢酶活性的增强与细胞葡萄糖代谢的变化和宫颈癌的发生有关[50]。其他研究发现,HPV E6/E7 能激活雷帕霉素相关途径的蛋白激酶 B 机制靶点等致癌信号[51],并使 p53 和 pRb 的肿瘤抑制途径失效[52]。这些证据表明,HPV E6/E7 可能参与调节 CC 的细胞葡萄糖代谢。研究发现,HPV 感染的 CC 更依赖于糖酵解,这可以从己糖激酶 2、乳酸脱氢酶和丙酮酸激酶肌同工酶 M2 活性的增强中得到证实[53]。HPV-16 E6/E7 过度表达刺激了葡萄糖的代谢,敲除 E6/E7 可显著降低宫颈癌细胞的葡萄糖代谢率。

多项研究报告称,癌细胞的高糖酵解会导致对氟尿嘧啶(fluorouracil,5-FU)的耐药性[54,55],这表明靶向糖酵解途径可能是一种有效的抗化疗耐药性方法。此外,抑制糖酵解可以克服 E6/E7 过表达的宫颈癌细胞对 5-FU 的耐药性,这提示糖酵解失调是 E6/E7 肿瘤蛋白的下游细胞途径。增加对 E6/E7 的抑制来对抗高糖酵解途径使 CC 细胞对 5-FU 敏感是一种新的治疗途径,靶向细胞葡萄糖代谢可能是减少或根除化疗耐药肿瘤的一种合适的有益途径。

参考文献

[1] Elfström KM, Arnheim-Dahlström L, von Karsa L, Dillner J. CC screening in Europe: quality assurance and organisation of programmes, Eur J Cancer 2015;51(8):950-68. https://doi.org/10.1016/j.ejca.2015.03.008. Epub 2015 Mar 25, 25817010.

[2] Sarkar K, Bhattacharya S, Bhattacharyya S, Chatterjee S, Mallick AH, Chakraborti S, Chatterjee D, Bal B. Oncogenic human papilloma virus and cervical pre-cancerous lesions in brothel-based sex workers in India, J Infect Public Health 2008;1(2):121-8. https://doi.org/10.1016/j.jiph.2008.09.01. Epub 2008 Nov 12, 20701853.

[3] Arbyn M, Weiderpass E, Bruni L, de Sanjosé S, Saraiya M, Ferlay J, Bray F. Estimates of incidence and mortality of CC in 2018: a worldwide analysis. Lancet Glob Health 2020; 8:e191-203.

[4] World Health Organization. Comprehensive CC control integrating health care for sexual and reproductive health care for sexual and reproductive health and chronic disease a guide to practice. Geneva: WHO Library Cataloguing; 2006, p. 3.

[5] Kaarthigeyan K. CC in India and HPV vaccination, Indian J Med Paediatr Oncol 2012;33 (1):7-12. https://doi.org/10.4103/0971-5851.96961. 22754202 PMC3385284.

[6] Panatto D, Amicizia D, Trucchi C, Casabona F, Lai PL, Bonanni P, Boccalini S, Bechini A, Tiscione E, Zotti CM, Coppola RC, Masia G, Meloni A, Castiglia P, Piana A, Gaspa-

rini R. Sexual behaviour and risk factors for the acquisition of human papillomavirus infections in young people in Italy: suggestions for future vaccination policies, BMC Public Health 2012; 12:623. https://doi.org/10.1186/1471-2458-12-623. 22871132 PMC3490840.

[7] Marx J. Cancer research. Obstacle for promising cancer therapy. Science 2002; 295 (5559):1444. https://doi.org/10.1126/science.295.5559.1444a.

[8] Meehan K, Vella LJ. The contribution of tumour-derived exosomes to the hallmarks of cancer. Crit Rev Clin Lab Sci 2016;53(2):121-31. https://doi.org/10.3109/10408363.2015.1092496.

[9] Zhou S, Huang C, Wei Y. The metabolic switch and its regulation in cancer cells. Sci China Life Sci 2010;53(8):942-58. https://doi.org/10.1007/s11427-010-4041-1.

[10] Huang YT, Wang CC, Tsai CS, Lai CH, Chang TC, Chou HH, Lee SP, Hong JH. Clinical behaviors and outcomes for adenocarcinoma or adenosquamous carcinoma of cervix treated by radical hysterectomy and adjuvant radiotherapy or chemoradiotherapy, Int J Radiat Oncol Biol Phys 2012;84(2):420-7. https://doi.org/10.1016/j.ijrobp.2011.12.013. Epub 2012 Feb 24, 22365621.

[11] Hoppe-Seyler K, Honegger A, Bossler F, Sponagel J, Bulkescher J, Lohrey C. Viral E6/E7 oncogene and cellular hexokinase 2 expressiom in HPV-positive cancer cell lines. Oncotarget 2017;8(63):106342-51.

[12] Kim MY, Kim YS, Kim M, Choi MY, Roh GS, Lee DH, Kim HJ, Kang SS, Cho GJ, Shin JK, Choi WS. Metformin inhibits CC cell proliferation via decreased AMPK O-GlcNAcylation, Anim Cells Syst (Seoul) 2019; 23(4): 302-9. https://doi.org/10.1080/19768354.2019.1614092. 31489252 PMC6711131.

[13] Tseng CH. Metformin use and CC risk in female patients with type 2 diabetes, Oncotarget 2016;7(37):59548-55. https://doi.org/10.18632/oncotarget.10934. 27486978 PMC5312330.

[14] Jin L, Alesi GN, Kang S. Glutaminolysis as a target for cancer therapy, Oncogene 2016; 35 (28): 3619-25. https://doi.org/10.1038/onc.2015.447. Epub 2015 Nov 23, 26592449 PMC5225500.

[15] Lunt SY, Vander Heiden MG. Aerobic glycolysis: meeting the metabolic requirements of cell proliferation, Annu Rev Cell Dev Biol 2011;27:441-64. https://doi.org/10.1146/annurev-cellbio-092910-154237. Review, 21985671.

[16] Newell K, Franchi A, Pouysségur J, Tannock I. Studies with glycolysis-deficient cells suggest that production of lactic acid is not the only cause of tumor acidity, Proc Natl Acad Sci U S A 1993;90(3):1127-31. 8430084 PMC45824.

[17] Shan L. Cy5.5-labeled pH low insertion peptide (pHLIP), In: Molecular imaging and contrast agent database (MICAD) [Internet]. Bethesda, MD: National Center for Biotechnology Information(US); 2009. p. 2004-13. Aug 8 [updated 2009 Nov 12]. Available from: http://www.ncbi.nlm.nih.gov/books/NBK23623/PubMed PMID: 20641819.

[18] Helmlinger G, Sckell A, Dellian M, Forbes NS, Jain RK. Acid production in glycolysis-

impaired tumors provides new insights into tumor metabolism, Clin Cancer Res 2002;8(4):1284-91. 11948144.

[19] Yamamoto M, Inohara H, Nakagawa T. Targeting metabolic pathways for head andneck cancers therapeutics, Cancer Metastasis Rev 2017;36(3):503-14. https://doi.org/10.1007/s10555-017-9691-z. Review, 28819926.

[20] Lu J, Tan M, Cai Q. The Warburg effect in tumor progression: mitochondrial oxidative metabolism as an anti-metastasis mechanism, Cancer Lett 2015;356(2 Pt A):156-64. https://doi.org/10.1016/j.can-let.2014.04.001. Epub 2014 Apr 13. Review, 24732809 PMC4195816.

[21] Chan B, VanderLaan PA, Sukhatme VP. 6-Phosphogluconate dehydrogenase regulates tumor cell migrationin vitro by regulating receptor tyrosine kinase c-Met. Biochem Biophys Res Commun 2013;439(2):247-51. https://doi.org/10.1016/j.bbrc.2013.08.048.

[22] Shen Z, Belinson J, Morton RE, Xu Y, Xu Y. Phorbol 12-myristate 13-acetate stimulates lysophosphatidic acid secretion from ovarian and CC cells but not from breast or leukemia cells, Gynecol Oncol 1998;71(3):364-8. ISSN 0090-8258. https://doi.org/10.1006/gyno.1998.5193.

[23] Kostenis E. Novel clusters of receptors for sphingosine-1-phosphate, sphingosylphosphorylcholine, and (lyso)-phosphatidic acid: new receptors for "old" ligands, J Cell Biochem 2004;92(5):923-36. Review, 15258916.

[24] Murray NR, Baumgardner GP, Burns DJ, Fields AP. Protein kinase C isotypes in human erythroleukemia (K562) cell proliferation and differentiation. Evidence that beta II protein kinase C is required for proliferation, J Biol Chem 1993;268(21):15847-53. 8340409.

[25] Chang MS, Chen BC, Yu MT, Sheu JR, Chen TF, Lin CH. Phorbol 12-myristate 13-acetate upregulates cyclooxygenase-2 expression in human pulmonary epithelial cells via Ras, Raf-1, ERK, and NF-kappaB, but not p38 MAPK, pathways, Cell Signal 2005;17(3):299-310. 15567061.

[26] Starzec AB, Spanakis E, Nehme A, Salle V, Veber N, Mainguene C, Planchon P, Valette A, Prevost G, Israel L. Proliferative responses of epithelial cells to 8-bromo-cyclic AMP and to a phorbol ester change during breast pathogenesis. J Cell Physiol 1994;161:31-8.

[27] Brueggemeier RW, Díaz-Cruz ES. Relationship between aromatase and cyclooxygenases in breast cancer: potential for new therapeutic approaches, Minerva Endocrinol 2006;31(1):13-26. Review, 16498361.

[28] Orsó E, Schmitz G. Lipoprotein(a) and its role in inflammation, atherosclerosis and malignancies, Clin Res Cardiol Suppl 2017;12(Suppl 1):31-7. https://doi.org/10.1007/s11789-017-0084-1. 28188431 PMC5352764.

[29] Westermann AM, Havik E, Postma FR, Beijnen JH, Dalesio O, Moolenaar WH, et al. Malignant effusions contain lysophosphatidic acid (LPA)-like activity. Ann Oncol 1998;9:437-42. https://doi.org/10.1023/A:1008217129273.

[30] Xu Y, Shen Z, Wiper DW, Wu M, Morton RE, Elson P, et al. Lysophosphatidic acid as a potential biomarker for ovarian and other gynecologic cancers. JAMA 1998;280:719-23. https://doi.org/10.1001/jama.280.8.719.

[31] Eder AM, Sasagawa T, Mao M, Aoki J, Mills GB. Constitutive and lysophosphatidic acid (LPA)-induced LPA production: role of phospholipase D and phospholipase A2. Clin Cancer Res 2000;6:2482-91.

[32] Hoogendam JP, Klerkx WM, de Kort GA, Beepat S, Zweemer RP, Sie-Go DM, et al. The influence of the b-value combination on apparent diffusion coefficient based differentiation between malignant and benign tissue in CC. J Magn Reson Imaging 2010;32:376-82.

[33] Xue HD, Li S, Sun F, Sun HY, Jin ZY, Yang JX, et al. Clinical application of body diffusion weighted MR imaging in the diagnosis and preoperative N staging of CC. Chin Med Sci J 2008;23:133-7.

[34] Chen YB, Hu CM, Chen GL, Hu D, Liao J. Staging of uterine cervical carcinoma: whole-body diffusion-weighted magnetic resonance imaging. Abdom Imaging 2011;36:619-26.

[35] Schalkwijk CG, van der Heijden MA, Bunt G, Maas R, Tertoolen LG, van Bergen Henegouwen PM, Verkleij AJ, van den Bosch H, Boonstra J. Maximal epidermal growth-factor-induced cytosolic phospholipase A2 activation in vivo requires phosphorylation followed by an increased intracellular calcium concentration, Biochem J 1996;313(Pt 1):91-6. https://doi.org/10.1042/bj3130091. 8546715 PMC1216914.

[36] Sato T, Nakajima H, Fujio K, Mori Y. Enhancement of prostaglandin E2 production by epidermal growth factor requires the coordinate activation of cytosolic phospholipase A2 and cyclooxygenase 2 in human squamous carcinoma A431 cells. Prostaglandins 1997;53(5): 355-69. https://doi.org/10.1016/0090-6980(97)00036-1.

[37] MacGregor DR, Gould P, Foreman J, Griffiths J, Bird S, Page R, Stewart K, Steel G, Young J, Paszkiewicz K, Millar AJ, Halliday KJ, Hall AJ, Penfield S. High expression of osmotically responsive genes1 is required for circadian periodicity through the promotion of nucleo-cytoplasmic mRNA export in Arabidopsis, Plant Cell 2013;25(11):4391-404. https://doi.org/10.1105/tpc.113.114959. Epub 2013 Nov 19, 24254125 PMC3875725.

[38] Kilickesmez O, Bayramoglu S, Inci E, Cimilli T, Kayhan A. Quantitative diffusion-weighted magnetic resonance imaging of normal and diseased uterine zones. Acta Radiol 2009; 50:340-7.

[39] Payne GS, Schmidt M, Morgan VA, Giles S, Bridges J, Ind T, et al. Evaluation of magnetic resonance diffusion and spectroscopy measurements as predictive biomarkers in stage 1 CC. Gynecol Oncol 2010;116:246-52.

[40] Liu Y, Bai R, Sun H, Liu H, Wang D. Diffusion-weighted magnetic resonance imaging of CC. J Comput Assist Tomogr 2009;33:858-62.

[41] Delikatny EJ, Russell P, Hunter JC, Hancock R, Atkinson AH, Van Haften-Day C, et al. Proton MR and human cervical neoplasia:*ex vivos* pectroscopy allows distinction of in-

vasive carcinoma of the cervix from carcinoma *in situ* and other preinvasive lesions. Radiology 1993;188:791-6.

[42] Mahon MM, Cox IJ, Dina R, Soutter WP, McIndoe GA, Williams AD, et al. (1)H magnetic resonance spectroscopy of preinvasive and invasive CC: *in vivo-ex vivo* profiles and effect of tumor load. J Magn Reson Imaging 2004;19:356-64.

[43] Manoharan D, Das CJ, Aggarwal A, Gupta AK. Diffusion weighted imaging in gynecological malignancies—present and future, World J Radiol 2016;8(3):288-97. https://doi.org/10.4329/wjr. v8. i3. 288. 27027614 PMC4807338.

[44] Oh JW, Rha SE, Oh SN, Park MY, Byun JY, Lee A. Diffusion-weighted MRI of epithelial ovarian cancers: correlation of apparent diffusion coefficient values with histologic grade and surgical stage, Eur J Radiol 2015;84(4):590-5. https://doi. org/10. 1016/j. ejrad. 2015. 01. 005. Epub 2015 Jan 16, 25623826.

[45] Kidd EA, Siegel BA, Dehdashti F, Grigsby PW. The standardized uptake value for F-18 fluorodeoxyglucose is a sensitive predictive biomarker for CC treatment response and survival. Cancer 2007;110(8):1738-44. https://doi. org/10. 1002/cncr. 22974.

[46] Pavlova NN, Thompson CB. The emerging hallmarks of cancer metabolism. Cell Metab 2016;23:27-47. https://doi. org/10. 1016/j. cmet. 2015. 12. 006.

[47] Kalyanaraman B. Teaching the basics of cancer metabolism: developing antitumor strategies by exploiting the differences between normal and cancer cell metabolism. Redox Biol 2017;12:833-42. https://doi. org/10. 1016/j. redox. 2017. 04. 018.

[48] Otto AM. Warburg effect(s)—a biographical sketch of Otto Warburg and his impacts on tumor metabolism. Cancer Metab 2016; 4: 5. https://doi. org/10. 1186/s40170-016-0145-9.

[49] Zhang R, Su J, Xue SL, et al. HPV E6/p53 mediated down-regulation of miR-34a inhibits Warburg effect through targeting LDHA in CC. Am J Cancer Res 2016;6:312-20.

[50] Zeng Q, Chen J, Li Y, et al. LKB1 inhibits HPV-associated cancer progression by targeting cellular metabolism. Oncogene 2017; 36: 1245-55. https://doi. org/10. 1038/onc. 2016. 290.

[51] Pastrez PRA, Mariano VS, Da Costa AM, et al. The relation of HPV infection and expression of p53 and p16 proteins in esophageal squamous cells carcinoma. J Cancer 2017;8:1062-70. https://doi. org/10. 7150/jca. 17080.

[52] Hoppe-Seyler K, Honegger A, Bossler F, et al. Viral E6/E7 oncogene and cellular hexokinase 2 expression in HPV-positive cancer cell lines. Oncotarget 2017;8:106342-51. https://doi. org/10. 18632/oncotarget. 22463.

[53] Wang T, Ning K, Sun X, Zhang C, Jin LF, Hua D. Glycolysis is essential for chemoresistance induced by transient receptor potential channel C5 in colorectal cancer. BMC Cancer 2018;18:207. https://doi. org/10. 1186/s12885-018-4242-8.

[54] Grasso C, Jansen G, Giovannetti E. Drug resistance in pancreatic cancer: impact of altered

energy metabolism. Crit Rev Oncol Hematol 2017;114:139-52. https://doi.org/10.1016/j.critrevonc.2017.03.026.

[55] He J, Xie G, Tong J, et al. Overexpression of microRNA-122 resensitizes 5-FU-resistant colon cancer cells to 5-FU through the inhibition of PKM2 *in vitro* and in vivo. Cell Biochem Biophys 2014;70:1343-50. https://doi.org/10.1007/s12013-014-0062.

第 13 章
乳腺癌和宫颈癌相关治疗的药物经济学和成本效益

Mohan Krishna Ghanta[a], Santosh C. Gursale[b], Narayan P. Burte[c], L. V. K. S. Bhaskar[d]

[a] Department of Pharmacology, SRMC & RI, Sri Ramachandra Institute of Higher Education and Research, Chennai, Tamil Nadu, India
[b] Department of Pharmacology, BKL Walawalkar Rural Medical College, Sawarde, Ratnagiri, Maharashtra, India
[c] Department of Pharmacology, Viswabharathi Medical College, Kurnool, Andhra Pradesh, India
[d] Department of Zoology, Guru Ghasidas Vishwavidyalaya, Bilaspur, Chhattisgarh, India

摘要

乳腺癌和宫颈癌是女性的常见疾病,其发病率在全球范围内不断增加。除疾病负担外,与乳腺癌和宫颈癌的治疗和诊断相关的费用也给患者的健康及其所在国家的经济带来了沉重压力。在大多数中低收入国家,这些疾病的治疗给患者造成了更沉重的经济负担。药物经济学的引入减轻了患者和政府疾病管理的经济负担。本章将从药物经济学的角度讨论乳腺癌和宫颈癌的全球治疗成本和成本效益疗法。

关键词

宫颈癌,乳腺癌,药物经济学概念,成本效益疗法,治疗费用负担

缩略词

BRCA1	人类肿瘤抑制基因(译者注:勘误,应为乳腺癌易感基因1)
CBA	成本效益分析
CEA	成本效果分析
CMA	最小费用分析
CRT	放化疗
CT	计算机 X 射线断层
CUA	成本效用分析
ER	雌激素受体
GDP	国内生产总值

HER2	人表皮生长因子受体 2
HPV	人乳头状瘤病毒
INR	印度卢比
IV	静脉注射
NAC	新辅助化疗
QALY	质量生命调整年
TNM	肿瘤淋巴结转移
USD	美元

一、概述

女性占全球总人口的 49.5%。最新研究揭示，癌症已成为全球女性死亡的第二大原因。我们需要高度重视女性癌症负担的不断增加，因为这不仅影响患者本身，还会对其家庭和照料者产生影响。女性特有的肿瘤类型给社会、家庭及个人均带来了沉重的经济负担。在女性最常见的癌症中，乳腺癌、子宫体癌、宫颈癌、卵巢癌、肺癌、肝癌和结直肠癌合计占所有癌症的 60%。本章节将详细探讨药物经济学及其在全球的应用现状，以及乳腺癌和宫颈癌的治疗成本和成本效益疗法[1-3]。

二、药物经济学

药物经济学涉及健康经济学，它将临床治疗和手术结果与经济成本措施相结合[4]。药物经济学指对医疗保健系统和社会的药物治疗成本的描述和分析[5]。药物经济学也称为"药物治疗的经济评价"[6]。

药物经济学的作用是确保一个国家的国内生产总值（gross domestic product，GDP）不受医疗保健政策的影响，根据临床疗效合理化药物的使用和费用，为卫生系统分配资源，鉴别低效和有效的治疗方案，决策药品补助、提供药品定价和报销决策、统一药品出口价格、保证卫生服务质量、改善医患关系、规范药品最高报销定价、评估优先药品清单、规范报销政策，并根据成本效益规范将药品添加到基本药物清单中。

为了量化药物治疗的药物经济学状况，人们已经发展出多种方法，包括成本最小化分析（cost-minimization analysis，CMA）、成本效益分析（cost-benefit analysis，CBA）、成本效果分析（cost-effective analysis，CEA）、成本效用分析（cost-utility analysis，CUA）和敏感性分析。CMA 是在 2 种临床结果相似的药物之间进行，旨在找到基于成本最优的治疗方案,还用于制定处方决策和药物治疗指南的制定。CBA用来评估治疗相关的成本和经济效益,适用于医保项目的制定政策决策。CEA是评估治疗成本及其对患者的临床效果,例如,以花费单位货币对单个患者产生的单位疗效衡量的一种治疗的临床效果。该方法用于确定个体患者的医保干预措施[7]及帮助制定处方决策。CUA以每单位健康的货币单位[质量调整生存年(quality adjusted life years,QALY)]来评估医疗保健干预措施和生活质量,适用于比较慢性病中采取的不同干预措施[8]。

三、乳腺癌

乳腺癌是女性常见的癌症,占女性所有癌症发病率的25%以上[9]。2012年,全球有1 671 100例新发乳腺癌病例,521 900例乳腺癌死亡病例[1]。澳大利亚、新西兰,以及欧洲和北美地区的乳腺癌发病率较高。美国、澳大利亚、巴西、以色列,以及欧洲地区患者的5年生存率为85%,印度、南非和阿尔及利亚患者的5年生存率为60%[10]。

(一)乳腺癌的病理分类与诊断

根据激素受体的表达情况,乳腺癌分为雌激素受体(estrogen receptor,ER)阳性、人表皮生长因子受体2(human epidermal growth factor receptor 2,HER2)阳性或三阴性乳腺癌。ER阳性癌与HER2受体无关,HER2阳性癌可能是也可能不是ER阳性,三阴性癌不涉及ER、孕激素受体(progesterone receptor,PR)或HER2。另一种基于分子亚型的乳腺癌替代分类揭示了4种类型的乳腺癌,分别是:Luminal A型乳腺癌,即ER阳性(低级别)和HER2阴性;Luminal B型乳腺癌,即ER阳性(高级别)且HER2阳性;HER2富集型乳腺癌,即HER2过度表达且ER阴性;基底样型乳腺癌,即ER和HER2均为阴性[11]。

从形态学上来说,乳腺癌分为非浸润性和浸润性。非浸润性乳腺癌包括导管原位癌和小叶原位癌。导管原位癌使受影响的小叶扩大,小叶原位癌使小叶变形为管状空间。浸润性乳腺癌包括浸润性导管癌、浸润性小叶癌、髓样癌、黏液性癌、管状癌和其他类型。浸润性导管癌在显微镜下的范围从完全发育的具有低级细胞核的小管到具有间变细胞层的肿瘤,并且表现为坚硬的、可触及的、不规则的肿块。这种类型的癌症大多为ER阳性,但也可能为HER2阳性,或者为ER和HER2阴性。浸润性小叶癌在形态学上与原位小叶癌相似。间质侵犯表现为"单列"且ER阳性。HER2上调很少见。髓样癌表现为圆形肿块,具有大的间变细胞层和淋巴细胞浸润,这在种系BRCA1突变中很常见。黏液癌或胶样癌表现为ER阳性和

HER2 阴性的软凝胶状肿瘤。管状癌表现为小的不规则肿瘤,具有发达的小管和低级别的细胞核,呈 ER 阳性和 HER2 阴性。炎性乳腺癌临床上表现为肿大的红斑性乳房,没有可触及的肿瘤或肿块[12-14],这种癌症既呈 ER 阳性,又呈 HER2 阳性。疾病的临床分期基于肿瘤淋巴结转移(tumor node metastasis,TNM)分类(表 13-1)。

表 13-1 乳腺癌的 TNM 分期[15]

分期	乳腺癌
肿瘤	
Tx	无法评估原发肿瘤
T0	无原发肿瘤证据
T1	肿瘤大小＜20 mm
T2	肿瘤大小 20～50 mm
T3	肿瘤大小＞50 mm
T4	肿瘤侵入胸壁和/或皮肤
Tis	原位癌
Tis(DCIS)	导管原位癌
Tis(LCIS)	原位小叶原位癌
淋巴结	
Nx	无法评估区域淋巴结
N0	无区域淋巴结受累
N1	累及同侧腋窝淋巴结且可活动
N2	累及同侧腋窝淋巴结并黏附于周围结构
N3	同侧锁骨、乳腺、腋窝淋巴结受累
转移	
M0	没有远处转移的临床或放射学证据
M1	通过临床或放射学检查结果诊断出远处转移

乳腺癌的诊断基于临床检查、乳房 X 线检查、超声检查、活检(细针穿刺细胞学检查或组织活检)、胸部、腹部 CT、同位素骨扫描和分子分型[13]。

(二)乳腺癌的治疗和费用

乳腺癌患者的主要治疗方法是手术治疗,包括乳房肿瘤切除术或乳房切除术。对于有复发风险的患者,建议进行辅助放疗和化疗。对于 ER 阴性乳腺癌患者或腋窝淋巴结受累的患者,均应接受化疗。对于已经发生转移的患者,治疗策略通常包括放射治疗和内分泌治疗。根据乳腺癌的分期及分子分型,制定相应的治疗方案,如表 13-2 所示。标准化疗方案包含蒽环类药物和紫杉烷类药物。蒽环类药物和环磷酰胺-紫杉烷方案包括使用 4 个周期的多柔比星和环磷酰胺,然后使用 4 个周期的紫杉醇[20]。

表 13-2 基于乳腺癌分期的当前治疗方法

分期	治疗
HR 阳性肿瘤	阿那曲唑、来普唑、他莫昔芬[16]
HER2 阳性肿瘤	曲妥珠单抗、帕妥珠单抗和拉帕替尼;Ⅱ/Ⅲ期应用曲妥珠单抗及蒽环类药物和环磷酰胺-紫杉烷方案[17,18]
三阴性肿瘤	化疗药物的单一或联合方案[19]

其他方案包括先使用蒽环类药物和环磷酰胺,然后使用紫杉醇 12 周或多西紫杉醇,每周 3 次,持续 4 个周期[21,22]。与乳腺癌治疗相关的不良事件包括认知障碍、骨质疏松症、慢性疲劳和阴道干燥[23]。

一项欧洲研究揭示了乳腺癌治疗的总费用(包括治疗后随访费用)。结果显示,诊断支出(平均成本)为 414 欧元,治疗平均费用为 8780 欧元,后续平均成本为 2351 欧元,总直接平均成本为 10 970 欧元,后续费用变化很大。印度旁遮普邦的一项研究报道,诊断或筛查的总成本为 4 147 700 印度卢比(Indian rupee,INR),总医疗成本为 79 080 682 INR,总直接成本为 82 639 662 INR,总间接成本为 21 594 507.97 INR[24]。一项荟萃分析报道了各阶段乳腺癌的累计治疗费用。Ⅰ期乳腺癌治疗的平均费用为 20 852 美元,Ⅱ期为 29 430 美元,Ⅲ期为 40 211 美元,Ⅳ期为 41 560 美元[25]。加拿大和意大利这一治疗费用更高[26,27]。

(三)具有成本效益的疗法

随着乳腺癌的疾病负担和治疗费用的持续上升,引入成本效益高的疗法和诊断模型对于预防癌症死亡至关重要。腋下淋巴结取样技术作为一种经济实惠的诊断方法,与前哨淋巴结活检相比,显示出更好的效果[28,29]。Lairson 等进行乳腺癌化疗的 CEA,比较了基于蒽环类药物的方案与非蒽环类药物的方案。他们发现,基于蒽环类药物的方案具有 12.05QALY,总治疗成本为 119 055 美元;而非基于蒽环类药物的方案具有 9.56QALY,总治疗成本为 86 383 美元。在这项比较研究中,基于蒽环类药物的化疗方案相对于非蒽环类药物方案在成本效益上显示出优势[30]。辅助曲妥珠单抗的较短治疗时间显示出不劣于 1 年治疗的疗效[31]。西班牙的一项 CMA 研究报告称,与静脉注射相比,皮下注射曲妥珠单抗更具成本效益[32]。术前孕酮治疗被证实是对于淋巴结阳性乳腺癌患者的一种经济有效的干预措施[33]。Palbociclib 被发现在治疗晚期乳腺癌方面具有成本效益优势,其与来曲唑辅助治疗的治疗费用为 768 498 美元/QALY,与氟维司群辅助治疗的治疗费用为 918 166 美元/QALY[34]。周期性化疗被认为是乳腺癌的另一种经济有效的治疗方法[35]。

四、宫颈癌

宫颈癌的发病率和死亡率在全世界女性癌症中排名第四,在发展中国家排名第二。2012 年,全球有 527 600 例宫颈癌患者,265 700 例死亡;在撒哈拉以南非洲、亚洲和南美洲的发病率最高。与其他发展中国家相比,印度的宫颈癌负担更大(90%)。在高收入国家中,宫颈癌患者的 5 年生存率为 60%~70%;而在低收入和中等收入国家(如印度)中,这一数字为 46%。宫颈癌通常通过异常的宫颈涂片检查、阴道出血的临床表现,以及与膀胱、直肠和盆腔有关的其他症状来诊断。远处转移主要发生在骨骼和肺部[13]。

从病理学上讲,宫颈癌可以是鳞状细胞癌、腺癌、混合性腺鳞癌或小细胞神经内分泌癌。针对宫颈癌患者的各种筛查包括细胞学检查和锥切、HPV 检测、膀胱镜检查、灵活的乙状结肠镜检查、磁共振成像、胸部 X 线检查,以及腹部和骨盆 CT[13]。宫颈癌的分期见表 13-3[37]。

表 13-3　宫颈癌分期(FIGO)和管理

肿瘤分期			描述	治疗
Stage 0			子宫颈上皮内癌或原位癌	化疗
Stage I			宫颈癌局限于子宫颈	
	Ⅰa		浸润性癌(仅通过显微镜诊断)	
		Ⅰa1	微浸润性或间质浸润深度<3 mm,延伸深度<7 mm	
		Ⅰa2	基质浸润深度>3 mm,延伸范围 5~7 mm	
	Ⅰb		临床可见病变局限于子宫颈	外科治疗和放射治疗
		Ⅰb1	肿瘤/病变<4 cm	
		Ⅰb2	肿瘤/病变>4 cm	
Stage Ⅱ			癌症超过子宫颈,但不超过骨盆侧壁或阴道下 1/3 癌至阴道上 2/3	

续表

肿瘤分期			描述	治疗
	Ⅱa			
		Ⅱa1	可见肿瘤/病变<4 cm	
		Ⅱa2	可见肿瘤/病变>4 cm	
	Ⅱb		伴有骨旁侵犯的病变	仅放射治疗
StageⅢ	Ⅲa		阴道下1/3以上的病变没有延伸至盆腔侧壁	
	Ⅲb		病变/肿瘤延伸至盆腔侧壁	
StageⅣ			病变/肿瘤延伸至真正的骨盆或活检显示累及膀胱或直肠黏膜	
	Ⅳa		直肠或膀胱侵犯	
	Ⅳb		远处转移	基于顺铂的化疗和放疗仅限于受影响的部位[13,36]

(一)宫颈癌的治疗和费用

手术、放疗和化疗是宫颈癌治疗的常见方式。宫颈癌的治疗取决于疾病的分期(表 13-3)。Liu 等[38]揭示了宫颈癌治疗的费用负担,诊断前阶段的平均治疗费用为 3155 加元,治疗初始阶段为 17 938 美元,生命最后 1 年的治疗费用为 58 319 美元[38]。巴西的一项研究显示,放射治疗的成本(直接成本)较高,为 199 794.32 美元,其次的成本负担是化疗 143 268.17 美元,手术治疗费用为 44 431.43 美元,诊断方法的直接成本是总计实验室检验成本和影像成本(19 714.81 美元),宫颈癌患者的总费用负担为 523 218.22 美元。美国一些关于医疗保险理赔的研究揭示了宫颈癌治疗的成本。结果显示,1990—1991 年期间,宫颈癌治疗的平均费用为 30 136 美元[39]。McCrory 等发现按分期评估宫颈癌治疗的平均成本为,Ⅰ期、Ⅱ/Ⅲ期和Ⅳ期分别为 17 645 美元、27 069 美元、40 280 美元[40]。Insinga 等的回顾性研究预估了平均死亡率调整成本为 29 649 美元[41]。Cromwell 等计算出患者从诊断到死亡的总体平均费用为 19 153±3484 美元[42]。另一项研究估计了加拿大安大略省宫颈癌诊断后前 5 年内治疗的直接费用,每个患者的成本负担在第 1~5 年期间分别为 39 187 美元、14 425 美元、11 280 美元、8444 美元和 5480 美元[43]。Oliveira 等报道 2013 年安大略省治疗费用估算为 4272 美元,远低于 2016 年报告的数字(13 697 美元)[43,44]。Subramanian 等计算了宫颈癌治疗在最初 6 个月内的费用,原位癌阶段为 3807 美元,局部癌为 23 187

美元,区域转移癌为 35 853 美元,远处转移癌为 45 028 美元[45]。

(二)成本效益疗法

基于人均 GDP 阈值的成本效益分析受到了批判[46],并从 WHO 建议中被撤回。建议采用替代方法,例如,比较新干预措施与现有干预措施之间的增量成本效益,以及评估为健康福利支付的意愿。预防 HPV 感染可以减轻宫颈癌患者的健康和经济负担。许多来自不同国家的成本效益研究证明,为青少年接种 HPV 疫苗具有成本效益优势[47]。在晚期宫颈癌患者中,使用贝伐珠单抗的成本是单独化疗的 13 倍[48]。使用醋酸进行宫颈癌筛查是一种成本效益高的筛查方法,每增加一个生命年的增量成本效益为 87 美元。新辅助化疗(neoadjuvant chemotherapy,NAC)方案包括在每个 21 天周期的第 1 天通过静脉输注顺铂 80 mg/m^2、静推博来霉素 30 mg,以及静脉输注长春新碱 1.4 mg/m^2,连续进行 3 个周期。放化疗方案包括从外照射放疗的第 1 天开始,每周 1 次静脉输注顺铂 40 mg/m^2,持续 5 周。NAC 方案在减少胃肠和血液毒性方面显示出不劣于放化疗的优势,但尚无研究对比这 2 种方案的成本效益[50]。

五、结论

本章阐述了乳腺癌和宫颈癌治疗给患者和国家带来的沉重经济负担。这可能为使用药物经济学工具选择具有成本效益的治疗方案提供数据,而这些工具目前在世界许多地区,特别是在中、低收入国家实施不力。本章的结论是,需要在全国范围内对癌症的成本效益、预算影响及成本进行更多研究。

参 考 文 献

[1] Torre LA, Islami F, Siegel RL, Ward EM, Jemal A. Global cancer in women: burden and trends. Cancer Epidemiol Biomarkers Prev 2017;26(4):444-57.

[2] United Nations. World population prospects: the 2015 revision. U N Econ Soc Aff 2015; 33(2):1-66.

[3] World Health Organization. Women and health: today's evidence tomorrow's agenda. World Health Organization; 2009.

[4] Bakst A. Pharmacoeconomics and the formulary decision-making process. Hosp Formul 1995;30(1): 42-50.

[5] Richardson J. Cost utility analysis: what should be measured? Soc Sci Med 1994;39(1):7-21.

[6] Arenas-Guzman R, Tosti A, Hay R, Haneke E. Pharmacoeconomics—an aid to better decision-making. J Eur Acad Dermatol Venereol 2005;19(s1):34-9.

[7] Hill SR. Cost-effectiveness analysis for clinicians. BMC Med 2012;10(1):10.

[8] Reimbursement decisions and the implied value of life: cost effectiveness analysis and decisions to reimburse pharmaceuticals in Australia 1993-1996. George B, Harris A, Mitchell A, editors. Economics and Health: 1997 proceedings of the nineteenth Australian conference of health economists. Sydney, Australia: School of Health Services Management, University of New South Wales; 1998.

[9] Ferlay J, Soerjomataram I, Dikshit R, Eser S, Mathers C, Rebelo M, et al. Cancer incidence and mortality worldwide: sources, methods and major patterns in GLOBOCAN 2012. Int J Cancer 2015;136(5):E359-86.

[10] Allemani C, Weir HK, Carreira H, Harewood R, Spika D, Wang XS, et al. Global surveillance of cancer survival 1995-2009: analysis of individual data for 25,676,887 patients from 279 population-based registries in 67 countries (CONCORD-2). Lancet 2015;385(9972):977-1010.

[11] Kumar V, Abbas AK, Aster JC. Robbins basic pathology e-book. Elsevier Health Sciences; 2017.

[12] Sinn H-P, Kreipe H. A brief overview of the WHO classification of breast tumors, 4th edition, focusing on issues and updates from the 3rd edition. Breast Care 2013;8(2):149-54.

[13] Ralston SH, Penman ID, Strachan MW, Hobson R. Davidson's principles and practice of medicine E-book. Elsevier Health Sciences; 2018.

[14] Eliyatkın N, Yalçın E, Zengel B, Aktaş S, Vardar E. Molecular classification of breast carcinoma: from traditional, old-fashioned way to a new age, and a new way. J Breast Health 2015;11(2):59-66.

[15] Koh J, Kim MJ. Introduction of a new staging system of breast cancer for radiologists: an emphasis on the prognostic stage. Korean J Radiol 2019;20(1):69-82.

[16] Davies C, Godwin J, Gray R, Clarke M, Cutter D, Darby S, et al. Relevance of breast cancer hormone receptors and other factors to the efficacy of adjuvant tamoxifen: patient-level meta-analysis of randomised trials. Lancet 2011;378(9793):771-84.

[17] Gianni L, Pienkowski T, Im YH, Roman L, Tseng LM, Liu MC, et al. Efficacy and safety of neoadjuvant pertuzumab and trastuzumab in women with locally advanced, inflammatory, or early HER2-positive breast cancer (NeoSphere): a randomised multicentre, open-label, phase 2 trial. Lancet Oncol 2012;13(1):25-32.

[18] Tolaney SM, Barry WT, Dang CT, Yardley DA, Moy B, Marcom PK, et al. Adjuvant paclitaxel and trastuzumab for node-negative, HER2-positive breast cancer. N Engl J Med 2015;372(2):134-41.

[19] Gogate A, Rotter JS, Trogdon JG, Meng K, Baggett CD, Reeder-Hayes KE, et al. An

updated systematic review of the cost-effectiveness of therapies for metastatic breast cancer. Breast Cancer Res Treat 2019;174(2):343-55.

[20] Citron ML, Berry DA, Cirrincione C, Hudis C, Winer EP, Gradishar WJ, et al. Randomized trial of dose-dense versus conventionally scheduled and sequential versus concurrent combination chemotherapy as postoperative adjuvant treatment of node-positive primary breast cancer: first report of Intergroup Trial C9741/Cancer and Leukemia Group B Trial 9741. J Clin Oncol 2003;21(8):1431-9.

[21] Sparano JA, Wang M, Martino S, Jones V, Perez EA, Saphner T, et al. Weekly paclitaxel in the adjuvant treatment of breast cancer. N Engl J Med 2008;358(16):1663-71.

[22] Sparano JA, Zhao F, Martino S, Ligibel JA, Perez EA, Saphner T, et al. Long-term follow-up of the E1199 phase III trial evaluating the role of taxane and schedule in operable breast cancer. J Clin Oncol 2015;33(21):2353-60.

[23] Pinto AC, de Azambuja E. Improving quality of life after breast cancer: dealing with symptoms. Maturitas 2011;70(4):343-8.

[24] Jain M, Mukherjee K. Economic burden of breast cancer to the households in Punjab, India. Int J Med Public Health 2016;6(1):13-8.

[25] Sun L, Legood R, Dos-Santos-Silva I, Gaiha SM, Sadique Z. Global treatment costs of breast cancer by stage: a systematic review. PLoS One 2018;13(11). e0207993-e.

[26] Capri S, Russo A. Cost of breast cancer based on real-world data: a cancer registry study in Italy. BMC Health Serv Res 2017;17(1):84.

[27] Mittmann N, Porter JM, Rangrej J, Seung SJ, Liu N, Saskin R, et al. Health system costs for stage-specific breast cancer: a population-based approach. Curr Oncol 2014;21(6):281-93.

[28] Radhakrishna S. Cost-effective breast cancer care in India. Int J Adv Med Health Res 2018;5(1):1.

[29] Parmar V, Hawaldar R, Nadkarni MS, Badwe RA. Low axillary sampling in clinically node-negative operable breast cancer. Natl Med J India 2009;22(5):234-6.

[30] Lairson DR, Parikh RC, Cormier JN, Chan W, Du XL. Cost-effectiveness of chemotherapy for breast cancer and age effect in older women. Value Health 2015;18(8):1070-8.

[31] Earl HM, Hiller L, Vallier A-L, Loi S, Howe D, Higgins HB, et al. PERSEPHONE: 6 versus 12 months(m) of adjuvant trastuzumab in patients (pts) with HER2 positive (+) early breast cancer (EBC): randomised phase 3 non-inferiority trial with definitive 4-year (yr) disease-free survival (DFS) results. J Clin Oncol 2018;36(15_suppl):506.

[32] Lopez-Vivanco G, Salvador J, Diez R, Lopez D, De Salas-Cansado M, Navarro B, et al. Cost minimization analysis of treatment with intravenous or subcutaneous trastuzumab in patients with HER2-positive breast cancer in Spain. Clin Transl Oncol 2017;19(12):1454-61.

[33] Badwe R, Hawaldar R, Parmar V, Nadkarni M, Shet T, Desai S, et al. Single-injection

depot progesterone before surgery and survival in women with operable breast cancer: a randomized controlled trial. J Clin Oncol 2011;29(21):2845-51.

[34] Mamiya H, Tahara RK, Tolaney SM, Choudhry NK, Najafzadeh M. Cost-effectiveness of palbociclib in hormone receptor-positive advanced breast cancer. Ann Oncol 2017;28(8): 1825-31.

[35] Simsek C, Esin E, Yalcin S. Metronomic chemotherapy: a systematic review of the literature and clinical experience. J Oncol 2019;2019:5483791.

[36] Eaker S, Adami H-O, Sparén P. Reasons women do not attend screening for cervical cancer: a population-based study in Sweden. Prev Med 2001;32(6):482-91.

[37] Šarenac T, Mikov M. Cervical cancer, different treatments and importance of bile acids as therapeutic agents in this disease. Front Pharmacol 2019;10(484):1-29.

[38] Liu N, Mittmann N, Coyte PC, Hancock-Howard R, Seung SJ, Earle CC. Phase-specific healthcare costs of cervical cancer: estimates from a population-based study. Am J Obstet Gynecol 2016;214(5): e1-e11. 615.

[39] Helms LJ, Melnikow J. Determining costs of health care services for cost-effectiveness analyses: the case of cervical cancer prevention and treatment. Med Care 1999;37(7): 652-61.

[40] McCrory DC, Matchar DB, Bastian L, Datta S, Hasselblad V, Hickey J, et al. Evaluation of cervical cytology. Evid Rep Technol Assess (Summ) 1999;(5):1-6.

[41] Insinga RP, Ye X, Singhal PK, Carides GW. Healthcare resource use and costs associated with cervical, vaginal and vulvar cancers in a large U.S. health plan. Gynecol Oncol 2008; 111(2):188-96.

[42] Cromwell I, Ferreira Z, Smith L, van der Hoek K, Ogilvie G, Coldman A, et al. Cost and resource utilization in cervical cancer management: a real-world retrospective cost analysis. Curr Oncol 2016;23(Suppl 1):S14-22.

[43] Pendrith C, Thind A, Zaric GS, Sarma S. Costs of cervical cancer treatment: population-based estimates from Ontario. Curr Oncol 2016;23(2):e109-15.

[44] de Oliveira C, Bremner KE, Pataky R, Gunraj N, Chan K, Peacock S, et al. Understanding the costs of cancer care before and after diagnosis for the 21 most common cancers in Ontario: a population-based descriptive study. CMAJ Open 2013;1(1):E1-8.

[45] Subramanian S, Trogdon J, Ekwueme DU, Gardner JG, Whitmire JT, Rao C. Cost of cervical cancer treatment: implications for providing coverage to low-income women under the Medicaid expansion for cancer care. Womens Health Issues 2010;20(6):400-5.

[46] Newall AT, Jit M, Hutubessy R. Are current cost-effectiveness thresholds for low-and middle-income countries useful? Examples from the world of vaccines. Pharmacoeconomics 2014;32(6):525-31.

[47] Van Minh H, My NTT, Jit M. Cervical cancer treatment costs and cost-effectiveness analysis of human papillomavirus vaccination in Vietnam: a PRIME modeling study. BMC

Health Serv Res 2017;17(1):353.

[48] Minion LE, Bai J, Monk BJ, Robin Keller L, Ramez EN, Forde GK, et al. A Markov model to evaluate cost-effectiveness of antiangiogenesis therapy using bevacizumab in advanced cervical cancer. Gynecol Oncol 2015;137(3):490-6.

[49] Ralaidovy AH, Gopalappa C, Ilbawi A, Pretorius C, Lauer JA. Cost-effective interventions for breast cancer, cervical cancer, and colorectal cancer: new results from WHO-CHOICE. Cost Eff Resour Alloc 2018;16:38.

[50] Dastidar GA, Gupta P, Basu B, Basu A, Shah JK, Seal SL. Is neo-adjuvant chemotherapy a better option for management of cervical cancer patients of rural India? Indian J Cancer 2016;53(1):56-9.

第 14 章
针对女性特异性肿瘤的精准医疗：策略、挑战和解决方案

Rama Rao Malla[a], Ganji Purnachandra Nagaraju[b]

[a] Cancer Biology Lab, Department of Biochemistry and Bioinformatics, Institute of Science, GITAM (Deemed to be University), Visakhapatnam, Andhra Pradesh, India
[b] Department of Hematology and Medical Oncology, Winship Cancer Institute, Emory University, Atlanta, GA, United States

摘要

女性特异性肿瘤（female-specific cancers, FSC）是一组妇科肿瘤，是世界癌症死亡率和发病率的重要组成部分。FSC 的病因主要与生活方式有关。畸形、遗传和表观遗传改变也会引起 FSC。手术（包括机器人辅助腹腔镜手术）切除受累器官和放化疗是有效的治疗方法。这些治疗方法虽然提高了 5 年生存率，但并不能达到治愈目标，肿瘤仍然容易复发和/或转移。这对研究人员来说仍是一个挑战。靶向治疗能够针对肿瘤病灶进行杀伤，对正常细胞毒性小，被认为是有效的治疗手段。精准医疗的出现则取代了单一疗法，且其能克服化疗药物耐药的弊端。根据癌症的期别和类型而进行个体化的治疗方法已被证明有效。诱变疗法可能是治疗癌症的新策略之一。此外，再生医学技术被认为是治疗 FSC 的新治疗选择，包括工程肿瘤干细胞和肿瘤微环境中的细胞外基质，其中细胞外基质在肿瘤转移中发挥着重要作用。另外，建议接种 HPV 疫苗和口服避孕药有助于防止 FSC 的发生。本章重点介绍 FSC 新的治疗策略。

关键词

女性特异性肿瘤，肿瘤微环境，耐药，转移，精准医疗

缩略词

BRCA	乳腺癌易感基因 1
FOX	大鼠
FSC	女性特异性肿瘤
HER	人表皮生长因子受体
KRAS	Kirsten 大鼠肉瘤

G. P. Nagaraju, R. R. Malla (eds.)
A Theranostic and Precision Medicine Approach for Female-Specific Cancers
ISBN 978-0-12-822009-2
https://doi.org/10.1016/B978-0-12-822009-2.00014-5

© 2021 Elsevier Inc.
All rights reserved.

PM 精准医疗
PTEN 磷酸酶-张力蛋白基因
TME 肿瘤微环境

在全球范围内,尽管治疗技术已取得进步,但女性特异性肿瘤(female-specific cancers,FSC)如乳腺癌、宫颈癌、卵巢癌和子宫内膜癌的发病率仍在上升。在过去10年中,研究者已经进行了多次通过使用靶向药物来改善女性特异性肿瘤治疗效果的尝试。然而,由于缺乏有效和特异性的早期检测方法,使得FSC的治疗更具挑战性。此外,肿瘤微环境(tumor microenvironments,TME)的重构、化疗药耐性和放疗不敏感的加剧,以及对抗肿瘤的有效免疫系统的缺乏,导致FSC患者的死亡率增加。到目前为止,尽管治疗方法对正常组织的影响已经逐渐降低,但最终的疗效仍令人失望。

针对表型和基因型相似的肿瘤,单一药物疗法的时代正在迅速衰落,并逐渐被精准医疗(precision medicine,PM)所取代[1]。肿瘤的精准医疗是指诊断、治疗、维持治疗、生存期内的预防复发[2]。当前,精准医疗被认为是选择性靶向肿瘤细胞而对正常细胞无损失或损失最小的解决方案[3]。精准医疗的目标是为每例患者提供最有效的特异性治疗,降低治疗风险和不良反应,并开发针对肿瘤生长关键细胞和分子途径的治疗方法[4]。

针对乳腺癌[5]和妇科肿瘤的个体化医疗是一个不断发展的领域[6]。以精准医疗为基础的治疗是针对一组特定癌症的治疗,而不是针对一个特定癌症的治疗[7]。例如,同一治疗方案可应用于不同诊断的乳腺癌患者,如人表皮生长因子受体2(human epidermal growth factor receptor2,HER2)阳性的患者、淋巴结肿瘤患者,以及使用曲妥珠单抗进行HER2靶向治疗的绝经前期女性[8]。但是,科研逻辑的挑战阻碍了这些研究临床层面的实施[9]。例如,由于需要对大量患者进行筛查,进行基因突变率低的随机对照试验较为困难[10]。只有扩大基因突变患者的筛查规模,并将同类基因组突变聚类在一起,才能解决这一问题。

精准医疗治疗妇科肿瘤的研究仍在进行中。目前已经发现了一些突变驱动因素。例如,卵巢癌中的 BRCA 突变、NOTCH、p13k、BRAS/MEK、FOX 1、p53,子宫内膜癌中的 TP53、PTEN、P1K3CA 和 KRAS,宫颈癌中的 P1K3CA、TP53、RB1 等[11]。靶向突变驱动因子的治疗方法正在快速发展,即通过利用肿瘤-基质相互作用、脉管系统和异常信号轴途径治疗肿瘤[12]。

卵巢癌患者精准医疗肿瘤委员会推荐了靶向异常组织和靶向治疗[13]。对基因型匹配的临床试验患者来说,精准医疗变得越来越重要[14]。为识别那些易受特定治疗影响的关键通路,必须进行进一步的研究。癌症和癌前蛋白质组学、表观基因组学和基因组学信息定义了 HPV 介导的癌变分子机制,并为诊断提供了个性化的生物标志物[15]。为了实现宫颈癌的早诊断、早治疗,还需要对宫颈癌的亚型和 PM 进行更加深入的研究。

表观遗传修饰是肿瘤发生和发展的关键因素。表观遗传学是精准医疗领域的一门创新学科,它揭示了新的遗传学过程,并发现了有前景的生物标志物、靶标和治疗方法,具有一定的应用前景[16]。近年来,TME 被认为是一个具有异质性、动态性和复杂性的多面系统[17]。通过免疫组织化学、流式和质谱法、高通量 RNA 测序[18]、分子成像和多组学分析对 TME 进行定量分析,为开展 FSC 的精确免疫治疗铺平了道路[19]。使用有监督和无监督模式分析数据集的机器学习方法也为 FSC 的精准医疗提供了帮助[20]。各种基于分子体外诊断的测试也支持精准医疗的发展,为癌症治疗提供了可行的替代方案[16]。

在实施精准医疗方面仍存在诸多挑战,但都能够克服。同时,也应理性展望,因为精准医疗不会在一夜之间自动发展起来。医疗保健利益相关者,包括政府、研究机构和制药行业、生物医学界、患者社区和监管机构,有能力通过制定严格的法律、提供平等社会经济环境、开发早期诊断工具,并提供保护患者的监管框架来解决这些困难。

参 考 文 献

[1] Dalby M, Cree IA, Challoner BR, Ghosh S, Thurston DE. The precision medicine approach to cancer therapy: part 1—solid tumours. Acute Pain 2019;15:44.

[2] Harris EE. Precision medicine for breast cancer: the paths to truly individualized diagnosis and treatment. Int J Breast Cancer 2018;2018:1-8.

[3] Penet M-F, Krishnamachary B, Chen Z, Jin J, Bhujwalla ZM. Molecular imaging of the tumor microenvironment for precision medicine and theranostics. Adv Cancer Res 2014;124:235-56.

[4] Lumachi F, Chiara GB, Foltran L, Basso SM. Proteomics as a guide for personalized adjuvant chemotherapy in patients with early breast cancer. Cancer Genomics Proteomics 2015;12(6):385-90.

[5] (a) Odle TG. Precision medicine in breast cancer. Radiol Technol 2017;88(4):401m-421m. (b) Cheng L, Majumdar A, Stover D, Wu S, Lu Y, Li L. Computational cancer cell models to guide precision breast cancer medicine. Genes 2020;11(3):263.

[6] Corey L, Valente A, Wade K. Personalized medicine in gynecologic cancer: fact or fiction? Obstet Gynecol Clin North Am 2019;46(1):155-63.

[7] (a) Montemurro F, Valabrega G, Aglietta M. Trastuzumab treatment in breast cancer. N Engl J Med 2006;354(20):2186. author reply 2186. (b) Xuhong JC, Qi XW, Zhang Y, Jiang J.

Mechanism, safety and efficacy of three tyrosine kinase inhibitors lapatinib, neratinib and pyrotinib in HER2-positive breast cancer. Am J Cancer Res 2019;9(10):2103-19.

[8] (a)Adamczyk A, Niemiec J, Janecka A, Harazin-Lechowska A, Ambicka A, Grela-Wojewoda A, Domagala-Haduch M, Cedrych I, Majchrzyk K, Kruczak A, Rys J, Jakubowicz J. Prognostic value of PIK3CA mutation status, PTEN and androgen receptor expression for metastasis-free survival in HER2-positive breast cancer patients treated with trastuzumab in adjuvant setting. Pol J Pathol 2015;66(2):133-41. (b)Harbeck N. Insights into biology of luminal HER2 vs. enriched HER2 subtypes: therapeutic implications. Breast 2015;24(Suppl 2):S44-8.

[9] Sachdev JC, Sandoval AC, Jahanzeb M. Update on precision medicine in breast cancer. Cancer Treat Res 2019;178:45-80.

[10] (a)Arnedos M, Vicier C, Loi S, Lefebvre C, Michiels S, Bonnefoi H, Andre F. Precision medicine for metastatic breast cancer—limitations and solutions. Nat Rev Clin Oncol 2015; 12(12):693-704. (b)Low SK, Zembutsu H, Nakamura Y. Breast cancer: the translation of big genomic data to cancer precision medicine. Cancer Sci 2018;109(3):497-506.

[11] Corey L, Valente A, Wade K. Personalized medicine in gynecologic cancer: fact or fiction? Surg Oncol Clin 2020;29(1):105-13.

[12] Horowitz N, Matulonis UA. New biologic agents for the treatment of gynecologic cancers. Hematol Oncol Clin North Am 2012;26(1):133-56.

[13] Sanchez NS, Mills GB, Mills Shaw KR. Precision oncology: neither a silver bullet nor a dream. Pharmacogenomics 2017;18(16):1525-39.

[14] Ray-Coquard I, Pujade Lauraine E, Le Cesne A, Pautier P, Vacher Lavenue MC, Trama A, Casali P, Coindre JM, Blay JY. Improving treatment results with reference centres for rare cancers: where do we stand? Eur J Cancer 2017;77:90-8.

[15] (a)Wilting SM, Steenbergen RDM. Molecular events leading to HPV-induced high grade neoplasia. Papillomavirus Res 2016;2:85-8. (b)Mirnezami R, Nicholson J, Darzi A. Preparing for precision medicine. N Engl J Med 2012;366(6):489-91.

[16] Beltran-Garcia J, Osca-Verdegal R, Mena-Molla S, Garcia-Gimenez JL. Epigenetic IVD tests for personalized precision medicine in cancer. Front Genet 2019;10:621.

[17] Petitprez F, Sun CM, Lacroix L, Sautes-Fridman C, de Reynies A, Fridman WH. Quantitative analyses of the tumor microenvironment composition and orientation in the era of precision medicine. Front Oncol 2018;8:390.

[18] Lau D, Bobe AM, Khan AA. RNA sequencing of the tumor microenvironment in precision cancer immunotherapy. Trends Cancer 2019;5(3):149-56.

[19] Finotello F, Eduati F. Multi-omics profiling of the tumor microenvironment: paving the way to precision immuno-oncology. Front Oncol 2018;8:430.

[20] Azuaje F. Artificial intelligence for precision oncology: beyond patient stratification. NPJ Precis Oncol 2019;3:6.

第 15 章
环境致癌物及其对女性特异性肿瘤的影响

N. Srinivas[a], Rama Rao Malla[b], K. Suresh Kumar[a], A. Ram Sailesh[a]

[a] Department of Environmental Science, Institute of Science, GITAM (Deemed to be University), Visakhapatnam, India
[b] Cancer Biology Lab, Department of Biochemistry and Bioinformatics, Institute of Science, GITAM (Deemed to be University), Visakhapatnam, Andhra Pradesh, India

摘要

环境致癌物是指能够通过食物、空气或材料进入人体的环境衍生物质或化学物质。2/3 的癌症是由环境中存在的各种自然和人为物质导致的。环境因素可分为物理、化学和生物因素,不同的环境暴露因素与特定的癌症类型有关。基因毒性物质有可能损害细胞的遗传物质,引起基因突变导致癌症的发生。有一些癌症通常只发生于女性,如乳腺癌(译者注:勘误,男性乳腺癌也存在)、子宫内膜癌、卵巢癌和宫颈癌。

关键词

乳腺癌,环境,基因毒性,突变,持久性有机污染物

缩略词

AhR	芳烃受体
DDT	二氯二苯三氯乙烷;滴滴涕(杀虫剂)
DDE	二氯二苯二氯乙烯
DNA	脱氧核糖核酸
EDC	内分泌干扰物
ER	雌激素受体
FDA	美国食品药品监督管理局
GLOBOCAN	全球癌症发病率、死亡率和患病率
HPV	人乳头状瘤病毒
OCP	有机氯农药
PAH	多环芳烃
PCB	多氯联苯

PFC	全氟化合物
POP	持久性有机污染物
PR	孕激素受体
UV	紫外线
VOC	挥发性有机化合物

一、概述

多年来,受人体内外因素或环境因素的影响,癌症的发病率持续升高。目前,恶性肿瘤分子机制的相关学说认为:环境因素,包括对人体健康有害的高浓度化学物质,可以直接或间接导致肿瘤的发生,这些物质统称为致癌物[1]。根据全球癌症发病率、死亡率和患病率(global cancer incidence, mortality, and prevalence, GLOBOCAN) 2018年的数据,1/3的女性和1/2的男性在其一生中有患上癌症的可能。

二、致癌因素

癌症是一种因细胞DNA受损致其发生突变的疾病,变异细胞生长失控,进而从原发部位转移到身体其他部位。基因突变是一种永久性变化,使细胞中存在的遗传物质数量或结构发生改变。导致突变发生的物质称为诱变剂,致突变物质大多是致癌物质,但并非所有致癌物质都会引起突变[2,3]。

环境致癌物

长期接触化学物质、物理因素(如放射线和阳光)可导致人体发生癌症,这些物质被称为一般致癌物。能够通过食物、空气或材料进入人体的环境衍生物质或化学物质被称为环境致癌物。实验证据表明,并非任何情况下接触致癌物都会致癌,不同的暴露水平、强度和时间,以及个体的遗传物质特性等许多因素都可能影响癌症的发生风险[4]。在医学文献中,环境是一个更广泛的概念,包括许多与人类主要类型的癌症发生有关的非遗传因素(生活方式、饮食和感染因素)[5]。

当前生物学相关机制研究表明,大多数癌症起源于遗传因素和环境。干扰细胞机制和信号处理可能有助于预防由外部因素引发的癌症[6]。

三、致癌物质

癌症可由存在于人体内外的某种物质诱发。因此,科学家们把所有在人体外相互作用的因素称为环境。有很多因素会增加癌症的发生风险，包括衰老、家族史、吸烟、饮酒、有机和无机化学品、电离辐射、阳光、细菌、病毒、空气和水污染。这些因素根据来源可分为物理因素、化学因素和生物因素（图 15-1）。本章将讨论存在于人体内外的这些因素。

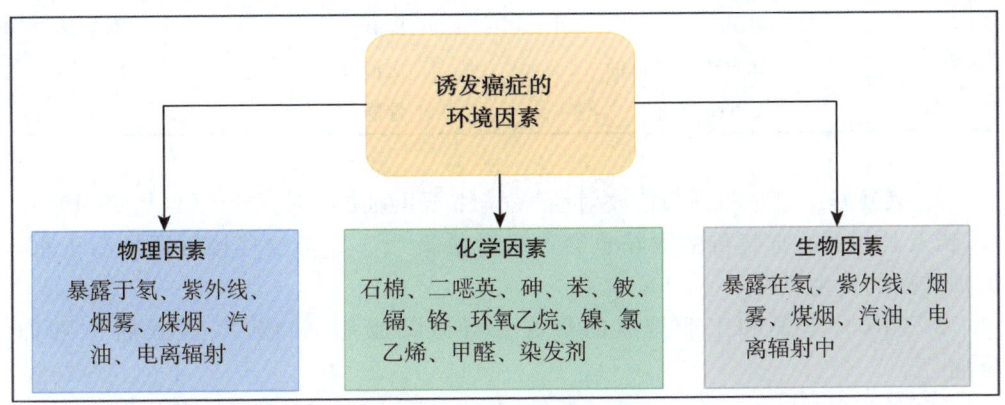

图 15-1　不同环境因素

（一）内在因素

人体内存在一些可以致癌的因素，例如，血液中激素水平异常、基因改变或免疫系统薄弱都可能导致癌症[7]。由于 DNA 的暴露或损伤，人们清除体内癌细胞或致癌物质的能力可能存在差异[8]，这些差异可能通过家族遗传，也可能与饮食或接触致癌物有关[9]。

（二）外在因素

因环境中存在的各种自然和人为因素导致的癌症约占 2/3[10]。这可能与个人习惯有关，如生活方式、饮酒、吸烟、不健康的饮食、缺乏锻炼等[11]。不健康的饮食、超重和缺乏锻炼是导致乳腺癌和前列腺癌的主要因素。接触石棉可导致肺癌，接触联苯胺可导致膀胱癌[12]。吸烟与口腔癌、肺癌、肾癌、食管癌直接相关，与胃癌、乳腺癌、宫颈癌、胰腺癌、肝癌间接相关[13]。致癌的环境因素可分为物理因素、化学因素和生物因素[14]。

（三）物理因素（表 15-1）

1. 紫外线辐射　黑色素瘤是由于暴露在来自阳光、日光浴和日光灯的紫外线辐射下而产生，这些辐射都会导致 DNA 损伤及皮肤过早老化[15]。

表 15-1　致癌因素:物理因素

致癌物名称	来源	影响部位	参考文献
氡暴露	矿物质衰变	肺	[1]
烟雾	汽车尾气,吸烟和空气污染	结肠和肺	[21]
煤烟	烟囱	皮肤	[22]
汽油	石油产品和石油	血液和肺	[23]
电离辐射	X射线照射	骨髓	[24]

2. 氡暴露　氡是一种惰性放射性气体,主要由铀的衰变和地下自然沉积物释放,铅及其相关的空气传播颗粒也会产生微量氡[16]。它与空气接触后易溶于水,增加肺癌的发生风险[17]。

3. 烟雾　车辆和工业排放的烟雾会导致结肠癌、肺癌[18]、乳腺癌[19]和卵巢癌[20]。

(四)化学因素(表 15-2)

1. 金属　据报道,被砷污染的水与肝癌、肺癌、膀胱癌、肾癌和皮肤癌的发生有关。肺癌主要发生在生产铍、镉化合物和镉金属行业的工作人员中[25],特别是国防、核能和航空航天行业。铬主要用于钢铁工业,与从事钢铁工业工人的肺癌发生有关。磷酸铅和醋酸铅是棉花染料和金属涂层的主要成分,会导致肾癌和脑癌[26]。镍用于电池、釉料、牙齿填充物和钢铁制造,鼻癌和肺癌与接触镍有关[27]。铁路和公路工程、车库工程、汽车修理和矿山排放的柴油废气也是潜在的致癌物,会增加患肺癌的风险[28]。

表 15-2　致癌因素:化学因素

致癌物名称	来源	影响部位
石棉	瓦片(地板及屋顶)	肺(间质瘤)
二噁英	冶炼和电气活动,药物处理	皮肤和肺
砷		
苯	洗涤剂,油漆,橡胶和石油	淋巴结和血液
铍	核反应堆,导弹燃料	肺
镉	涂料,油漆,电池	前列腺
铬	油漆、防腐剂和颜料	肺

续表

致癌物名称	来源	影响部位
乙烯	催熟剂,气体	血液
二氧化物		
镍	铁合金、陶瓷和电池	肺和鼻腔
氯乙烯	胶水和制冷剂	肝
甲醛	胶水和制冷剂	咽和鼻腔
染发剂	理发师和美发师	膀胱

2. 杀虫剂 常见的杀虫剂如滴滴涕(dichlorodiphenyltrichloroethane,DDT)、六氯苯、醋酸铅、杀草强、毒杀芬和环氧乙烷等,已因其具有致癌性而被禁止使用。数十年来的研究表明,农民、制造商、施用者和作物喷粉机驾驶员因接触农药而导致患淋巴癌、白血病、胃癌、脑癌、前列腺癌和黑色素瘤的风险增高[29]。

3. 二噁英 二噁英是碳氢化合物和含氯化合物化学加工过程中的副产品,它们通过纸浆和纸张漂白,以及医院和城市废物释放。有研究表明,二噁英会导致癌症[30]。

4. 多环芳烃 燃烧木材和燃料等含碳物质,车辆排放尾气和香烟的烟雾,会向空气中释放多芳烃(releases polyaromatic hydrocarbons,PAH)。暴露于 PAH 会导致皮肤癌、肺癌和泌尿系统癌症[31]。

5. 医疗药品 治疗癌症的药物氯苯、环磷酰胺和美法兰与白血病等继发性癌症的发生风险相关[32]。在器官移植中用作免疫抑制剂的硫唑嘌呤和环孢素与淋巴瘤的发生风险相关[33]。美国食品药品监督管理局(Food and Drug Administration,FDA)明确指出,使用这些治疗药物的患者在多年后患其他癌症的风险升高。

(五)生物因素(表 15-3)

1. 病毒和细菌 病毒和细菌与各种类型的癌症有关。例如,HPV 是一种性传播病毒,是导致肛门癌和宫颈癌的主要病因[34]。尽管携带 HPV 很常见,但 HPV 在初次性生活年龄过小或多个性伴侣的女性中携带率更高[35]。

2. 真菌毒素 生长在花生和谷物等常见食物上的某些真菌会产生一种称为黄曲霉毒素的致癌物质[36],被黄曲霉素污染的食物可被视为暴露源。

表 15-3 致癌因素:生物因素

致癌物名称	来源	影响部位	参考文献
肝炎病毒(B,C)	吸毒,医务人员	肝	[1,37]
Burkitt 淋巴瘤	南非人	淋巴结	[38]
幽门螺杆菌	严重细菌感染	胃	[39]
人乳头状瘤病毒	不止 1 个性伴侣	皮肤、宫颈和头/颈部	[40]

四、其他致癌因素

(一)烟草

接触含烟草产品,如雪茄、香烟和鼻烟,以及接触烟草烟雾引起死亡的人数占美国每年癌症死亡人数的 1/3。不同的烟草制品与肺癌、肾癌、口腔癌、结肠癌、咽喉癌、食管癌、胃癌及唇癌有关[41]。

(二)饮食/体重/缺乏运动

肥胖和超重被认为是某些癌症的主要原因[42]。缺乏运动的人容易患乳腺癌和结肠癌,而老年肥胖女性特别容易罹患子宫内膜癌、食管癌、肾癌和结肠癌[43]。

(三)酒精饮料

饮酒与食管癌、肝癌、口腔癌和喉癌有直接关系。与只吸烟的人群相比,经常饮酒(通常每天 2 杯)的人群患上述癌症的风险增加[44]。

人们发现,在所有的物理、化学和生物因素中,持久性有机污染物是导致各种类型癌症的突出因素,尤其是在女性中[45]。

五、女性特异性肿瘤

正常情况下,人体需要一定数量的细胞更新,旧细胞分解,新细胞在有序过程中再生。癌症发生始于细胞内部[46],当出现癌症迹象时,新细胞停止再生,现有细胞开始分裂,这种异常的细胞分裂也可以导致肿瘤发生。随着时间的推移,这些肿瘤细胞会干扰正常和健康细胞的发育进程并侵入其中。肿瘤最初可能并无症状,它的发展和转移需要数年时间[47]。肿瘤可分为良性和恶性两种,良性肿瘤具有部位特异性,不易扩散到身体其他部位;恶性肿瘤则可以从其原发部位逃逸,进入淋巴系统或血液，扩散到身体其他部位。随着时间的推移，一些良性肿瘤也可能变成恶性肿瘤。

癌症以其生长的特定器官或细胞类型命名[48]。结肠癌、乳腺癌、肺癌和胃癌是一些常见的癌症。发生在皮肤、黏膜组织和眼睛的黑色素细胞的癌症被称为黑色素瘤，黑色素细胞负责皮肤色素。淋巴瘤是在淋巴系统中发展并导致白血病（血细胞癌）的肿瘤（译者注：勘误，淋巴瘤是发生于淋巴系统的恶性肿瘤）。发生在肝、肺、乳腺或皮肤等上皮组织的肿瘤被称为癌。肉瘤是发生于骨骼细胞、脂肪、肌肉、结缔组织和软骨的恶性肿瘤。

有少数癌症通常只发生于女性，包括乳腺癌（译者注：勘误，男性乳腺癌也存在）、子宫内膜癌、卵巢癌和宫颈癌[49]。

（一）乳腺癌

乳腺癌是女性最常见的癌症之一，在世界范围内乳腺癌的发病率正以惊人的速度增长[50]。乳腺癌可以发生在任何年龄，但老年女性更常见。由于某些因素，一些女性可能比其他女性更容易患乳腺癌。因此，每位女性都应该知晓患乳腺癌的风险，以及如何减少接触环境致癌物从而降低患癌风险。有多项研究表明，环境中存在的某些化学物质在导致乳腺癌发生方面起着重要作用。因此，对化学物质诱发乳腺癌发病机制的研究是一个重要领域[51]。基因毒性物质更有可能对细胞的遗传物质造成损害，从而导致基因突变和癌症发生[52]。幼年时期接触电离辐射和医疗辐射，成年后患乳腺癌的风险显著提高[53]。

（二）子宫内膜癌

子宫内膜癌是一种发生于子宫内膜的癌症，子宫内膜癌的发病率随着女性年龄的增加而升高。他莫昔芬的应用可能会降低乳腺癌的风险，但会影响女性的激素水平[54]。月经初潮早、绝经晚、不孕症家族史或产次少和未生育均可增加患内膜癌的风险[55]。个人或家族有遗传性非息肉病性结直肠癌、多囊卵巢综合征或肥胖病史的女性患子宫内膜癌的风险也增加[56]。既往有乳腺癌或卵巢癌病史也可能增加患子宫内膜癌的风险[57]。

（三）宫颈癌

已知慢性 HPV 感染是宫颈癌最重要的危险因素之一[58]。HPV 通过阴道、不洁性生活等接触传播[59]。宫颈癌的其他危险因素包括吸烟、感染导致的免疫功能低下、肥胖和环境污染物[60]。

六、接触持久性有机污染物对女性健康的影响

持久性有机污染物(persistent organic pollutants,POP)是一种有机化合物,其中含有许多人工产生的化合物,如多氯联苯(polychlorinated biphenyls,PCB)、二噁英和有机氯农药(organochlorine pesticides,OCP)、全氟化合物(perfluorinated compounds,PFC)和多环芳烃(polyaromatic hydrocarbons,PAH),这些化合物由于耐光解和生化过程而留在环境中[61]。它们在机体的脂肪组织中累积,并最终转移到更高层次的食物链中[62]。工业活动中的技术进步导致每天向环境中释放的不同化学物质越来越多,这些化学物质和污染物对人类和生态系统都构成威胁。数十年来的流行病学研究报道显示,意外或职业暴露于金属和有机化合物会引发癌症[63]。

七、持久性有机污染物的作用机制

POP 暴露的细胞和分子机制与多种受体途径相关,其在不同器官中的毒性作用反映出影响疾病结果的不同机制。芳烃受体(aryl hydrocarbon receptor,AhR)途径的激活是介导 POP 不良影响的基本机制[64],它们会模拟人类内分泌激素的作用并破坏内分泌稳态[65]。DDT、二氯二苯二氯乙烯(dichlorodiphenyldichloro-ethylene,DDE)、多氯联苯和二噁英是主要的干扰内分泌的化学物质(endocrine-disrupting chemicals,EDC)[66]。

接触 POP 所涉及的化学物质可能与多个生物靶标相互作用,从而导致癌症易感性,以及内分泌和心血管系统的功能紊乱[67]。此外,女性、婴儿、儿童和老年人更容易受到 POP 的影响。例如,甲状腺疾病在女性中更为常见,而痴呆症常见于老年人或老年女性[68]。

八、持久性有机污染物对癌症的影响

关于女性接触 POP 的各种研究尤其侧重于乳腺癌。研究发现,患有乳腺癌的女性体内 PCB 含量较高,而乳腺癌的发生与全氟烷基酸和 PCB 之间存在显著关联[69]。

一项针对印度女性的研究报告称,乳腺癌与通过食用受污染食品摄入的 OCP 之间存在关联。此外,与老年患者相比,年轻患者体内的农药含量更高[70]。清除 POP,只能通过分娩和哺乳进行[71]。对阿拉斯加本土雌激素受体(estrogen receptor，ER)或孕激素受体(progesterone receptor，PR)阳性的乳腺癌女性患者的类似研究发现，这些女性体内的农药浓度很高[72]。西班牙的一项研究检测了乳腺癌患者血清和脂肪组织中的 POP 含量，证实某些 POP 可能导致了乳腺癌的侵袭性[73]。

一项针对日本女性的研究表明，其血清中一些 PCB 水平的升高与白细胞 DNA 的低甲基化有关。另一项针对格陵兰岛因纽特人的研究表明，血清 POP 高水平与白细胞 DNA 的低甲基化呈负相关，表明 POP 可以介导表观遗传，这可能是其致癌机制[74]。

一研究小组发现，居住在危险化学品废物场附近的居民中，女性乳腺癌的发病率和住院率会显著升高，这些危险化学品包括 POP 和挥发性有机化合物[75]。五大湖地区食用鱼类可使血清总 PCB 浓度升高，并与子宫肌瘤的发生呈正相关[76]。子宫肌瘤又称子宫平滑肌瘤，是由子宫平滑肌组织发展而来的良性肿瘤。检测子宫肌瘤患者相关的环境致癌物结果显示，PCB、POP 及其代谢物在皮下脂肪中的平均浓度较高。检验接受子宫肌瘤切除术的绝经前女性的子宫内膜也显示其对应浓度升高[76,77]。

九、结论

研究表明，OCP 与女性特异性癌症(包括宫颈癌、卵巢癌、子宫内膜癌和乳腺癌)的发生呈正相关。患有子宫体癌的女性血液中含有更高水平的 OCP(如狄氏剂)。

致谢

作者感谢 GITAM 提供的基础设施。

利益冲突

作者声明不存在利益冲突。

资助信息

RamaRao Malla(作者之一)感谢印度新德里的 DST-EMR(EMR/2016/002694)提供的财政支持。

参 考 文 献

[1] Parsa N. Environmental factors inducing human cancers. Iran J Public Health 2012;41

(11):1-9.

[2] Soto AM, Sonnenschein C. Environmental causes of cancer: endocrine disruptors as carcinogens. Nat Rev Endocrinol 2010;6(7):363-70.

[3] (a) Baccarelli A, Bollati V. Epigenetics and environmental chemicals. Curr Opin Pediatr 2009;21(2):243-51. (b) Ohshima H, Tatemichi M, Sawa T. Chemical basis of inflammation-induced carcino genesis. Arch Biochem Biophys 2003;417(1):3-11.

[4] Valavanidis A. Environmental carcinogenic substances, exposure and risk assessment for carcinogenci potential. Classifications and Regulations by International and National Institutions. Scientific reviews, Athens, Greece: Department of Chemistry, National and Kapodistrian University of Athens, University Campus Zografou; 2017.

[5] Tomatis L. Cancer: causes occurrence and control. IARC Scientific Publications; 1990.

[6] Sonnenschein C, Soto AM. Theories of carcinogenesis: an emerging perspective. Semin Cancer Biol 2008;18(5):372-7.

[7] Bardeesy N, DePinho RA. Pancreatic cancer biology and genetics. Nat Rev Cancer 2002;2 (12): 897-909.

[8] Ladiges W. Mouse models of XRCC1 DNA repair polymorphisms and cancer. Oncogene 2006; 25(11):1612-9.

[9] Salnikow K, Zhitkovich A. Genetic and epigenetic mechanisms in metal carcinogenesis and cocarcinogenesis: nickel, arsenic, and chromium. Chem Res Toxicol 2008;21(1):28-44.

[10] Wild CP. Environmental exposure measurement in cancer epidemiology. Mutagenesis 2009;24(2): 117-25.

[11] Weiderpass E. Lifestyle and cancer risk. J Prev Med Public Health 2010;43(6):459-71.

[12] Calle EE, Kaaks R. Overweight, obesity and cancer: epidemiological evidence and proposed mechanisms. Nat Rev Cancer 2004;4(8):579-91.

[13] Boyle P. Cancer, cigarette smoking and premature death in Europe: a review including the recommendations of European cancer experts consensus meeting, Helsinki, October 1996. Lung Cancer 1997; 17(1):1-60.

[14] Trosko JE, Chang C-C. Environmental carcinogenesis: an integrative model. Q Rev Biol 1978; 53(2):115-41.

[15] (a) Mead MN. Benefits of sunlight: a bright spot for human health. National Institute of Environmental Health Sciences; 2008. (b) Gasparro FP. Sunscreens, skin photobiology, and skin cancer: the need for UVA protection and evaluation of efficacy. Environ Health Perspect 2000;108(Suppl 1):71-8.

[16] Varshney R. Natural radioactivity and Radon/Thoron measurement in environment & quantification of heavy elements. Aligarh Muslim University; 2013.

[17] Darby S, Hill D, Auvinen A, Barros-Dios J, Baysson H, Bochicchio F, Deo H, Falk R, Forastiere F, Hakama M. Radon in homes and risk of lung cancer: collaborative analysis of individual data from 13 European case-control studies. BMJ 2005;330(7485):223.

[18] Kloog I, Haim A, Stevens RG, Portnov BA. Global co-distribution of light at night (LAN) and cancers of prostate, colon, and lung in men. Chronobiol Int 2009;26(1): 108-25.

[19] Matsumoto H, Adachi S, Suzuki Y. Bisphenol A in ambient air particulates responsible for the proliferation of MCF-7 human breast cancer cells and its concentration changes over 6 months. Arch Environ Contam Toxicol 2005;48(4):459-66.

[20] Hung L-J, Chan T-F, Wu C-H, Chiu H-F, Yang C-Y. Traffic air pollution and risk of death from ovarian cancer in Taiwan: fine particulate matter (PM2.5) as a proxy marker. J Toxicol Environ Health A 2012;75(3):174-82.

[21] Møller P, Folkmann JK, Forchhammer L, Bräuner EV, Danielsen PH, Risom L, Loft S. Air pollution, oxidative damage to DNA, and carcinogenesis. Cancer Lett 2008;266(1): 84-97.

[22] Hogstedt C, Jansson C, Hugosson M, Tinnerberg H, Gustavsson P. Cancer incidence in a cohort of Swedish chimney sweeps, 1958-2006. Am J Public Health 2013;103(9): 1708-14.

[23] Okoro A, Ani E, Ibu J, Akpogomeh B. Effect of petroleum products inhalation on some haematological indices of fuel attendants in Calabar metropolis, Nigeria. Niger J Physiol Sci 2006;21:1-2.

[24] Madani I, De Neve W, Mareel M. Does ionizing radiation stimulate cancer invasion and metastasis? Bull Cancer 2008;95(3):292-300.

[25] (a) Huff J, Lunn RM, Waalkes MP, Tomatis L, Infante PF. Cadmium-induced cancers in animals and in humans. Int J Occup Environ Health 2007;13(2):202-12. (b) Tchounwou PB, Yedjou CG, Patlolla AK, Sutton DJ. Heavy metal toxicity and the environment. In: Molecular, clinical and environmental toxicology. Springer; 2012. p. 133-64.

[26] (a) Alghazal M, Šutiaková I, Kovalkovičová N, Legath J, Falis M, Pistl J, Sabo R, Beňová K, Sabova L, Váczi P. Induction of micronuclei in rat bone marrow after chronic exposure to lead acetate trihydrate. Toxicol Ind Health 2008;24(9):587-93. (b) Naja GM, Volesky B. Metals in the environment: toxicity and sources. In: Wang LK, Chen JP, Hung YT, Shammas NK, editors. Handbook on heavy metals in the environment. Boca Raton, FL: Taylor & Francis and CRC Press; 2009. p. 13-61 [chapter 2].

[27] (a) Martin S, Griswold W. Human health effects of heavy metals. Environ Sci Technol Briefs Citizens 2009;15:1-6. (b) Goyer RA, Clarkson TW. Toxic effects of metals. In: Casarett and Doull's toxicology: the basic science of poisons. 5:Center for Hazardous Substance Research (CHSR), Kansas State University; 1996. p. 696-8.

[28] Boffetta P, Harris RE, Wynder EL. Case-control study on occupational exposure to diesel exhaust and lung cancer risk. Am J Ind Med 1990;17(5):577-91.

[29] (a) Blair A, Zahm SH. Agricultural exposures and cancer. Environ Health Perspect 1995; 103(Suppl 8):205-8. (b) Alavanja MC, Hoppin JA, Kamel F. Health effects of chronic

pesticide exposure: cancer and neurotoxicity. Annu Rev Public Health 2004;25:155-97.

[30] (a)Kogevinas M. Human health effects of dioxins: cancer, reproductive and endocrine system effects. APMIS 2001;109(S103):S223-32; (b)Cole P, Trichopoulos D, Pastides H, Starr T, Mandel JS. Dioxin and cancer: a critical review. Regul Toxicol Pharmacol 2003; 38(3):378-88.

[31] (a) Boffetta P, Jourenkova N, Gustavsson P. Cancer risk from occupational and environmental exposure to polycyclic aromatic hydrocarbons. Cancer Causes Control 1997;8(3): 444-72. (b) Mastrangelo G, Fadda E, Marzia V. Polycyclic aromatic hydrocarbons and cancer in man. Environ Health Perspect 1996;104(11):1166-70.

[32] Cuzick J, Erskine S, Edelman D, Galton D. A comparison of the incidence of the myelodysplastic syndrome and acute myeloid leukaemia following melphalan and cyclophosphamide treatment for myelomatosis. Br J Cancer 1987;55(5):523-9.

[33] Opelz G, Dohler B. Lymphomas after solid organ transplantation: a collaborative transplant study report. Am J Transplant 2004;4(2):222-30.

[34] (a) Burd EM. Human papillomavirus and cervical cancer. Clin Microbiol Rev 2003;16(1): 1-17. (b) Krzowska-Firych J, Lucas G, Lucas C, Lucas N, Pietrzyk Ł. An overview of human papillomavirus (HPV) as an etiological factor of the anal cancer. J Infect Public Health 2019;12(1):1-6.

[35] Castellsagué X. Natural history and epidemiology of HPV infection and cervical cancer. Gynecol Oncol 2008;110(3 Suppl 2):S4-7.

[36] (a) Wogan GN. Aflatoxins as risk factors for hepatocellular carcinoma in humans. Cancer Res 1992;52(7 Suppl):2114s-2118s. (b) Dvorackova I. Aflatoxin inhalation and alveolar cell carcinoma. Br Med J 1976;1(6011):691. (c) Pitt J. Toxigenic fungi and mycotoxins. Br Med Bull 2000;56(1):184-92.

[37] (a) Buendia M. Mammalian hepatitis B viruses and primary liver cancer. Semin Cancer Biol 1992; 3(5):309-20. (b) Perz JF, Armstrong GL, Farrington LA, Hutin YJ, Bell BP. The contributions of hepatitis B virus and hepatitis C virus infections to cirrhosis and primary liver cancer worldwide. J Hepatol 2006;45(4):529-38.

[38] Bornkamm GW, Hausen HZ, Stein H, Lennert K, Ruggeberg F, Bartels H. Attempts to demonstrate virus-specific sequences in human tumors. IV. EB viral DNA in European Burkitt lymphoma and immunoblastic lymphadenopathy with excessive plasmacytosis. Int J Cancer 1976;17(2):177-81.

[39] Song ZQ, Zhou LY. Helicobacter pylori and gastric cancer: clinical aspects. Chin Med J (Engl) 2015;128(22):3101-5.

[40] (a) Rettig EM, D'Souza G. Epidemiology of head and neck cancer. Surg Oncol Clin N Am 2015; 24(3):379-96. (b) Yete S, D'Souza W, Saranath D. High-risk human papillomavirus in oral cancer: clinical implications. Oncology 2018;94(3):133-41.

[41] Shiels MS, Gibson T, Sampson J, Albanes D, Andreotti G, Beane Freeman L, Berrington

de Gonzalez A, Caporaso N, Curtis RE, Elena J, Freedman ND, Robien K, Black A, Morton LM. Cigarette smoking prior to first cancer and risk of second smoking-associated cancers among survivors of bladder, kidney, head and neck, and stage Ⅰ lung cancers. J Clin Oncol Off J Am Soc Clin Oncol 2014;32(35):3989-95.

[42] Bianchini F, Kaaks R, Vainio H. Overweight, obesity, and cancer risk. Lancet Oncol 2002;3(9):565-74.

[43] Calle EE, Thun MJ. Obesity and cancer. Oncogene 2004;23(38):6365-78.

[44] (a) Pelucchi C, Gallus S, Garavello W, Bosetti C, La Vecchia C. Cancer risk associated with alcohol and tobacco use: focus on upper aero-digestive tract and liver. Alcohol Res Health 2006;29(3):193-8. (b) Elwood JM, Pearson JC, Skippen DH, Jackson SM. Alcohol, smoking, social and occupational factors in the aetiology of cancer of the oral cavity, pharynx and larynx. Int J Cancer 1984;34(5):603-12.

[45] Wikoff D, Fitzgerald L, Birnbaum L. Persistent organic pollutants: an overview. In: Dioxins and health, vol. 3; John Wiley & Sons, Inc.; 2012. p. 1-36

[46] Ewing J. Neoplastic diseases, a text-book on tumors: James Ewing... with 479 illustrations. WB Saunders Company; 1919.

[47] Nguyen DX, Bos PD, Massague J. Metastasis: from dissemination to organ-specific colonization. Nat Rev Cancer 2009;9(4):274-84.

[48] Lengauer C, Kinzler KW, Vogelstein B. Genetic instabilities in human cancers. Nature 1998; 396(6712):643-9.

[49] (a) Weiderpass E, Labrèche F. Malignant tumors of the female reproductive system. In: Occupational cancers. Springer; 2014. p. 409-22. (b) Pike MC, Pearce CL, Wu AH. Prevention of cancers of the breast, endometrium and ovary. Oncogene 2004;23(38):6379-91.

[50] Forouzanfar MH, Foreman KJ, Delossantos AM, Lozano R, Lopez AD, Murray CJ, Naghavi M. Breast and cervical cancer in 187 countries between 1980 and 2010: a systematic analysis. Lancet 2011; 378(9801):1461-84.

[51] Cancer IB, Committee ERC. Breast cancer and the environment: prioritizing prevention. National Institute of Environmental Health Sciences; 2013.

[52] Lee SJ, Yum YN, Kim SC, Kim Y, Lim J, Lee WJ, Koo KH, Kim JH, Kim JE, Lee WS, Sohn S, Park SN, Park JH, Lee J, Kwon SW. Distinguishing between genotoxic and non-genotoxic hepato-carcinogens by gene expression profiling and bioinformatic pathway analysis. Sci Rep 2013;3:2783.

[53] (a) Land CE, Tokunaga M, Koyama K, Soda M, Preston DL, Nishimori I, Tokuoka S. Incidence of female breast cancer among atomic bomb survivors, Hiroshima and Nagasaki, 1950-1990. Radiat Res 2003;160(6):707-17. (b) Henderson TO, Amsterdam A, Bhatia S, Hudson MM, Meadows AT, Neglia JP, Diller LR, Constine LS, Smith RA, Mahoney MC, Morris EA, Montgomery LL, Landier W, Smith SM, Robison LL, Oeffinger KC.

Systematic review: surveillance for breast cancer in women treated with chest radiation for childhood, adolescent, or young adult cancer. Ann Intern Med 2010;152(7):444-55 w144-54.

[54] van Leeuwen FE, Van den Belt-Dusebout A, Benraadt J, Diepenhorst F, Van Tinteren H, Coebergh J, Kiemeney L, Gimbrère C, Otter R, Schouten L. Risk of endometrial cancer after tamoxifen treatment of breast cancer. Lancet 1994;343(8895):448-52.

[55] (a) Ali AT. Reproductive factors and the risk of endometrial cancer. Int J Gynecol Cancer 2014; 24(3):384-93. (b) Modan B, Ron E, Lerner-Geva L, Blumstein T, Menczer J, Rabinovici J, Oelsner G, Freedman L, Mashiach S, Lunenfeld B. Cancer incidence in a cohort of infertile woman. Am J Epidemiol 1998;147(11):1038-42.

[56] (a) Bharati R, Jenkins MA, Lindor NM, Le Marchand L, Gallinger S, Haile RW, Newcomb PA, Hopper JL, Win AK. Does risk of endometrial cancer for women without a germline mutation in a DNA mismatch repair gene depend on family history of endometrial cancer or colorectal cancer? Gynecol Oncol 2014;133(2):287-92. (b) Schmeler KM, Soliman PT, Sun CC, Slomovitz BM, Gershenson DM, Lu KH. Endometrial cancer in young, normal-weight women. Gynecol Oncol 2005;99(2):388-92.

[57] Tulinius H, Egilsson V, Olafsdottir GH, Sigvaldason H. Risk of prostate, ovarian, and endometrial cancer among relatives of women with breast cancer. Br Med J 1992; 305 (6858):855-7.

[58] Bosch F, Munoz N, De Sanjosé S. Human papillomavirus and other risk factors for cervical cancer. Biomed Pharmacother 1997;51(6-7):268-75.

[59] Dietz CA, Nyberg CR. Genital, oral, and anal human papillomavirus infection in men who have sex with men. J Am Osteopath Assoc 2011;111(3_Suppl_2):S19-25.

[60] (a) Baay M, Verhoeven V, Avonts D, Vermorken J. Risk factors for cervical cancer development: what do women think? Sex Health 2004;1(3):145-9. (b) Wang LD-L, Lam WWT, Wu J, Fielding R. Hong Kong Chinese women's lay beliefs about cervical cancer causation and prevention. Asian Pac J Cancer Prev 2014;15(18):7679-86. (c) Scheurer ME, Danysh HE, Follen M, Lupo PJ. Association of traffic-related hazardous air pollutants and cervical dysplasia in an urban multiethnic population: a cross-sectional study. Environ Health 2014;13(1):52.

[61] (a) Ritter L, Solomon K, Forget J, Stemeroff M, O'Leary C. Persistent organic pollutants: an assessment report on: DDT, aldrin, dieldrin, endrin, chlordane, heptachlor, hexachlorobenzene, mirex, toxaphene, polychlorinated biphenyls, dioxins and furans. International Programme on Chemical Safety(IPCS); 1995. (b) Ritter L, Solomon K, Forget J, Stemeroff M, O'Leary C. In: Persistent organic pollutants. An assessment report on: DDT-aldrin-dieldrin-chlordane-heptachlor-hexachlorobenzene-mirex-toxaphene, polychlorinated biphenyls, dioxins and furans. Second Meeting of ISG, Canberra, Australia; 1996. p. 5-8. (c) El-Shahawi MS, Hamza A, Bashammakh AS, Al-Saggaf WT. An over-

view on the accumulation, distribution, transformations, toxicity and analytical methods for the monitoring of persistent organic pollutants. Talanta 2010;80(5):1587-97.

[62] Vallack HW, Bakker DJ, Brandt I, Broström-Lundén E, Brouwer A, Bull KR, Gough C, Guardans R, Holoubek I, Jansson B, Koch R, Kuylenstierna J, Lecloux A, Mackay D, McCutcheon P, Mocarelli P, Taalman RD. Controlling persistent organic pollutants—what next? Environ Toxicol Pharmacol 1998;6(3):143-75.

[63] Chow W-H, Dong LM, Devesa SS. Epidemiology and risk factors for kidney cancer. Nat Rev Urol 2010;7(5):245.

[64] Sorg O. AhR signalling and dioxin toxicity. Toxicol Lett 2014;230(2):225-33.

[65] (a) Geyer HJ, Rimkus GG, Scheunert I, Kaune A, Schramm K-W, Kettrup A, Zeeman M, Muir DC, Hansen LG, Mackay D. Bioaccumulation and occurrence of endocrine-disrupting chemicals (EDCs), persistent organic pollutants (POPs), and other organic compounds in fish and other organisms including humans. In: Bioaccumulation—new aspects and developments. Springer; 2000. p. 1-166. (b) De Coster S, Van Larebeke N. Endocrine-disrupting chemicals: associated disorders and mechanisms of action. J Environ Public Health 2012;2012:713696. https://doi.org/10.1155/2012/713696.

[66] (a) Aoki Y. Polychlorinated biphenyls, polychlorinated dibenzo-p-dioxins, and polychlorinated dibenzofurans as endocrine disrupters—what we have learned from Yusho disease. Environ Res 2001;86(1):2-11. (b) De Coster S, van Larebeke N. Endocrine-disrupting chemicals: associated disorders and mechanisms of action. J Environ Public Health 2012; 2012:713696. (c) Boverhof DR, Kwekel JC, Humes DG, Burgoon LD, Zacharewski TR. Dioxin induces an estrogen-like, estrogen receptor-dependent gene expression response in the murine uterus. Mol Pharmacol 2006;69(5): 1599-606.

[67] Khalil N, Chen A, Lee M. Endocrine disruptive compounds and cardio-metabolic risk factors in children. Curr Opin Pharmacol 2014;19:120-4.

[68] (a) Fantini F, Porta D, Fano V, De Felip E, Senofonte O, Abballe A, D'Ilio S, Ingelido AM, Mataloni F, Narduzzi S, Blasetti F, Forastiere F. Epidemiologic studies on the health status of the population living in the Sacco River Valley. Epidemiol Prev 2012;36(5 Suppl 4):44-52. (b) Lee DH, Lind PM, Jacobs Jr. DR, Salihovic S, van Bavel B, Lind L. Association between background exposure to organochlorine pesticides and the risk of cognitive impairment: a prospective study that accounts for weight change. Environ Int 2016; 89-90:179-84.

[69] Wielsøe M, Kern P, Bonefeld-Jørgensen EC. Serum levels of environmental pollutants is a risk factor for breast cancer in Inuit: a case control study. Environ Health 2017;16(1):56.

[70] Mathur V, Bhatnagar P, Sharma RG, Acharya V, Sexana R. Breast cancer incidence and exposure to pesticides among women originating from Jaipur. Environ Int 2002;28(5):331-6.

[71] Fernández-Rodríguez M, Arrebola JP, Artacho-Cordón F, Amaya E, Aragones N, Llorca J, Perez-Gomez B, Ardanaz E, Kogevinas M, Castano-Vinyals G, Pollan M, Olea N.

Levels and predictors of persistent organic pollutants in an adult population from four Spanish regions. Sci Total Environ 2015;538:152-61.

[72] (a) Holmes AK, Koller KR, Kieszak SM, Sjodin A, Calafat AM, Sacco FD, Varner DW, Lanier AP, Rubin CH. Case-control study of breast cancer and exposure to synthetic environmental chemicals among Alaska Native women. Int J Circumpolar Health 2014;73:25760. (b) Holmes AK, Koller KR, Kieszak SM, Sjodin A, Calafat AM, Sacco FD, Varner DW, Lanier AP, Rubin CH. Case-control study of breast cancer and exposure to synthetic environmental chemicals among Alaska Native women. Int J Circumpolar Health 2014;73(1):25760.

[73] Arrebola JP, Fernández-Rodríguez M, Artacho-Cordón F, Garde C, Perez-Carrascosa F, Linares I, Tovar I, González-Alzaga B, Expósito J, Torne P, Fernández MF, Olea N. Associations of persistent organic pollutants in serum and adipose tissue with breast cancer prognostic markers. Sci Total Environ 2016;566-567:41-9.

[74] (a) Itoh H, Iwasaki M, Kasuga Y, Yokoyama S, Onuma H, Nishimura H, Kusama R, Yoshida T, Yokoyama K, Tsugane S. Association between serum organochlorines and global methylation level of leukocyte DNA among Japanese women: a cross-sectional study. Sci Total Environ 2014;490:603-9. (b) Rusiecki JA, Baccarelli A, Bollati V, Tarantini L, Moore LE, Bonefeld-Jorgensen EC. Global DNA hypomethylation is associated with high serum-persistent organic pollutants in Greenlandic Inuit. Environ Health Perspect 2008;116(11):1547-52.

[75] Lu X, Lessner L, Carpenter DO. Association between hospital discharge rate for female breast cancer and residence in a zip code containing hazardous waste sites. Environ Res 2014;134:375-81.

[76] Lambertino A, Turyk M, Anderson H, Freels S, Persky V. Uterine leiomyomata in a cohort of Great Lakes sport fish consumers. Environ Res 2011;111(4):565-72.

[77] Schaefer WR, Hermann T, Meinhold-Heerlein I, Deppert WR, Zahradnik HP. Exposure of human endometrium to environmental estrogens, antiandrogens, and organochlorine compounds. Fertil Steril 2000;74(3):558-63.

第 16 章
CYP1B1 基因 rs1056836 位点多态性与子宫内膜癌风险的荟萃分析

Samrat Rakshit, L. V. K. S. Bhaskar

Department of Zoology, Guru Ghasidas Vishwavidyalaya, Bilaspur, Chhattisgarh, India

摘要

子宫内膜癌（endometrial cancer，EMC）是最常见的妇科肿瘤，占全球女性癌症死亡人数的 2% 以上。本文总结了 CYP1B1 rs1056836 变异与 EMC 风险之间的关系。为了收集数据，笔者严格检索了 Google Scholar、PubMed 和 Embase，以获取相关的已发表的文章。CYP1B1 rs1056836 与 EMC 之间的相关性通过计算 95% 置信区间（confidence intervals，CI）的比值比（odds ratios，OR）来评估。通过 Cochrane Q 检验计算 I^2 统计量的值，以确定研究的异质性。为了解研究间的异质性，笔者进行了亚组分析和敏感性分析，采用漏斗图和 Egger 检验来确定发表偏倚。17 项独立研究共调查了 4804 例 EMC 患者和 7185 例对照者 CYP1B1 rs1056836 多态性与 EMC 风险的关系。显性遗传模型的汇总分析显示，CYP1B1 rs1056836 多态性与 EMC（$OR=1.31$；95% CI 1.08～1.59；$P=0.005$）种族间存在显著异质性，未观察到发表偏倚。综上所述，本荟萃分析显示 rs1056836 变异是发生 EMC 的主要危险因素，还需要进一步的研究来探究这些关联的临床和生物学意义。

关键词

子宫内膜癌，单核苷酸多态性，荟萃分析，多态性，置信区间，比值比

缩略词

CI	置信区间
CYP1B1	细胞色素 P-450 1B1
EMC	子宫内膜癌
OR	比值比
SNP	单核苷酸多态性

一、概述

子宫内膜癌(endometrial cancer, EMC)是最常见的妇科肿瘤,占全球女性癌症死亡人数的2%以上,仅次于乳腺癌[1,2]。与世界其他地区相比,北美和欧洲部分地区的EMC患者人数更多[1,2],这是因为这些地区肥胖和代谢综合征的人群更多[1,3]。最近的报道表明,EMC的发病率和相关死亡率较前升高,并可能在未来10年内继续升高[1]。仅在2012年,全球就报告了319 605例新增EMC病例,其中包括死亡76 160例[2]。除遗传危险因素外,一些非遗传危险因素如肥胖、缺乏运动、外源性雌激素过度使用、胰岛素抵抗、乳腺癌后使用他莫昔芬等均与EMC风险增加有关[2]。EMC患者中高达81%合并肥胖,19%~36%为病态肥胖。除了目前EMC的标准治疗方法,包括切除子宫(子宫切除术)同时切除输卵管和卵巢外,还可以考虑其他治疗方法,如辅助放疗和化疗[4]。

细胞色素P-450 1B1(cytochrome P-450 1B1, $CYP1B1$)基因位于2号染色体p22-p21上,在人类恶性肿瘤中普遍过表达,并且可被多种致癌物激活。该酶在多环芳烃、前致癌物和某些抗癌药物的代谢中起主要作用,导致致癌物活化,最终引起肿瘤发生[5]。$CYP1B1$通过激活蛋白和改变组织对激素及抗癌药物的反应,可以促进癌症的发展。在人群中,迄今为止已报道了50多种$CYP1B1$单核苷酸多态性(single nucleotide polymorphism, SNP)[6-8]。$CYP1B1$在人类子宫内膜中的表达相对较高,但其作用机制尚不清楚。$CYP1B1$最常见的4种多态性[Gly在密码子48(rs10012)处的Arg、Ser在密码子119(rs1056827)处的Ala、Val在密码子432(rs1056836)处的Leu和Ser在密码子453(rs1800440)处的Asn]已在不同癌症中表达,其中包括EMC。$CYP1B1$的催化活性受到这4种多态性的影响[7,8]。$CYP1B1$基因编码一种羟化酶细胞色素P450 1B1,将雌激素转化为儿茶酚类雌激素或2-羟基雌激素[9]。$CYP1B1$基因rs1056836的多态性增加了EMC的风险[10]。此前进行的一些荟萃分析,目的在于研究$CYP1B1$多态性(rs1056836)和其他多态性与EMC之间的关系,但这些荟萃分析并未包含所有已发表的研究,包括一些已经发表的样本量更大的原始研究。为获得$CYP1B1$ Leu432Val与EMC风险之间相关性更确凿的证据,笔者进行了另一项荟萃分析。

二、材料和方法

(一)数据选择

截至2020年1月24日,笔者在PubMed、Google Scholar和EMbase数据库中对EMC和CYP1B1 rs1056836多态性的关联研究进行了全面检索。在考虑用于荟萃分析的任何报告之前,对已发表的符合条件文章的参考文献进行人工检索,检索持续进行至没有相关的研究为止,且只纳入英文文献[9-25]。

本荟萃分析纳入标准:①rs1056836 CYP1B1基因型多态性的病例对照研究;②rs1056836与EMC之间的相关性研究;③有足够数据计算95%CI和P值的OR的研究。排除标准:①数据重叠的研究;②病例研究;③没有CYP1B1 rs1056836多态性的研究;④以非英语语言发表的文章。笔者收集了每项研究的主要作者姓名、发表年份、原籍国、病例及对照组的种族和基因型。

(二)统计分析

为评估CYP1B1 rs1056836与EMC风险之间的关联强度,使用优势模型部署95%CI的粗略OR。采用Q检验和I^2统计量评估研究间异质性。由于存在显著的异质性($I^2>77\%$,$P<0.001$),采用随机效应模型评估合并的OR。采用Egger线性回归检验和Begg漏斗图评估发表偏倚,采用留一法进行敏感性分析。按种族进行亚组分析,$P<0.05$具有统计学意义。最后,使用MetaGenyo网络工具对数据进行分析[26]。

三、结果

如图16-1所示,基于搜索策略,通过在线数据库的严格搜索,确定了57篇可能相关的已发表文章。笔者发现并删除了14项重复研究,在检查这些研究的真实性时,排除了一篇已被撤回的研究。在仔细查看标题和摘要后,又排除25篇与其他SNP相关或数据无法使用的文章。最后,有17项符合标准的研究纳入了荟萃分析。目前的荟萃分析包括CYP1B1 rs1056836多态性,涉及4804例患者和7185例对照。所有研究中CYP1B1 rs1056836多态性的基因型频率见表16-1。在一些研究中已发现HardyWeinberg平衡偏差。

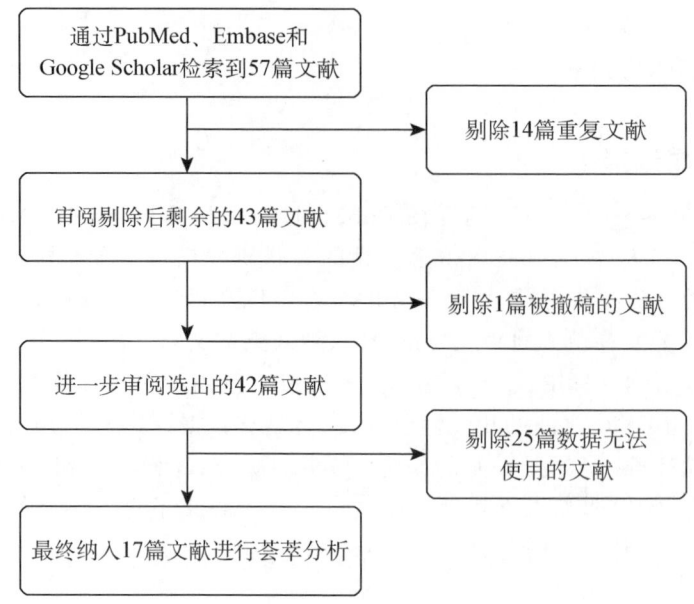

图 16-1　荟萃分析的研究特征流程图

表 16-1　rs1056836 SNP 基因型在 EMC 和对照组中的分布情况

参考文献	国家	种族	EMC			对照组			HW P 值
			CC	CG	GG	CC	CG	GG	
Sasaki 等[11]	中国	亚洲人	59	39	17	69	24	7	0.028
McGrath 等[12]	美国	白种人	61	113	45	193	316	146	0.441
Zimarina[13]	俄罗斯/挪威	白种人	25	62	34	37	73	22	0.166
Rylander-Rudqvist 等[14]	瑞典	白种人	195	336	134	425	676	279	0.733
Doherty 等[15]	美国	白种人	115	170	86	145	194	81	0.266
Rebbeck 等[16]	美国	白种人	119	371ª		376	877ª		NC
Tao 等[17]	中国	亚洲人	792	232	13	806	206	22	0.044
Cho 等[18]	韩国	亚洲人	160	25	3	178	41	2	0.831
Ye 等[19]	中国	亚洲人	71	29	0	70	40	0	0.020
Hirata 等[20]	美国	白种人	53	64	33	55	72	38	0.130
Ashton 等[21]	澳大利亚	亚洲人	32	88	71	50	139	101	0.854

续表

参考文献	国家	种族	EMC			对照组			HW P 值
			CC	CG	GG	CC	CG	GG	
Sliwinski 等[10]	波兰	白种人	29	37	34	33	31	36	<0.001
Rebbeck 等[22]	美国	白种人	77	107[a]		154	37[a]		NC
El-Shennawy 等[23]	埃及	白种人	96	59	5	74	19	7	0.002
Lundin 等[9]	瑞典/意大利/美国	白种人	126	189	76	221	352	131	0.659
Li 等[24]	中国	亚洲人	165	67	18	188	54	8	0.103
Zhou 等[25]	中国	亚洲人	34	26	12	55	19	6	0.032

注:EMC. 子宫内膜癌;NC. 未计算;[a]CG+GG(译者注:原文未标注)。

采用 Q 统计获得的研究间异质性表明,研究间存在显著异质性($I^2>77\%$;$P<0.001$)。图 16-2 显示了涉及 rs1056836 和 rs1056836 关联的每个单独研究,以及合并研究($n=17$)的森林图。

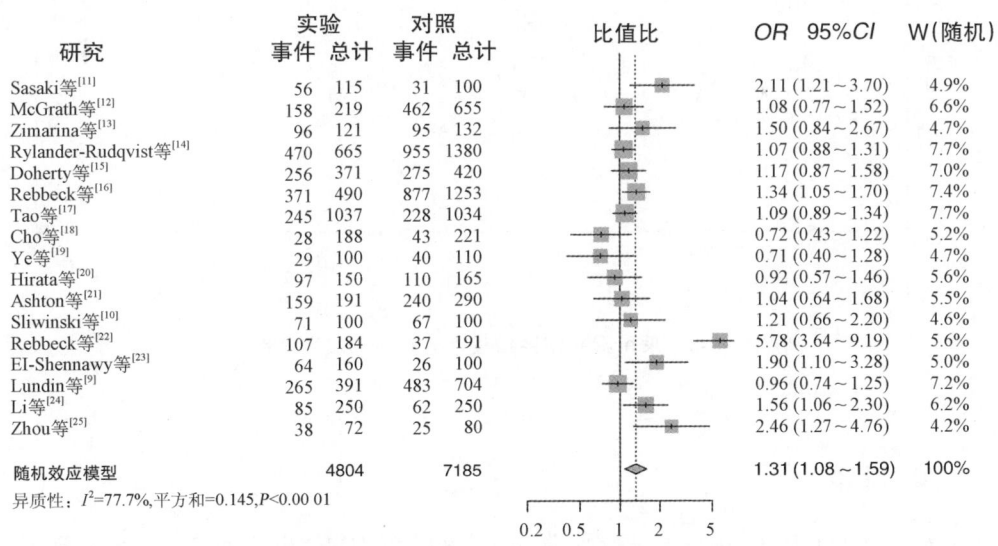

图 16-2 rs1056836 SNP 基因型在 EMC 和对照组中的分布情况

显性遗传模型的汇总分析显示,$CYP1B1$ rs1056836 多态性与 EMC 发生显著相关($OR=1.31,95\%CI\ 1.08\sim1.59;P<0.005$),如图 16-2 所示。亚组分析显示,rs1056836 多态性与高加索人群 EMC 风险显著相关($OR=1.38,95\%CI\ 1.05\sim1.80;P<0.019$),但在亚洲人群中没有显著相关($OR<1.22,95\%CI\ 0.91\sim1.64;P=0.174$)。在 Begg 漏斗图中未发现明显不对称,表明没有发表偏倚(图 16-3)。Egger 检验进一步证实无发表偏倚(优势模型,$P=0.211$)。笔者为证实研究的稳定性,通过逐一剔除每个独立研究来进行敏感性分析,结果显示,合并的 OR 没有任何实质性差异(图 16-4)。

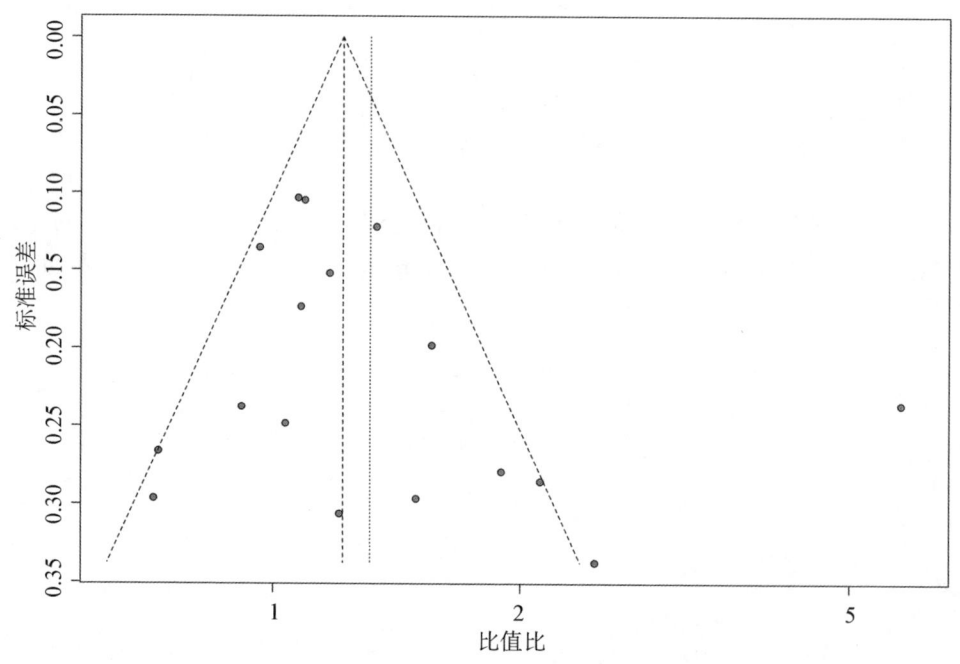

图 16-3 采用漏斗图评估荟萃分析中的发表偏倚

四、讨论

笔者分析了从 17 项独立研究中收集的 4804 例 EMC 患者和 7185 例对照,这些研究分析了 $CYP1B1$ rs1056836 多态性与 EMC 风险之间的相关性。在显性遗传模型中发现 $CYP1B1$ rs1056836 与 EMC 发病风险呈正相关,且观察到研究间存在显著的异质性。亚组分析显示 rs1056836 与高加索人 EMC 发病相关,而与亚洲人无关,未观察到发表偏倚。笔者的荟萃分析结果与之前报道的 $CYP1B1$

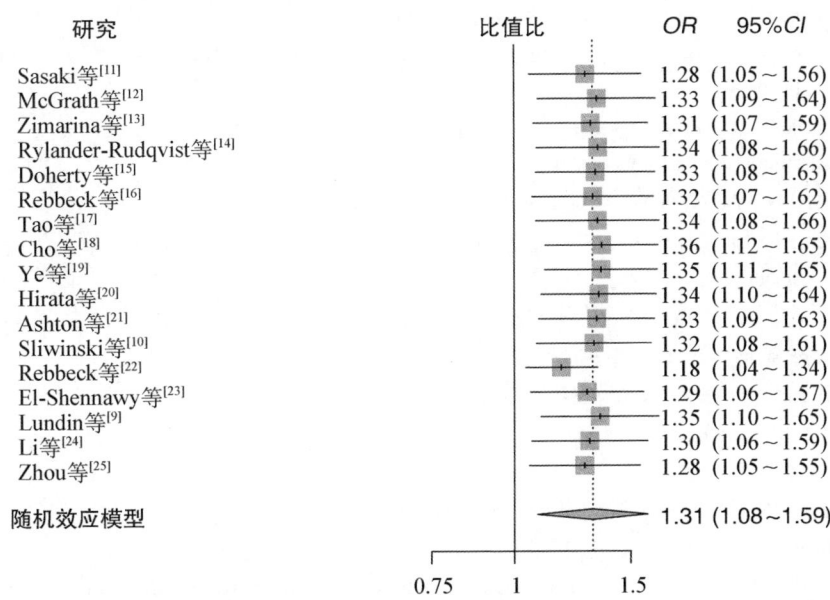

图 16-4 本荟萃分析的敏感性分析

rs1056836 多态性[6,27,28]增加 EMC 风险的部分荟萃分析一致。与此相反,其他荟萃分析显示 CYP1B1 rs1056836 多态性与 EMC 发病风险之间无相关性[29]。

CYP450 促进类固醇激素生物合成,并有助于致癌物的代谢活化。CYP1B1 是该系统的主要酶,有助于将雌激素转化为 4-羟基雌激素[23]。CYP1B1 在多种人类恶性肿瘤中过表达并激活多种致癌因子。CYP1B1 可以催化特定多环芳烃的二氢二醇形成并将其氧化为致癌性二氢二醇环氧化物。早期研究报道了 CYP1B1 Leu432Val 在所有癌症发病风险中的作用,但结果仍存在争议。Zhou 等报道 EMC 组 CYP1B1 rs1056836 多态性基因型 G/G 和 C/G 的频率高于对照组[25]。与此相反,其他一些研究发现,CYP1B1 rs1056836 多态性与人群 EMC 发病风险无显著相关性[21]。

综上所述,该荟萃分析发现 rs1056836 是 EMC 发生的主要危险因素,仍需要进一步的研究去揭示这些关联之间的临床和生物学意义。

参 考 文 献

[1] Clarke MA, Long BJ, Morillo ADM, Arbyn M, Bakkum-Gamez JN, Wentzensen N. Association of endometrial cancer risk with postmenopausal bleeding in women: a systematic review and meta-analysis. JAMA Intern Med 2018;178(9):1210-22.

[2] Raglan O, Kalliala I, Markozannes G, Cividini S, Gunter MJ, Nautiyal J, et al. Risk factors for endometrial cancer: an umbrella review of the literature. Int J Cancer 2019;145(7):1719-30.

[3] Morice P, Leary A, Creutzberg C, Abu-Rustum N, Darai E. Endometrial cancer. Lancet 2016;387(10023):1094-108.

[4] Galaal K, Donkers H, Bryant A, Lopes AD. Laparoscopy versus laparotomy for the management of early stage endometrial cancer. Cochrane Database Syst Rev 2018;10:CD006655.

[5] Li C, Long B, Qin X, Li W, Zhou Y. Cytochrome P1B1 (CYP1B1) polymorphisms and cancer risk: a meta-analysis of 52 studies. Toxicology 2015;327:77-86.

[6] Liu J-Y, Yang Y, Liu Z-Z, Xie J-J, Du Y-P, Wang W, et al. Association between the CYP1B1 polymorphisms and risk of cancer: a meta-analysis. Mol Genet Genomics 2015;290(2):739-65.

[7] Falero-Perez J, Song Y-S, Sorenson CM, Sheibani N. CYP1B1: a key regulator of redox homeostasis. Trends Cell Mol Biol 2018;13:27.

[8] van den Berg M, van Duursen MB. Mechanistic considerations for reduced endometrial cancer risk by smoking. Curr Opin Toxicol 2019;14:52-9.

[9] Lundin E, Wirgin I, Lukanova A, Afanasyeva Y, Krogh V, Axelsson T, et al. Selected polymorphisms in sex hormone-related genes, circulating sex hormones and risk of endometrial cancer. Cancer Epidemiol 2012;36(5):445-52.

[10] Sliwinski T, Sitarek P, Stetkiewicz T, Sobczuk A, Blasiak J. Polymorphism of the ERα and CYP1B1 genes in endometrial cancer in a Polish subpopulation. J Obstet Gynaecol Res 2010;36(2):311-7.

[11] Sasaki M, Tanaka Y, Kaneuchi M, Sakuragi N, Dahiya R. Alleles of polymorphic sites that correspond to hyperactive variants of CYP1B1 protein are significantly less frequent in Japanese as compared to American and German populations. Hum Mutat 2003;21(6):652.

[12] McGrath M, Hankinson SE, Arbeitman L, Colditz GA, Hunter DJ, De Vivo I. Cytochrome P450 1B1 and catechol-O-methyltransferase polymorphisms and endometrial cancer susceptibility. Carcinogenesis 2004;25(4):559-65.

[13] Zimarina T, Kristensen V, Imyanitov E, Berstein L. Polymorphisms of CYP1B1 and COMT in breast and endometrial cancer. Mol Biol 2004;38(3):322-8.

[14] Rylander-Rudqvist T, Wedren S, Jonasdottir G, Ahlberg S, Weiderpass E, Persson I, et al. Cytochrome P450 1B1 gene polymorphisms and postmenopausal endometrial cancer risk. Cancer Epidemiol Biomarkers Prev 2004;13(9):1515-20.

[15] Doherty JA, Weiss NS, Freeman RJ, Dightman DA, Thornton PJ, Houck JR, et al. Genetic factors in catechol estrogen metabolism in relation to the risk of endometrial cancer. Cancer Epidemiol Biomarkers Prev 2005;14(2):357-66.

[16] Rebbeck TR, Troxel AB, Wang Y, Walker AH, Panossian S, Gallagher S, et al. Estro-

gen sulfation genes, hormone replacement therapy, and endometrial cancer risk. J Natl Cancer Inst 2006;98(18):1311-20.

[17] Tao MH, Cai Q, Xu WH, Kataoka N, Wen W, Zheng W, et al. Cytochrome P450 1B1 and catechol-O-methyltransferase genetic polymorphisms and endometrial cancer risk in Chinese women. Cancer Epidemiol Biomarkers Prev 2006;15(12):2570-3.

[18] Cho YJ, Hur SE, Lee JY, Song IO, Moon H-S, Koong MK, et al. Single nucleotide polymorphisms and haplotypes of the genes encoding the CYP1B1 in Korean women: no association with advanced endometriosis. J Assist Reprod Genet 2007;24(7):271-7.

[19] Ye Y, Cheng X, Luo H-B, Liu L, Li Y-B, Hou Y-P, et al. CYP1A1 and CYP1B1 genetic polymorphisms and uterine leiomyoma risk in Chinese women. J Assist Reprod Genet 2008;25(8):389-94.

[20] Hirata H, Hinoda Y, Okayama N, Suehiro Y, Kawamoto K, Kikuno N, et al. CYP1A1, SULT1A1, and SULT1E1 polymorphisms are risk factors for endometrial cancer susceptibility. Cancer 2008;112(9):1964-73.

[21] Ashton KA, Proietto A, Otton G, Symonds I, McEvoy M, Attia J, et al. Polymorphisms in genes of the steroid hormone biosynthesis and metabolism pathways and endometrial cancer risk. Cancer Epidemiol 2010;34(3):328-37.

[22] Rebbeck TR, Su HI, Sammel MD, Lin H, Tran TV, Gracia CR, et al. Effect of hormone metabolism genotypes on steroid hormone levels and menopausal symptoms in a prospective population-based cohort of women experiencing the menopausal transition. Menopause 2010;17(5):1026.

[23] El-Shennawy GA, Elbialy A-AA, Isamil AE, El Behery MM. Is genetic polymorphism of ER-α, CYP1A1, and CYP1B1 a risk factor for uterine leiomyoma? Arch Gynecol Obstet 2011;283(6):1313-8.

[24] Li Y, Tan S-Q, Ma Q-H, Li L, Huang Z-Y, Wang Y, et al. CYP1B1 C4326G polymorphism and susceptibility to cervical cancer in Chinese Han women. Tumour Biol 2013;34(6):3561-7.

[25] Zhou J, Zhang L, Wei L, Wang J. Endometrial carcinoma-related genetic factors: application to research and clinical practice in China. BJOG 2016;123:90-6.

[26] Martorell-Marugan J, Toro-Dominguez D, Alarcon-Riquelme ME, Carmona-Saez P. MetaGenyo: a web tool for meta-analysis of genetic association studies. BMC Bioinformatics 2017;18(1):563.

[27] Teng Y, He C, Zuo X, Li X. Catechol-O-methyltransferase and cytochrome P-450 1B1 polymorphisms and endometrial cancer risk: a meta-analysis. Int J Gynecol Cancer 2013;23(3):422-30.

[28] Wang F, Zou Y-F, Sun G-P, Su H, Huang F. Association of CYP1B1 gene polymorphisms with susceptibility to endometrial cancer: a meta-analysis. Eur J Cancer Prev 2011;20(2):112-20.

[29] Wang X-W, Chen Y-L, Luo Y-L, Liu Q-Y. No association between the CYP1B1 C4326G polymorphism and endometrial cancer risk: a meta-analysis. Asian Pac J Cancer Prev 2011;12:2343-8.

第 17 章
纳米技术的发展在乳腺癌中的应用

Kiranmayi Patnala[a], Soumya Vishwas[a], Rama Rao Malla[b]

[a] Department of Biotechnology, Institute of Science, GITAM (Deemed to be University), Visakhapatnam, Andhra Pradesh, India
[b] Cancer Biology Lab, Department of Biochemistry and Bioinformatics, Institute of Science, GITAM (Deemed to be University), Visakhapatnam, Andhra Pradesh, India

摘要

癌症是人类死亡的主要原因之一，是一个全球关注的问题。过去10年在了解癌症发生、发展及其治疗方面取得了惊人进展。然而，随着癌症发病率的不断升高，临床上管理癌症仍是一个挑战。乳腺癌是发达国家及发展中国家最常见的女性恶性肿瘤，是20～59岁女性死亡的主要原因，也是60岁以上女性死亡的第二原因，仅次于肺癌。因此，更有效的治疗对晚期乳腺癌患者来说至关重要。纳米技术是化学、生物学、工程学和医学相结合的综合研究领域，是一项可以满足肿瘤检测和治疗需求的新兴技术。纳米技术正在用来开发女性特异性肿瘤的新型治疗，值得一提的是，基于纳米颗粒的给药系统为这种新型治疗策略提供了潜在益处。

关键词

乳腺癌，癌症管理，化疗，纳米技术，纳米疗法

缩略词

AAV2	腺相关病毒2型
ART	青蒿素
CDK4	细胞周期蛋白依赖性激酶4
CNT	碳纳米管
CPSNP	磷酸钙纳米颗粒
CPSNP	磷酸钙纳米颗粒药物递送系统
DOX	多柔比星
DTX	多西他赛
GNP	金纳米颗粒
H&E	苏木精和伊红

HER	人表皮生长因子受体
ICG	吲哚菁绿
LTNP	脂质纳米颗粒
MRI	磁共振成像
NDDS	基于纳米技术的给药
NIR	近红外
NP	纳米颗粒
PBS	磷酸盐缓冲液
PDT	光动力疗法
PEG	聚乙二醇
PINT	光免疫疗法
PTA	光热消融
QD	量子点
SERM	选择性雌激素受体调节剂
TAM	他莫昔芬
Tf	转铁蛋白
TNBC	三阴性乳腺癌
ZnMCPPc	含锌的单羧基苯氧基酞菁化合物

一、概述

癌症是全球人类死亡的主要原因[1,2]，它被定义为细胞的无节制生长和增殖，通常发生在基因突变的数年内[3,4]。癌细胞在分裂时,促进生长的基因不断复制而变得不稳定,从而获得致死性[5]。女性特有的肿瘤起源于女性的主要或次要生殖器官。女性肿瘤的主要种类包括卵巢癌、宫颈癌和乳腺癌,统称为妇科肿瘤。在过去,对癌症的发生、发展和治疗方面的研究已取得了重大进展,然而,随着癌症发病率的不断上升,临床上癌症的管理仍是一个巨大的挑战。大量研究表明,血管生成、细胞死亡、生长因子结合、转录或信号转导等一些生物学过程在肿瘤中都会受到干扰[6]。这些研究结果启发了人们去寻找对应合理的抗癌药物,从而产生了拉帕替尼、吉非替尼、利妥昔单抗、曲妥珠单抗、西妥昔单抗、贝伐珠单抗和伊马替尼等一些用于治疗肿瘤的新型药物,这些药物均已被批准用于常规临床试验。目前的治疗方法在于破坏肿瘤细胞、阻断其血液供应或改变基因受损机制[7]。手术切除癌变部位、化学治疗和放射治疗等常规治疗都有其自身的局限性[8]。手术治疗并不能使所有肿瘤患者受益,因为即使手术完全切除受累器官,后续肿瘤也可能复发。放疗虽然能成功破坏肿瘤细胞,但也对周围的健康细胞有害[7]。化疗是另一种通过药物毒性杀死肿瘤细胞的方式,通过抑制细胞分裂或阻止营养摄取等方式破坏肿瘤细胞[9],但治疗晚期肿瘤成功率很低。目前可用的化疗药物只能使患者实现短时间内无瘤生存。化疗失败的原因之一是化疗药物无法特异性到达肿瘤部位发挥作用,以及剂量限制性毒性[10]。因此,研发能够克服药物毒性和耐药性的先进的化疗药物或靶点特异性药物递送系统令人憧憬[11]。这些系统具有破坏肿瘤细胞而不损伤健康组织的潜能,并将药物高效、特异地递送到作用部位,以达到最佳的治疗效果。在这种背景下,基于纳米技术的治疗策略或许可能成为治疗肿瘤的有效方法。

二、纳米技术在癌症管理中的应用

纳米技术是一项将化学、生物学、工程学和医学相结合的综合研究领域。这一新兴领域满足了肿瘤检测和治疗创新性方法的需求[12]。纳米技术可以定义为在纳米级水平制造和/或利用材料。这项技术可以通过扩展一组原子来实现,也可以通过将大型材料缩小到纳米级粒子来实现。由于其可调的理化特性,纳米颗粒(nanoparticles,NP)在技术进步中占据重要位置。肿瘤诊断和治疗、成像和药物递送等不同的生物疗法使用多种生物纳米材料[13]。这些 NP 的径线可达数百纳米,容易与细胞表面或细胞内存在的生物分子相互作用[14]。设计 NP 用于肿瘤诊断、成像和治疗的纳米平台,它们通过克服许多物理、医学或生物障碍,可有效实现靶向给药。肿瘤纳米装置由金纳米粒子(gold NP,GNP)、顺磁性纳米粒子、碳纳米管(carbon nanotubes,CNT)、量子点(quantum dots,QD)、脂质体和 MRI 造影剂组成。基于 NP 的方法用于检测 DNA 和蛋白质具有较高的特异性,与传统方法相比具有明显优势[12,15-17]。生物亲和力 NP 探针的发展使分子和细胞成像、药物靶向和设计纳米设备用于肿瘤早期检测的方法变得更加容易。这些进展为肿瘤个体化治疗提供了合适机会,可以根据患者特征个体化使用蛋白质和遗传生物标志物[18]。关于药物有效载荷和稳定性的文献表明,NP 制剂具有较高的载药量,适用于通过各种途径分配疏水性和亲水性物质[19]。这些制剂可能通过选择性地利用肿瘤独特生理特性将活性药物转运到肿瘤细胞。与常规疗法相比,基于纳米技术明确靶向肿瘤细胞的给药系统(nanotechnology-based drug-delivery systems,NDDS)显示出更长的有效期,可以通过各种途径更好地给药(图 17-1)。

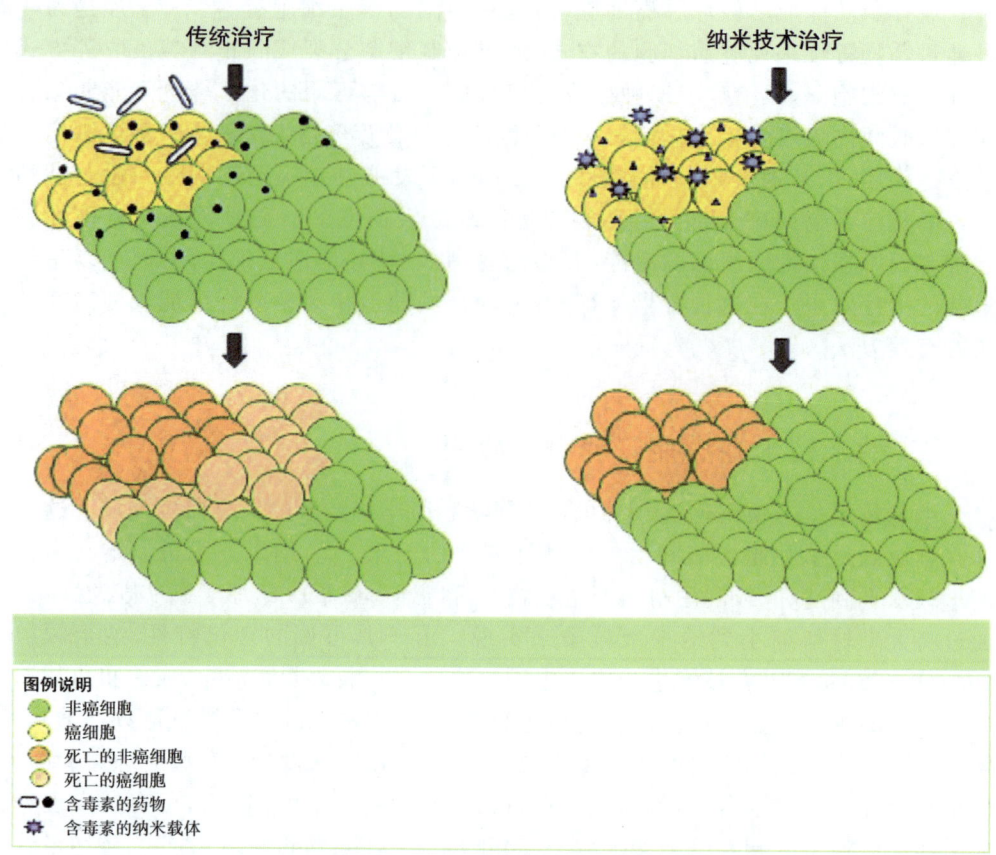

图 17-1　纳米技术相较于传统癌症治疗的优势

注：纳米制剂有可能通过选择性地利用肿瘤独特的病理生理学将活性药物运送到癌细胞中。这些基于纳米技术的药物递送系统或基于纳米技术的给药系统（NDDS）明确针对癌细胞，对邻近的非癌细胞无影响。与传统化疗相比，该系统表现出更长的有效期并实现更佳的药物分布。

NP 系统材料特性的发展直接改善了其向效应部位的分布[20]。目前使用的肿瘤治疗 NP 包括胶束、脂质体树状大分子、脂质纳米颗粒、蛋白质纳米颗粒、金属纳米颗粒、病毒纳米颗粒、陶瓷纳米颗粒、聚合物纳米颗粒（polymeric NP, PNP）和碳纳米管[21]。脂质体是大小为 50～450 nm 的球形囊泡，由类固醇和磷脂组成。脂质体的结构与细胞膜的结构相当，这种结构特性可以促进药物有效进入细胞[22]。脂质体可与疏水性或亲水性药物一起使用。这些脂质体能够使治疗药物结构更加稳定并改善其分布。此外，它们具有生物相容性和生物降解性。传统脂质体由 2 种材料填充，聚乙二醇（polyethylene glycol, PEG）结合到聚乙二醇化脂质体表面达到空间平衡。碳水化合物、肽和抗体等配体与配体靶向脂质体的外部连接,或者尾端与先前连接的聚乙二醇链连接。治疗性脂质体是传统脂质体、聚乙二醇化脂质体和配体靶向脂质体的融合[23]。

聚合物胶束(<100 nm)是一种自组装结构,由具有两亲性质的聚合物分子链卷曲形成。疏水性药物如紫杉醇、多西他赛或喜树碱可装载到疏水核心中,亲水外壳可将该系统溶于水中从而稳定核心颗粒。由于其分布范围有限,肾脏排泄缓慢,从而渗透性和滞留性作用增强(enhanced permeability and retention,EPR),容易在受累组织中蓄积。此外,其聚合物外壳可防止与生物因子产生不明的相互作用[24,25]。树枝状大分子是一种具有高度分支、单分散性和明显球状结构的化合物,因其表面可以很容易地添加功能性分子,而被认为是药物递送的杰出制剂[26]。这种结构特征可在其边缘添加和呈现抗原分子,从而具有多功能性。通常通过氢键、疏水作用、化学键或与聚合物支架偶联将药物装载到核心腔中[27]。

无机 NP 包括二氧化硅、氧化铁、金和银颗粒。大多数 NP 正处于临床试验阶段,只有少数已真正用于临床。银和金纳米颗粒与脂质体、树状大分子和胶束的不同点在于,其具有表面等离子体共振(surface plasmon resonance,SPR)的特殊性质。它们具有良好的生物相容性和表面功能化的通用性[28]。纳米晶体是一种小于 1000 nm 的非合金颗粒药物,这些药物不需要连接载体分子,通过使用表面活性剂或聚合物空间稳定剂达到稳定。加入纳米混悬液能够减轻纳米晶体在任何边缘液体介质(如水或液体聚乙二醇和油)中的悬浮[29]。纳米晶体的特性使其能够克服诸如膜的黏附力增加、溶解速度增加和饱和溶解度增加等难题。

QD 是大小为 2~10 nm 的半导体纳米晶体,其大小决定了其发光和吸光度等光学性质。其发射波长<650 nm,这是生物医学成像的关键特征,因为生物组织表现出光散射减少和光吸收降低,所以,量子点超越了纳米医学领域常规使用的有机材料[30]。此外,使用相同光源可将不同组成和大小的量子点激发到广泛的光谱范围内[31,32]。因此,量子点对集体成像非常有吸引力。量子点作为造影剂,也被广泛研究用于药物递送成像和传感[30,33,34]。生物聚合物 NP 包括生物来源的多糖和蛋白质[35],作为基于蛋白质的 NP,它们可以很容易地分解并附着在特定药物或预制的配体上。

三、乳腺癌

乳腺癌是全球女性最常见的肿瘤,也是所有年龄段女性死亡的主要原因。已知乳腺癌患者的死亡原因是肿瘤转移至淋巴结、肺、肝、骨和脑,因此,更有效的治疗对晚期患者的生存至关重要。目前的治疗手段包括手术、放疗、激素治疗和化疗[36]。这些治疗的局限性是缺乏特异性，因此，基于 NP 的给药系统提供了潜在获益的可能。

四、纳米技术在化疗中的应用

紫杉烷类和蒽环类药物是晚期乳腺癌的关键性化疗药物[37]。他莫昔芬-NP、氟维司群和芳香化酶抑制剂是众所周知的激素药物。他莫昔芬是一种"抗雌激素"药物，通过与乳腺癌细胞中的 ER 受体结合来阻断雌激素的作用。目前，大多数乳腺癌都会使用他莫昔芬治疗[38]。

Doxil 是一种包裹多柔比星的聚乙二醇化脂质体，是美国 FDA 批准使用的药物，它通过嵌入 DNA 碱基对来抑制 DNA 的合成和转录，可用于治疗肉瘤、乳腺癌和卵巢癌[39]。有研究表明，每个月使用剂量 $50~mg/m^2$ 的多柔比星脂质体与每 21 天给予相同剂量的普通多柔比星可获得同样的疗效。值得注意的是，多柔比星脂质体显著降低了游离多柔比星峰值浓度相关的心脏毒性风险[40]。

Genexol-PM 是目前正在进行临床试验的纳米药物。它是一种新型紫杉醇聚合物胶束制剂，临床证实其可递送比常规化疗剂量更高剂量的紫杉醇[41]。Ⅱ期临床试验中使用 Genexol-PM 治疗转移性乳腺癌总缓解率为 $43.5\%\sim73.7\%$。新型制剂的全身毒性和不良反应降低可能要归功于缺少了聚氧乙基化蓖麻油，这种物质用于增加紫杉醇的溶解度，并与超敏反应有关[42]。

紫杉醇与微管结合并促进微管蛋白聚合，从而在细胞分裂期间稳定微管聚合物并抑制聚合物解体[43]。因此，癌细胞内的微管运动、有丝分裂和转运被阻断，从而导致细胞凋亡[44]。Abraxane 是一种获得美国 FDA 批准的药物，其粒径为 130 nm，由紫杉醇和人血清白蛋白在高压下均质化后制成[45,46]。在 NP 白蛋白结合型紫杉醇中，白蛋白和紫杉醇通过可逆的非共价键连接构成复合物，与细胞表面的 gp60 受体结合，随后通过质膜微囊转运至血管外[47]。

在生理盐水中，白蛋白结合型紫杉醇可以复溶至剂量 $<10~mg/ml$，这远大于 Cremophor-EL 紫杉醇。因此，白蛋白结合型紫杉醇可以安全地使用更大剂量，并显著缩短注射时间，而且无须留置导管，无须为预防超敏反应提前用药[45,48]。在一项针对转移性乳腺癌患者的Ⅲ期临床试验中，白蛋白结合型紫杉醇注射剂量比紫杉醇耐受剂量高出约 50%，结果显示，与紫杉醇相比，白蛋白结合型紫杉醇的清除率和分布容积更高，缓解率也更高（$34\%~vs.~19\%$）。

纳米医学相关的研究表明，多西他赛（docetaxel，DTX）、紫杉醇（paclitaxel，Taxol）和多柔比星（doxorubicin，DOX）等药物可以通过石墨烯、富勒烯和 CNT 等有效靶向或以受控方式递送至受累部位[49-54]。当富勒烯 C60 与多西他赛（C60/DTX）联合用于系统构象时,多西他赛的生物利用度增加高达 4 倍,而清除率最高降低 50%[51]。此外,该 C60/DTX 复合物与红细胞相容,在 2 h 内以受控方式释放多西他赛,疗效达 84.32%。此外,与使用游离多西他赛相比,C60/DTX 复合物对 MCF-7 和 MDA-MB-231 细胞系表现出更高的细胞毒性。HA-MWCNT/Tf@ART 是 Zhang 等开发的一种靶向肿瘤 MCF-7 细胞的给药系统,该系统在体外处理这些细胞[55]。在这个系统中,用透明质酸功能化的 MWCNT 作为青蒿素（artemisinin,ART）药物靶向转铁蛋白（targeting transferrin,Tf）配体的载体,即使在辐射下,ART 也可以通过其在癌细胞内的蓄积而表现出抑瘤作用。

有研究表明,功能化的 MWCNT 可作为 MRI 中有效的细胞探针,因为 CNT 可以携带成像[56,57]。也有研究表明,钆（gadolinium,Gd）碳纳米管可作为高质量试剂用于小鼠体内 MRI 检查[58]。在网状内皮系统的循环过程中,磷脂功能化的 CNT 具有更高的生物相容性和稳定性[59]。单羧基苯氧基酞菁锌（Zinc mono carboxy phenoxy phthalocyanine,ZnMCPPc）与亚精胺偶联并吸附到单臂碳纳米管（SWCNT）（即 ZnMCPPc-spermine-SWCNT）上,对 MCF-7 细胞表现出光动力疗法（photodynamic therapy,PDT）的活性[60]。当 ZnMCPPc-spermine-SWCNT 在这些 MCF-7 细胞系上测试而不暴露在光照下时,它对测试的乳腺癌细胞表现出无毒性。此外,40 mM 精胺试验结果显示可以改善 PDT 的疗效。另外,开发了一种可以用于癌症诊断、磁性靶向、PDT 和射频辅助热疗的多功能系统[61]。该系统是利用叶酸、PEG、氧化铁 NP 和富勒烯 C60 建立的,此外,针对该系统的研究并未显示体内或体外的显著毒性。石墨烯纳米点可有效用于内脏器官或深部组织的癌症成像。当在 MDA-MB231 细胞系上进行测试时,这些羧基功能化的石墨烯纳米点可有效杀死 70% 以上的乳腺癌细胞,进而证明它们在光动力疗法中的潜在用途[62]。

Hwang 等开发了一个识别早期乳腺癌的系统,该系统使用石墨烯传感器,不仅有助于检测早期肿瘤,还有助于检测肿瘤可能发生的任何突变[63]。曼彻斯特大学的研究人员表示,石墨烯可以靶向选择肿瘤干细胞,而对正常细胞无毒性[64]。Hwang 等开发了一种可以灵敏识别突变和早期乳腺癌的石墨烯传感器[63],该项成果也得到了其他研究人员的支持。研究结果表明,氧化石墨烯对健康细胞无毒性,可作为特异性靶向肿瘤干细胞的抗癌药物[64]。虽然这些技术较新颖,但它们在预防或治疗乳腺癌方面展现出的结果令人期待。各种纳米药物治疗乳腺癌的临床试验列于表 17-1。

表 17-1　纳米药物治疗乳腺癌的临床试验

药物	美国生产商	平台型临床试验	美国的使用动态
Abraxane	Abraxis Bioscience	纳米颗粒白蛋白结合型紫杉醇	2005年获批
多柔比星	Janssen Products	PEG化脂质体/盐酸多柔比星	1995年获批
NK-105 临床试验信息库：NCT01644890	Nippon Kayaku	PEG-聚天冬氨酸/紫杉醇	Ⅲ期
Genexol-PM 临床试验信息库：NCT00876486	Samyang Biopharmaceuticals	PEG-聚(D,L-丙交酯)/紫杉醇	Ⅲ期
Myocet 临床试验信息库：NCT00294996	Sopherion Therapeutics	非PEG化脂质体/多柔比星	Ⅲ期
NK-012 临床试验信息库：NCT00951054	Nippon Kayaku	PEG-聚谷氨酸/SN-38	Ⅱ期
LEP-ETU	INSYS Therapeutics	脂质体/紫杉醇	Ⅱ期
Xyotax 临床试验信息库：NCT00148707	Dana-Farber Cancer Institute	紫杉醇-聚谷氨酸	Ⅱ期
Liposomal Annamycin（阿霉素脂质体） 临床试验信息库：NCT00012129	New York University, School of Medicine	脂质体/半合成多柔比星类似物	Ⅰ/Ⅱ期
ThermoDox 临床试验信息库：NCT00826085	Celsion	热激活脂质体/多柔比星	Ⅰ/Ⅱ期
Rexin-G 临床试验信息库：NCT00505271	Epeius Biotechnologies	靶向蛋白标记的磷脂/microRNA122	Ⅰ/Ⅱ期
SPI-077 临床试验信息库：NCT01861496	LiPlasome Pharma	隐形脂质体顺铂	Ⅰ期

续表

药物	美国生产商	平台型临床试验	美国的使用动态
BIND-014 临床试验信息库： NCT01300533	BIND	PEG-聚乳酸-羟基乙酸共聚物/多西他赛	Ⅰ期
Nanoxel 临床试验信息库： NCT00915369	Fresenius Kabi Oncology	PEG-聚(D,L-丙交酯)/多西他赛	Ⅰ期
S-CKD602 临床试验信息库： NCT00177281	Alza	聚乙二醇脂质体/CKD602	Ⅰ期

五、纳米技术在新型疗法中的应用

HER2是一种受体酪氨酸激酶，在调节基因、细胞生长及其迁移、增殖、凋亡和癌细胞的其他反应中发挥重要作用[65]。HER2/HER3是效应最强的肿瘤激活的二聚化组合[66]，在大多数乳腺肿瘤中过表达[65,67]。HER2的过表达可用于靶向治疗乳腺癌的纳米药物的开发。第一种临床HER2靶向药物是曲妥珠单抗[68]，它有2个抗原特异性位点可以黏附HER2，从而阻止酪氨酸激酶的激活和HER2二聚化[69]。曲妥珠单抗可激活免疫细胞，产生细胞介导的细胞毒性，从而促进癌细胞死亡[70]。曲妥珠单抗的应用也会增强其他化疗药物的治疗效果[71]。曲妥珠单抗被广泛应用，可以单药使用或与其他化疗药物联合用于辅助治疗，以减少癌症复发并在临床上改善HER2阳性患者的整体生存期[72]。

曲妥珠单抗中2个抗原特异性位点的识别和结合，使其能够直接靶向识别HER2过表达的癌细胞[69]。Anhorn等开发了表面功能化的负载多柔比星的纳米颗粒(doxorubicin-doped albumin NP,DOX-NP)和曲妥珠单抗的联合物(DOX-NP-曲妥珠单抗)。这种DOX-NP-曲妥珠单抗可与乳腺癌细胞(SK-Br-3)中73%的HER2结合，这种细胞结合的增加依赖于曲妥珠单抗的浓度，在HER2低表达的细胞系MCF-7细胞中未观察到这种结合的增加[73]。不幸的是，部分患者在使用曲妥珠单抗后达到初始缓解1年内出现了曲妥珠单抗耐药[65]。因此，研究者们开发了其他HER2靶向治疗的策略。帕妥珠单抗是另一种与HER2结合并阻断HER受体同源和异源二聚化的单克隆抗体。目前，关于帕妥珠单抗的临床试验主要集中在评价帕妥珠单抗与其他药物联合治疗乳腺癌的疗效[74-76]。酪氨酸激酶拮抗剂拉帕替尼(Tykerb)是另一种类型的HER2抑制剂。近期一项体内研究表明，脂质纳米颗粒(lipid nanoparticles,LTNP)拉帕替尼比游离拉帕替尼和拉帕替尼混悬液的有效率高3~5倍[77]。此外,乳腺癌细胞摄取LTNP后可以导致细胞凋亡[78]。

乳腺癌的一个重要亚型是三阴性乳腺癌(triple-negative breast cancer,TNBC),是依据孕激素受体、雌激素受体和HER2的低表达或完全缺失来进行分类的,具有高侵袭性和高转移性特点,近15%的女性乳腺癌患者是此种类型[79]。由于癌细胞的增殖率高、复发早和生存率低,TNBC的治疗是目前临床面临的重大挑战之一。治疗TNBC的化疗药物包括顺铂、紫杉烷类和蒽环类药物[80],但TNBC患者的总体预后不佳[81]。TNBC患者1年、3年和5年的估计总生存率分别为90%、74%和64%,而非TNBC患者分别为97%、89%和81%[82]。研究TNBC的新型有效的疗法是当务之急。Alam等报道了一种利用腺相关病毒2型(adeno-associated virus type 2,AAV2)在体内诱导癌细胞坏死性死亡和抑制TNBC肿瘤生长的TNBC新疗法。将三阴性MDA-MB-435细胞植入皮下,在接受AAV2治疗后观察到肿瘤生长被显著抑制[83]。这种新型病毒感染治疗乳腺癌的方案显示出很大的潜力。

在体外条件下,载有针对细胞周期蛋白依赖性激酶4(cyclin-dependent kinase 4,CDK4)的小干扰RNA(siRNA)的脂质纳米粒使MDA-MB-468乳腺癌细胞摄取siRNA的能力增加16倍[84]。LNP-siRNA可有效诱导MDA-MB-468细胞发生CDK4抑制和G1细胞周期阻滞(13.8%),而与游离CDK4 siRNA孵育后未发生CDK4 mRNA或G1细胞周期的下调。这表明,LNP-siRNA有可能抑制癌细胞生长,且无不良反应[84]。Honma等制备了稳定的核蛋白Ⅱ小干扰RNA(RPN2 siRNA)-去端肽胶原复合物,并检测了针对多种药物耐药的MCF-7-ADR乳腺癌细胞系使用该复合物是否可改善其对多西他赛的敏感性[85]。在MCF-7-ADR细胞体外研究中,与游离siRNA的多西他赛相比,RPN2 siRNA-去端肽胶原复合物显著抑制细胞生长并诱导细胞凋亡。经RPN2 siRNA-去端肽胶原复合物处理的MCF-7-ADR细胞对紫杉醇和多西他赛的敏感性均高于转染非靶向siRNA的细胞,分别为2.6倍和3.5倍。使用这种复合物联合多西他赛治疗1周后,有效缩小了种植MCF-7-ADR细胞小鼠的乳腺肿瘤大小。当分别用多西他赛、RPN2 siRNA或siRNA-去端肽胶原复合物处理小鼠时,结果并无明显改善。Li等还报道了该复合物可增强多柔比星、紫杉醇和顺铂的化疗敏感性,促进靶siRNA的递送[86]。

在NP介导的光热消融(photothermal ablation,PTA)中,NP表现出光热效应,它们将近红外(near-infrared,NIR)辐射吸收的能量转化为热能[87]。用于该治疗的纳米材料大多是金属纳米颗粒,在体内表现出无效清除[88]。基于金和银颗粒的纳米材料在近红外区域具有较高的吸收电位,从而表现出较高的光热效应[89]。Carpin等报道了与抗HER2抗体偶联的二氧化硅-金纳米壳用于乳腺癌细胞的光热消融[90],与HER2阴性乳腺癌细胞MCF-10A相比,抗HER2纳米壳与SK-BR-3(曲妥珠单抗敏感)和BT474 AZ LR(曲妥珠单抗耐药)的结合显著增加。

基于磷酸钙纳米颗粒的药物递送系统(calcium phosphosilicate NP-based drug-delivery system,CPSNP)被认为是封装各种化疗药物的主要方法[91]。磷酸钙(calcium phosphate,CP)在生理pH值(pH 7.4)下相对不溶,但在实体瘤微环境(pH 5.8~7.8)和后期内溶酶体中(pH 4.8~5.5)释放后更易溶解[92,93]。多西他赛结合的CPSNP是另一组治疗乳腺癌的新型纳米药物。可通过使用聚乙二醇表面功能化的多西他赛,增加渗透性和滞留力来实现被动生长。同样,多西他赛与CD71抗体联合使用可主动靶向乳腺癌细胞[94,95]。Barth等的研究证明了这一点,他们针对无胸腺裸鼠模型的研究结果表明,CD71 CPSNP可以有效靶向乳腺癌细胞[95]。

结合吲哚菁绿的CPSNP(indocyanine green-CPSNP,ICG-CPSNP)作为新型光免疫纳米治疗(photo immuno nano therapy,PINT)的光敏剂,可用于近红外生物成像[96,97]。给含MDA-MB-231乳腺癌肿瘤细胞(T细胞缺陷)的无胸腺裸鼠和含鼠410.4乳腺癌细胞(T细胞活性)的BALB/cJ小鼠分别注射聚乙二醇化ICG-CPSNP、游离ICG、无封装剂的聚乙二醇化CPNSP和枸橼酸盐表面功能化ICG-CPSNP后进行近红外激光治疗,结果显示,通过聚乙二醇化ICG-CPSNP介导的PINT治疗后,2种模型鼠中的肿瘤生长均被有效抑制。PINT首次用于治疗非实体瘤慢性髓细胞性白血病,预示着其在转移性乳腺癌治疗中的应用潜能(表17-2)。

表17-2 乳腺癌新型纳米疗法的总结

活性药物	方案	纳米疗法
曲妥珠单抗、帕妥珠单抗和拉帕替尼	通过抑制酪氨酸激酶活性和HER2的同源或异源二聚化靶向过表达的HER2乳腺癌细胞	靶向纳米疗法
纳米包裹的AAV2	通过诱导坏死抑制乳腺癌肿瘤生长	基因治疗
siRNA-去端肽胶原复合物	通过改善siRNA-去端肽胶原复合物的摄取抑制肿瘤细胞的生长并诱导细胞凋亡	基因治疗
金属基纳米材料(AU或Ag)或具有高光热转换效应的纳米材料	通过释放高于热消融阈值的热能靶向乳腺癌细胞	光热消融(PTA)
CPSNP掺杂多西他赛,吲哚菁绿(光敏剂)	通过释放活性药物靶向后期内溶酶体形成的乳腺癌细胞	光动力疗法

六、结论

肿瘤纳米技术是肿瘤生物医学中快速发展的领域之一,在乳腺癌的诊断和治疗方面有着广泛应用。与乳腺癌其他常规治疗相比,使用 NP 更有效,也可能更安全。多种 FDA 批准的可能有效治疗肿瘤的方案也是在 NP 的基础上开展的,并且也有其他基于 NP 的治疗方案正在进行临床试验。肿瘤疗法中使用的 NP 可塑性很强,能够很容易地靶向不同类型的肿瘤位点,并有可能将各种活性制剂递送到靶向位点。虽然不同 NP 的特性差异使纳米医学的研究有些艰难,但它们具有巨大潜力改善患者病情。未来,人类需要努力的不仅仅是进一步改善治疗乳腺癌的技术,更要控制肿瘤的复发和转移。

资助信息

作者感谢 DST-EMR(研究数字信号技术和电磁辐射的一个机构)(EMR/2016/002694,2017 年 8 月 21 日),印度新德里,支持该项目。

利益冲突

作者声明无利益冲突。

致谢

作者感谢印度安得拉邦维沙卡帕特南甘地技术和管理研究所、科学研究所生物技术系。

参 考 文 献

[1] Siegel RL, Miller KD, Jemal A. Cancer statistics, 2015. CA Cancer J Clin 2015;65(1):5-29.

[2] Arnold R. Prospective cancer treatment found in the Cowpea Mosaic Virus. Microrev Cell Mol Biol 2016;1(1):1-3.

[3] Anand P, Kunnumakkara AB, Sundaram C, Harikumar KB, Tharakan ST, Lai OS, Sung B, Aggarwal BB. Cancer is a preventable disease that requires major lifestyle changes. Pharm Res 2008;25(9):2097-116.

[4] Duncan R. Polymer conjugates as anticancer nanomedicines. Nat Rev Cancer 2006;6(9):688-701.

[5] Couvreur P, Vauthier C. Nanotechnology: intelligent design to treat complex disease. Pharm Res 2006;23(7):1417-50.

[6] Sikora K. The impact of future technology on cancer care. Clin Med 2002;2(6):560-8.

[7] Singh OP, Nehru R. Nanotechnology and cancer treatment. Asian J Exp Sci 2008;22(2):6.
[8] Rajitha B, Malla RR, Vadde R, Kasa P, Prasad GLV, Farran B, Kumari S, Pavitra E, Kamal MA, Raju GSR, Peela S, Nagaraju GP. Horizons of nanotechnology applications in female specific cancers. Semin Cancer Biol 2019;19:30090-2.
[9] Chidambaram M, Manavalan R, Kathiresan K. Nanotherapeutics to overcome conventional cancer chemotherapy limitations. Int J Pharm Pharm Sci 2011;14(1):67-77.
[10] Sinha R, Kim GJ, Nie S, Shin DM. Nanotechnology in cancer therapeutics: bioconjugated nanoparticles for drug delivery. Mol Cancer Ther 2006;5(8):1909-17.
[11] Ranganathan R, Madanmohan S, Kesavan A, Baskar G, Krishnamoorthy YR, Santosham R, Ponraju D, Rayala SK, Venkatraman G. Nanomedicine: towards development of patient-friendly drug-delivery systems for oncological applications. Int J Nanomedicine 2012;7:1043-60.
[12] Cai W, Gao T, Hong H, Sun J. Applications of gold nanoparticles in cancer nanotechnology. Nanotechnol Sci Appl 2008;1:17-32.
[13] Ghanbari H, de Mel A, Seifalian AM. Cardiovascular application of polyhedral oligomeric silsesquioxane nanomaterials: a glimpse into prospective horizons. Int J Nanomedicine 2011;6:775-86.
[14] Elsersawi A. World of nanobioengineering: potential big ideas for the future. Author House.
[15] Kircher MF, Mahmood U, King RS, Weissleder R, Josephson L. A multimodal nanoparticle for preoperative magnetic resonance imaging and intraoperative optical brain tumor delineation. Cancer Res 2003;63(23):8122-5.
[16] Ferrari M. Cancer nanotechnology: opportunities and challenges. Nat Rev Cancer 2005;5(3):161-71.
[17] Jamieson T, Bakhshi R, Petrova D, Pocock R, Imani M, Seifalian AM. Biological applications of quantum dots. Biomaterials 2007;28(31):4717-32.
[18] Cai W, Chen X. Multimodality molecular imaging of tumor angiogenesis. J Nucl Med 2008;49(Suppl. 2):113s-128s.
[19] Gelperina S, Kisich K, Iseman MD, Heifets L. The potential advantages of nanoparticle drug delivery systems in chemotherapy of tuberculosis. Am J Respir Crit Care Med 2005;172(12):1487-90.
[20] Byrne JD, Betancourt T, Brannon-Peppas L. Active targeting schemes for nanoparticle systems in cancer therapeutics. Adv Drug Deliv Rev 2008;60(15):1615-26.
[21] Hahn MA, Singh AK, Sharma P, Brown SC, Moudgil BM. Nanoparticles as contrast agents for in-vivo bioimaging: current status and future perspectives. Anal Bioanal Chem 2011;399(1):3-27.
[22] Bozzuto G, Molinari A. Liposomes as nanomedical devices. Int J Nanomedicine 2015;10:975.

[23] Sercombe L, Veerati T, Moheimani F, Wu SY, Sood AK, Hua S. Advances and challenges of liposome assisted drug delivery. Front Pharmacol 2015;6:286.

[24] Xu W, Ling P, Zhang T. Polymeric micelles, a promising drug delivery system to enhance bioavailability of poorly water-soluble drugs. J Drug Deliv 2013;2013:340315.

[25] Miyata K, Christie RJ, Kataoka K. Polymeric micelles for nano-scale drug delivery. React Funct Polym 2011;71(3):227-34.

[26] Zhu J, Shi X. Dendrimer-based nanodevices for targeted drug delivery applications. J Mater Chem B 2013;1(34):4199-211.

[27] Ordikhani F, Erdem Arslan M, Marcelo R, Sahin I, Grigsby P, Schwarz JK, Azab AK. Drug delivery approaches for the treatment of cervical cancer. Pharmaceutics 2016;8(3):23.

[28] Choi S-J, Lee JK, Jeong J, Choy J-H. Toxicity evaluation of inorganic nanoparticles: considerations and challenges. Mol Cell Toxicol 2013;9(3):205-10.

[29] Du J, Li X, Zhao H, Zhou Y, Wang L, Tian S, Wang Y. Nanosuspensions of poorly water-soluble drugs prepared by bottom-up technologies. Int J Pharm 2015;495(2):738-49.

[30] Volkov Y. Quantum dots in nanomedicine: recent trends, advances and unresolved issues. Biochem Biophys Res Commun 2015;468(3):419-27.

[31] Liu J, Lau SK, Varma VA, Moffitt RA, Caldwell M, Liu T, Young AN, Petros JA, Osunkoya AO, Krogstad T, Leyland-Jones B, Wang MD, Nie S. Molecular mapping of tumor heterogeneity on clinical tissue specimens with multiplexed quantum dots. ACS Nano 2010;4(5):2755-65.

[32] Xu G, Zeng S, Zhang B, Swihart MT, Yong KT, Prasad PN. New generation cadmium-free quantum dots for biophotonics and nanomedicine. Chem Rev 2016;116(19):12234-327.

[33] Shi Y, Pramanik A, Tchounwou C, Pedraza F, Crouch RA, Chavva SR, Vangara A, Sinha SS, Jones S, Sardar D, Hawker C, Ray PC. Multifunctional biocompatible graphene oxide quantum dots decorated magnetic nanoplatform for efficient capture and two-photon imaging of rare tumor cells. ACS Appl Mater Interfaces 2015;7(20):10935-43.

[34] Han HS, Niemeyer E, Huang Y, Kamoun WS, Martin JD, Bhaumik J, Chen Y, Roberge S, Cui J, Martin MR, Fukumura D, Jain RK, Bawendi MG, Duda DG. Quantum dot/antibody conjugates for in vivo cytometric imaging in mice. Proc Natl Acad Sci U S A 2015;112(5):1350-5.

[35] Bassas-Galia M, Follonier S, Pusnik M, Zinn M. Natural polymers: a source of inspiration. In: Bioresorbable polymers for biomedical applications. Elsevier; 2017. p. 31-64.

[36] Hortobagyi GN. Treatment of breast cancer. N Engl J Med 1998;339(14):974-84.

[37] Peto R, Davies C, Godwin J, Gray R, Pan HC, Clarke M, Cutter D, Darby S, McGale P, Taylor C, Wang YC, Bergh J, Di Leo A, Albain K, Swain S, Piccart M, Pritchard K. Comparisons between different polychemotherapy regimens for early breast cancer: meta-

analyses of long-term outcome among 100,000 women in 123 randomised trials. Lancet 2012;379(9814):432-44.

[38] Davies C, Godwin J, Gray R, Clarke M, Cutter D, Darby S, McGale P, Pan HC, Taylor C, Wang YC, Dowsett M, Ingle J, Peto R. Relevance of breast cancer hormone receptors and other factors to the efficacy of adjuvant tamoxifen: patient-level meta-analysis of randomised trials. Lancet 2011; 378(9793):771-84.

[39] Barenholz Y. Doxil®-the first FDA-approved nano-drug: lessons learned. J Control Release 2012; 160(2):117-34.

[40] O'Brien ME, Wigler N, Inbar M, Rosso R, Grischke E, Santoro A, Catane R, Kieback D, Tomczak P, Ackland S. Reduced cardiotoxicity and comparable efficacy in a phase III trial of pegylated liposomal doxorubicin HCl (CAELYX™/Doxil®) versus conventional doxorubicin for first-line treatment of metastatic breast cancer. Ann Oncol 2004;15(3):440-9.

[41] Tang X, Loc WS, Dong C, Matters GL, Butler PJ, Kester M, Meyers C, Jiang Y, Adair JH. The use of nanoparticulates to treat breast cancer. Nanomedicine 2017;12(19):2367-88.

[42] Gelderblom H, Verweij J, Nooter K, Sparreboom A. Cremophor EL: the drawbacks and advantages of vehicle selection for drug formulation. Eur J Cancer 2001;37(13):1590-8.

[43] Mackler NJ, Pienta KJ. Drug insight: use of docetaxel in prostate and urothelial cancers. Nat Clin Pract Urol 2005;2(2):92-100 quiz 1 p following 112.

[44] Jordan MA, Wilson L. Microtubules as a target for anticancer drugs. Nat Rev Cancer 2004;4(4):253-65.

[45] Ibrahim NK, Desai N, Legha S, Soon-Shiong P, Theriault RL, Rivera E, Esmaeli B, Ring SE, Bedikian A, Hortobagyi GN, Ellerhorst JA. Phase I and pharmacokinetic study of ABI-007, a Cremophor-free, protein-stabilized, nanoparticle formulation of paclitaxel. Clin Cancer Res 2002; 8(5):1038-44.

[46] Miele E, Spinelli GP, Miele E, Tomao F, Tomao S. Albumin-bound formulation of paclitaxel(Abraxane ABI-007) in the treatment of breast cancer. Int J Nanomedicine 2009;4:99-105.

[47] Hawkins MJ, Soon-Shiong P, Desai N. Protein nanoparticles as drug carriers in clinical medicine. Adv Drug Deliv Rev 2008;60(8):876-85.

[48] Sparreboom A, Scripture CD, Trieu V, Williams PJ, De T, Yang A, Beals B, Figg WD, Hawkins M, Desai N. Comparative preclinical and clinical pharmacokinetics of a cremophor-free, nanoparticle albumin-bound paclitaxel (ABI-007) and paclitaxel formulated in Cremophor (Taxol). Clin Cancer Res 2005;11(11):4136-43.

[49] Hashemi M, Yadegari A, Yazdanpanah G, Omidi M, Jabbehdari S, Haghiralsadat F, Yazdian F, Tayebi L. Normalization of doxorubicin release from graphene oxide: new approach for optimization of effective parameters on drug loading. Biotechnol Appl Biochem

2017;64(3):433-42.

[50] Shi J, Wang B, Wang L, Lu T, Fu Y, Zhang H, Zhang Z. Fullerene (C60)-based tumor-targeting nanoparticles with "off-on" state for enhanced treatment of cancer. J Control Release 2016;235:245-58.

[51] Raza K, Thotakura N, Kumar P, Joshi M, Bhushan S, Bhatia A, Kumar V, Malik R, Sharma G, Guru SK. C60-fullerenes for delivery of docetaxel to breast cancer cells: a promising approach for enhanced efficacy and better pharmacokinetic profile. Int J Pharm 2015;495(1):551-9.

[52] Jiang T, Sun W, Zhu Q, Burns NA, Khan SA, Mo R, Gu Z. Furin-mediated sequential delivery of anticancer cytokine and small-molecule drug shuttled by graphene. Adv Mater 2015;27(6):1021-8.

[53] Xu Z, Zhu S, Wang M, Li Y, Shi P, Huang X. Delivery of paclitaxel using PEGylated graphene oxide as a nanocarrier. ACS Appl Mater Interfaces 2015;7(2):1355-63.

[54] Zhou T, Zhou X, Xing D. Controlled release of doxorubicin from graphene oxide based charge-reversal nanocarrier. Biomaterials 2014;35(13):4185-94.

[55] Zhang H, Ji Y, Chen Q, Jiao X, Hou L, Zhu X, Zhang Z. Enhancement of cytotoxicity of artemisinin toward cancer cells by transferrin-mediated carbon nanotubes nanoparticles. J Drug Target 2015;23(6): 552-67.

[56] Hernández-Rivera M, Zaibaq NG, Wilson LJ. Toward carbon nanotube-based imaging agents for the clinic. Biomaterials 2016;101:229-40.

[57] Servant A, Jacobs I, Bussy C, Fabbro C, Da Ros T, Pach E, Ballesteros B, Prato M, Nicolay K, Kostarelos K. Gadolinium-functionalised multi-walled carbon nanotubes as a T1 contrast agent for MRI cell labelling and tracking. Carbon 2016;97:126-33.

[58] Marangon I, Menard-Moyon C, Kolosnjaj-Tabi J, Béoutis ML, Lartigue L, Alloyeau D, Pach E, Ballesteros B, Autret G, Ninjbadgar T. Covalent functionalization of multi-walled carbon nanotubes with a gadolinium chelate for efficient T1-weighted magnetic resonance imaging. Adv Funct Mater 2014;24(45):7173-86.

[59] Mallick K, Strydom AM. Biophilic carbon nanotubes. Colloids Surf B Biointerfaces 2013;105:310-8.

[60] Ogbodu RO, Limson JL, Prinsloo E, Nyokong T. Photophysical properties and photodynamic therapy effect of zinc phthalocyanine-spermine-single walled carbon nanotube conjugate on MCF-7 breast cancer cell line. Synth Met 2015;204:122-32.

[61] Shi J, Wang L, Gao J, Liu Y, Zhang J, Ma R, Liu R, Zhang Z. A fullerene-based multifunctional nanoplatform for cancer theranostic applications. Biomaterials 2014;35(22): 5771-84.

[62] Nurunnabi M, Khatun Z, Reeck GR, Lee DY, Lee YK. Photoluminescent graphene nanoparticles for cancer phototherapy and imaging. ACS Appl Mater Interfaces 2014;6(15): 12413-21.

[63] Hwang MT, Landon PB, Lee J, Choi D, Mo AH, Glinsky G, Lal R. Highly specific SNP detection using 2D graphene electronics and DNA strand displacement. Proc Natl Acad Sci U S A 2016;113(26):7088-93.

[64] Fiorillo M, Verre AF, Iliut M, Peiris-Pagés M, Ozsvari B, Gandara R, Cappello AR, Sotgia F, Vijayaraghavan A, Lisanti MP. Graphene oxide selectively targets cancer stem cells, across multiple tumor types: implications for non-toxic cancer treatment, via "differentiation-based nano-therapy". Oncotarget 2015;6(6):3553-62.

[65] Meric-Bernstam F, Hung MC. Advances in targeting human epidermal growth factor receptor-2 signaling for cancer therapy. Clin Cancer Res 2006;12(21):6326-30.

[66] Pinkas-Kramarski R, Lenferink AE, Bacus SS, Lyass L, van de Poll ML, Klapper LN, Tzahar E, Sela M, van Zoelen EJ, Yarden Y. The oncogenic ErbB-2/ErbB-3 heterodimer is a surrogate receptor of the epidermal growth factor and betacellulin. Oncogene 1998;16(10):1249-58.

[67] Tan M, Yao J, Yu D. Overexpression of the c-erbB-2 gene enhanced intrinsic metastasis potential in human breast cancer cells without increasing their transformation abilities. Cancer Res 1997; 57(6):1199-205.

[68] Carter P, Presta L, Gorman CM, Ridgway JB, Henner D, Wong WL, Rowland AM, Kotts C, Carver ME, Shepard HM. Humanization of an anti-p185HER2 antibody for human cancer therapy. Proc Natl Acad Sci U S A 1992;89(10):4285-9.

[69] Hudis CA. Trastuzumab—mechanism of action and use in clinical practice. N Engl J Med 2007; 357(1):39-51.

[70] Park S, Jiang Z, Mortenson ED, Deng L, Radkevich-Brown O, Yang X, Sattar H, Wang Y, Brown NK, Greene M, Liu Y, Tang J, Wang S, Fu YX. The therapeutic effect of anti-HER2/neu antibody depends on both innate and adaptive immunity. Cancer Cell 2010;18(2):160-70.

[71] Pegram M, Hsu S, Lewis G, Pietras R, Beryt M, Sliwkowski M, Coombs D, Baly D, Kabbinavar F, Slamon D. Inhibitory effects of combinations of HER-2/neu antibody and chemotherapeutic agents used for treatment of human breast cancers. Oncogene 1999;18(13):2241-51.

[72] Romond EH, Perez EA, Bryant J, Suman VJ, Geyer Jr. CE, Davidson NE, Tan-Chiu E, Martino S, Paik S, Kaufman PA, Swain SM, Pisansky TM, Fehrenbacher L, Kutteh LA, Vogel VG, Visscher DW, Yothers G, Jenkins RB, Brown AM, Dakhil SR, Mamounas EP, Lingle WL, Klein PM, Ingle JN, Wolmark N. Trastuzumab plus adjuvant chemotherapy for operable HER2-positive breast cancer. N Engl J Med 2005;353(16):1673-84.

[73] Anhorn MG, Wagner S, Kreuter J, Langer K, von Briesen H. Specific targeting of HER2 overexpressing breast cancer cells with doxorubicin-loaded trastuzumab-modified human serum albumin nanoparticles. Bioconjug Chem 2008;19(12):2321-31.

[74] Baselga J, Cortes J, Kim SB, Im SA, Hegg R, Im YH, Roman L, Pedrini JL, Pienkows-

ki T, Knott A, Clark E, Benyunes MC, Ross G, Swain SM. Pertuzumab plus trastuzumab plus docetaxel for metastatic breast cancer. N Engl J Med 2012;366(2):109-19.

[75] Gianni L, Pienkowski T, Im YH, Roman L, Tseng LM, Liu MC, Lluch A, Staroslawska E, de la Haba-Rodriguez J, Im SA, Pedrini JL, Poirier B, Morandi P, Semiglazov V, Srimuninnimit V, Bianchi G, Szado T, Ratnayake J, Ross G, Valagussa P. Efficacy and safety of neoadjuvant pertuzumab and trastuzumab in women with locally advanced, inflammatory, or early HER2-positive breast cancer(NeoSphere): a randomised multicentre, open-label, phase 2 trial. Lancet Oncol 2012;13(1):25-32.

[76] Baselga J, Gelmon KA, Verma S, Wardley A, Conte P, Miles D, Bianchi G, Cortes J, McNally VA, Ross GA, Fumoleau P, Gianni L. Phase II trial of pertuzumab and trastuzumab in patients with human epidermal growth factor receptor 2-positive metastatic breast cancer that progressed during prior trastuzumab therapy. J Clin Oncol Off J Am Soc Clin Oncol 2010;28(7):1138-44.

[77] Gao H, Chen C, Xi Z, Chen J, Zhang Q, Cao S, Jiang X. In vivo behavior and safety of lapatinib-incorporated lipid nanoparticles. Curr Pharm Biotechnol 2014;14(12):1062-71.

[78] Gao H, Cao S, Chen C, Cao S, Yang Z, Pang Z, Xi Z, Pan S, Zhang Q, Jiang X. Incorporation of lapatinib into lipoprotein-like nanoparticles with enhanced water solubility and anti-tumor effect in breast cancer. Nanomedicine 2013;8(9):1429-42.

[79] Foulkes WD, Smith IE, Reis-Filho JS. Triple-negative breast cancer. N Engl J Med 2010;363(20):1938-48.

[80] Hudis CA, Gianni L. Triple-negative breast cancer: an unmet medical need. Oncologist 2011;16(Suppl. 1):1-11.

[81] Tan DS, Marchió C, Jones RL, Savage K, Smith IE, Dowsett M, Reis-Filho JS. Triple negative breast cancer: molecular profiling and prognostic impact in adjuvant anthracycline-treated patients. Breast Cancer Res Treat 2008;111(1):27-44.

[82] Liedtke C, Mazouni C, Hess KR, Andre F, Tordai A, Mejia JA, Symmans WF, Gonzalez-Angulo AM, Hennessy B, Green M, Cristofanilli M, Hortobagyi GN, Pusztai L. Response to neoadjuvant therapy and long-term survival in patients with triple-negative breast cancer. J Clin Oncol Off J Am Soc Clin Oncol 2008;26(8):1275-81.

[83] Alam S, Bowser BS, Israr M, Conway MJ, Meyers C. Adeno-associated virus type 2 infection of nude mouse human breast cancer xenograft induces necrotic death and inhibits tumor growth. Cancer Biol Ther 2014;15(8):1013-28.

[84] Wang X, Yu B, Wu Y, Lee RJ, Lee LJ. Efficient down-regulation of CDK4 by novel lipid nanoparticle-mediated siRNA delivery. Anticancer Res 2011;31(5):1619-26.

[85] Honma K, Iwao-Koizumi K, Takeshita F, Yamamoto Y, Yoshida T, Nishio K, Nagahara S, Kato K, Ochiya T. RPN2 gene confers docetaxel resistance in breast cancer. Nat Med 2008;14(9):939-48.

[86] Li YT, Chua MJ, Kunnath AP, Chowdhury EH. Reversing multidrug resistance in breast

cancer cells by silencing ABC transporter genes with nanoparticle-facilitated delivery of target siRNAs. Int J Nanomedicine 2012;7:2473-81.

[87] Guo Y, Zhang Z, Kim DH, Li W, Nicolai J, Procissi D, Huan Y, Han G, Omary RA, Larson AC. Photothermal ablation of pancreatic cancer cells with hybrid iron-oxide core gold-shell nanoparticles. Int J Nanomedicine 2013;8:3437-46.

[88] Longmire M, Choyke PL, Kobayashi H. Clearance properties of nano-sized particles and molecules as imaging agents: considerations and caveats. Nanomedicine 2008;3(5):703-17.

[89] Huang X, Jain PK, El-Sayed IH, El-Sayed MA. Gold nanoparticles: interesting optical properties and recent applications in cancer diagnostics and therapy. Nanomedicine 2007;2(5):681-93.

[90] Carpin LB, Bickford LR, Agollah G, Yu TK, Schiff R, Li Y, Drezek RA. Immunoconjugated gold nanoshell-mediated photothermal ablation of trastuzumab-resistant breast cancer cells. Breast Cancer Res Treat 2011;125(1):27-34.

[91] Altinoǧlu EI, Adair JH. Near infrared imaging with nanoparticles. Wiley Interdiscip Rev Nanomed Nanobiotechnol 2010;2(5):461-77.

[92] Panyam J, Labhasetwar V. Biodegradable nanoparticles for drug and gene delivery to cells and tissue. Adv Drug Deliv Rev 2003;55(3):329-47.

[93] Pinto O, Tabakovic A, Goff T, Liu Y, Adair J. Calcium phosphate and calcium phosphosilicate mediated drug delivery and imaging. In: Intracellular delivery. Springer; 2011. p. 713-44.

[94] Altinoǧlu EI, Russin TJ, Kaiser JM, Barth BM, Eklund PC, Kester M, Adair JH. Near-infrared emitting fluorophore-doped calcium phosphate nanoparticles for in vivo imaging of human breast cancer. ACS Nano 2008;2(10):2075-84.

[95] Barth BM, Sharma R, Altinoǧlu EI, Morgan TT, Shanmugavelandy SS, Kaiser JM, McGovern C, Matters GL, Smith JP, Kester M, Adair JH. Bioconjugation of calcium phosphosilicate composite nanoparticles for selective targeting of human breast and pancreatic cancers in vivo. ACS Nano 2010;4(3):1279-87.

[96] Barth BM, Erhan IA, Shanmugavelandy SS, Kaiser JM, Crespo-Gonzalez D, DiVittore NA, McGovern C, Goff TM, Keasey NR, Adair JH, Loughran Jr. TP, Claxton DF, Kester M. Targeted indocyanine-green-loaded calcium phosphosilicate nanoparticles for in vivo photodynamic therapy of leukemia. ACS Nano 2011;5(7):5325-37.

[97] Barth BM, Shanmugavelandy SS, Kaiser JM, McGovern C, Altınoǧlu E, Haakenson JK, Hengst JA, Gilius EL, Knupp SA, Fox TE, Smith JP, Ritty TM, Adair JH, Kester M. PhotoImmunoNanoTherapy reveals an anticancer role for sphingosine kinase 2 and dihydrosphingosine-1-phosphate. ACS Nano 2013;7(3):2132-44.